Advances in Vascular Surgery - From the Diagnostic Phase to the Use of Hybrid and Endovascular Techniques in the Management of Aortic Dissection

Edited by Dario Buioni and Carlo Bassano

Published in London, United Kingdom

Advances in Vascular Surgery - From the Diagnostic Phase to the Use of Hybrid and Endovascular Techniques in the Management of Aortic Dissection
http://dx.doi.org/10.5772/intechopen.1003456
Edited by Dario Buioni and Carlo Bassano

Contributors
Ahmed Elsharkawy, Alessandro Cristian Salvati, André Timóteo Sapalo, Antonio Nenna, Babak Abai, Boris Kozlov, Chiara Ferrisi, Chika Sato, Ciro Mastroianni, Claudia Altieri, David Tang, Diletta Corrado, Dmitri Panfilov, Francesco Loreni, Gennaro Sorrentino, Giulio Pellegrini, Hiroyasu Tsukaguchi, James Hu, Jin Park, Kamaraj Radhakrishnan, Kazumasa Orihashi, Laura De Felice, Lorenzo Terzano, Manuela Moresco, Mario Lusini, Marzia Flaminio, Massimo Chello, Matthew Carnevale, Mattia Scognamiglio, Natalie Lukasik, Nicola Habash, Nikhil Chandra, Omar Giacinto, Paolo Nardi, Paul Lajos, Phạm Thị Xuyên, Pier Luigi Stefàno, Raffaele Barbato, Saki Shimada, Sayoko Haruyama, Sean D. Galvin, Shuo Huang, Tadaaki Koyama, Takayuki Okada, Thierry Carrel, Valentina Ajello

First published in London, United Kingdom, 2025 by IntechOpen
IntechOpen is the global imprint of INTECHOPEN LIMITED, registered in England and Wales, registration number: 11086078, 167-169 Great Portland Street, London, W1W 5PF, United Kingdom

For EU product safety concerns: IN TECH d.o.o., Prolaz Marije Krucifikse Kozulić 3, 51000 Rijeka, Croatia, info@intechopen.com or visit our website at intechopen.com.

British Library Cataloguing-in-Publication Data
A catalogue record for this book is available from the British Library

Advances in Vascular Surgery - From the Diagnostic Phase to the Use of Hybrid and Endovascular Techniques in the Management of Aortic Dissection
Edited by Dario Buioni and Carlo Bassano
p. cm.
Print ISBN 978-0-85466-077-3
Online ISBN 978-0-85466-076-6
eBook (PDF) ISBN 978-0-85466-078-0

Meet the editors

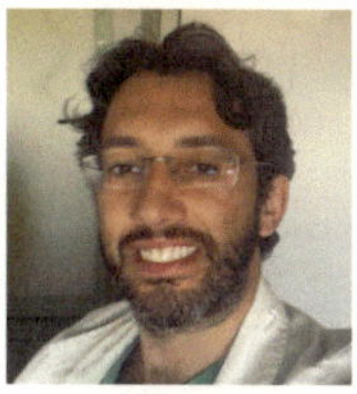

Dario Buioni completed the residency program in Cardiac Surgery at Sapienza University of Rome in 2014 and is a Ph.D. student at the University of Tor Vergata in Rome, analyzing the genetic aspects of aortic pathologies. He is currently a tutor in the Residency Program in Cardiac Surgery at the University of Tor Vergata. He has more than 10 years of experience in cardiac surgery, particularly interested in acute and chronic aortopathies, minimally invasive approaches, transcatheter aortic valve replacement and aortic insufficiency. He works in academia and has published research articles, book chapters and conference proceedings.

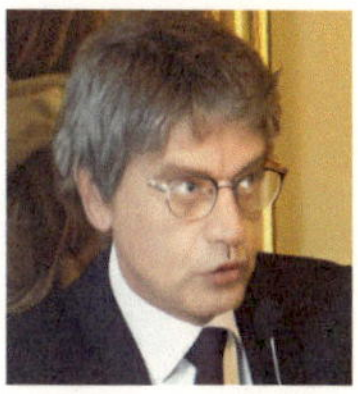

Dr. Carlo Bassano is a professor of Cardiac Surgery and vice director of the Residency Program in Cardiac Surgery at Tor Vergata University in Rome. He is also a senior surgeon and manager of the Unit of Cardiac Surgical Emergencies at Tor Vergata University Hospital. He obtained his Ph.D. in Cardiac Surgical Pathophysiology with a thesis about retrograde cerebral perfusion for central nervous system protection during surgery on the aortic arch (1994). His fields of interest include acute and chronic aortic dissection, off-pump coronary artery bypass grafting, minimally invasive aortic valve and proximal aorta replacement, complex aortic surgery, and bioprostheses.

Contents

Preface

The aim of this book, *Advances in Vascular Surgery – From the Diagnostic Phase to the Use of Hybrid and Endovascular Techniques in the Management of Aortic Dissection*, is to provide the reader with a broad vision of the progress achieved so far in the treatment of one of the aortic syndromes, aortic dissection. Aortic dissection still represents a huge challenge for cardiac surgeons and vascular surgeons, as it is characterized by high mortality and morbidity perioperative. The book is aimed at both colleagues dealing with this pathology for the first time and expert colleagues. Various aspects were addressed, including epidemiology, screening, surgical techniques, cerebral protection, and endovascular approaches. Each procedure was evaluated in terms of its risks and benefits.

Dario Buioni and Carlo Bassano
Cardiac Surgery Unit,
Policlinico Tor Vergata,
University of Tor Vergata,
Rome, Italy

Chapter 1

Aortic Dissection

Shuo Huang, James Hu, Matthew Carnevale and Paul Lajos

Abstract

Aortic dissection is part of a spectrum of disorders known as acute aortic syndrome, which includes penetrating aortic ulcer, intramural hematoma, aortic transection, and aortic dissection. Aortic dissection occurs when there is separation of the media layer within the aortic wall, often triggered by the sheer force of pulsatile blood flow. The direction in which the dissection extends along the aorta and its branches plays a crucial role in determining treatment. Dissections extending into the ascending aorta require emergent surgery, while those confined to the descending aorta may initially be managed with medications. However, a subset of descending aortic dissections may also necessitate surgical intervention. During dissection, the separation of the media layer compresses the elastic fibers in the true lumen, while the rest of the aortic wall loses much of its structural integrity. Over time, this may lead to degeneration of the aorta. As our understanding of this disease process deepens, approaches to its management and surgical treatment continue to evolve. This chapter provides an overview of the current knowledge of aortic dissections.

Keywords: aortic dissection, type B aortic dissection, acute aortic dissection, thoracic endovascular aortic repair (TEVAR), chronic dissection

1. Introduction

Acute aortic dissection was first described in 1760 when King George II was witnessed straining on the commode and subsequently collapsed. This was documented by his personal physician, Frank Nicholls, who performed the autopsy and found a "transverse fissure ... in the trunk of the aorta" that led to the King's fatal demise by cardiac tamponade [1]. In 1761, Morgani provided the first pathologic description of aortic dissection; however, it was not until 1802 that Maunoir used the now familiar terminology of "aortic dissection" and in 1819 Laennec utilized the term "dissecting aneurysm" [2, 3].

On July 7th, 1954, DeBakey, Cooley, and Creech performed the first successful surgical resection of a dissecting thoracic aneurysm. An open descending thoracic repair was performed *via* a left posterolateral thoracotomy incision, where an aneurysmal descending aorta was noted. Proximal and distal clamps were placed around the aneurysm, and after resection of the aortic segment, a dissection flap was noted in the distal end (**Figure 1**). This was sutured using interrupted sutures and the ends reattached with an end-to-end anastomosis (**Figure 2**) [4].

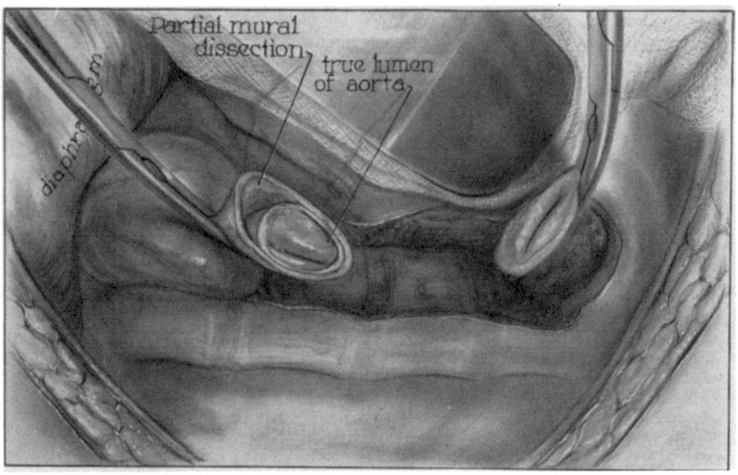

Figure 1.
Original drawing of first open aortic dissection repair with the demonstration of dissection flap in the distal segment of the aorta (permission pending).

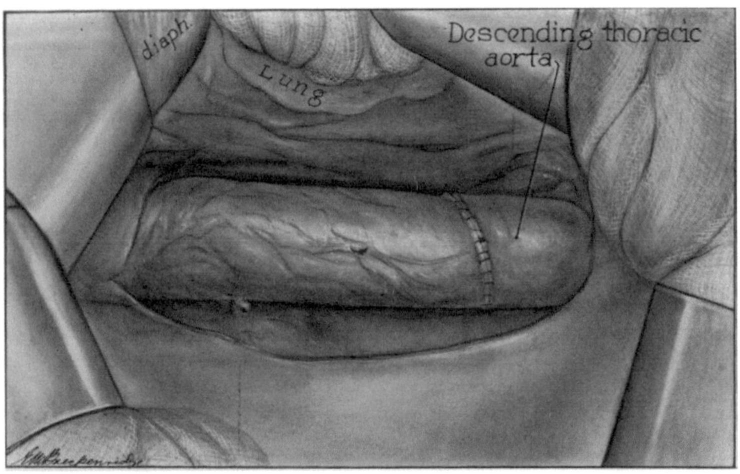

Figure 2.
Completed anastomosis of first aortic repair (permission pending).

In the last 50 years, the trend of aortic dissection repair has evolved from open surgical technique to minimally invasive endovascular stent grafting. Originally described in 1999, Nienaber et al. [5] found in their prospective study, with statistical significance, that endovascular stent graft repairs had shorter operative times, ICU stays, and lengths of hospital stay [6]. Thoracic aortic endovascular stent grafting (TEVAR) has all but replaced open repair and is now the standard of care.

2. Pathophysiology

Acute aortic dissection is a rare but highly morbid disorder in which a separation of the layers of the aortic wall propagates either circumferentially or longitudinally along the vessel axis. The intramural hemorrhage that occurs in aortic dissection creates a false lumen within the media. When the false lumen is continuous with the true aortic lumen, blood flow may occur, provided there is outflow. In the absence of flow, the false lumen will thrombose. The etiology of spontaneous aortic dissection remains unknown. Whether the disrupted vasa vasorum and resulting propagating column of blood results in or occurs because of an intimal tear is undetermined. When there is no communication between the false and true lumens and thus no resulting flow channel for the blood which results in thrombosis, the condition is known as intramural hemorrhage, which is also known as aortic dissection without an identified entry tear. These conditions exist on a spectrum. When dissection occurs, the septum typically forms when the intima and approximately two-thirds of the media separate from the remaining one-third of the media and the adventitia which make up the outer wall of the false lumen which is thinner and less elastic, thus requiring dilation to a greater extent to generate an equal amount of wall tension to the undissected aorta. The septum will recoil and collapse the true lumen resulting in the typically observed findings on imaging of false lumen expansion and true lumen compression.

3. Epidemiology

The incidence of aortic dissection is between 2.6 and 3.5 cases per 100,000 people per year; however, this is likely an underestimate due to the significant prehospital mortality rate [7]. Compared to aneurysmal disease, aortic dissection patients tend to be younger and 65% of them are male [8]. This condition may also present in much younger patients, typically in the setting of uncontrolled hypertension, catecholamine-releasing drugs use such as cocaine or amphetamines, and underlying connective tissue disorders (i.e., Marfans Syndrome or Ehler-Danlos Syndrome).

Up to 15% of aortic dissections are limited to the aortic root or ascending arch, 25 to 30% involve the descending thoracic aorta distal to the origin of the left subclavian artery, and 60% involve and extend beyond the ascending aorta and the aortic arch [9]. Presentation, treatment modality, and survivability differ greatly based on the anatomic origin of dissection.

4. Diagnosis

Most patients presenting with aortic dissection describe tearing chest pain, often radiating to the neck, back, or jaw. Ascending aortic dissection can result in aortic insufficiency and cardiac tamponade. Descending aortic dissections can similarly result in branch vessel malperfusion depending on the extent and location of the dissection flap. Peripheral malperfusion may be detected on physical exam by detecting a pulse differential in the extremities. Given the overlap in symptoms between aortic dissection and alternative life-threatening conditions like acute coronary syndromes, a high degree of suspicion should be maintained especially considering the consequences of missed or delayed diagnosis which can be fatal. This is compounded by the fact that up to 20% of aortic dissection patients have ST segment changes on electrocardiogram [10]. Various imaging modalities may be used to diagnose aortic dissection, including gated-computed tomographic angiography, magnetic resonance angiography and echocardiography, each with their advantages and disadvantages.

Gated-computed tomographic angiography is the gold standard imaging technique that is frequently easiest to obtain and paramount to operative case planning and long-term follow-up.

5. Classification

The treatment algorithms for management vary based on the anatomic location of the aortic dissection. There are two traditional classification systems commonly used, as well as a newly proposed classification system for aortic dissections. Aortic dissection is categorized anatomically, as well as by the presence or absence of branch vessel compromise. Although various classification schemes exist, the classically employed Stanford system categorizes aortic dissection into the more common type A, in which the ascending aorta or proximal arch is involved, or type B, in which the dissection plane is limited to the aorta distal to the left subclavian artery origin [11]. Alternatively, the original DeBakey classification categorizes the dissection into three schemas based on the proximal intimal tear and the distal extent of the dissection. DeBakey type I aortic dissections involve the ascending aorta and extent distal to the arch (**Figure 3**). Type II is limited to the ascending aorta and type III originates and is limited to the descending thoracic aorta [13].

A more contemporary classification scheme proposed by a joint committee of the societies of thoracic and vascular surgery provides a more detailed anatomical description of the aortic dissection [14]. In this classification system, the proximal and distal aortic extent of the tear are denoted as subscripts relating to the aortic zone after the A of B determination based on the Stanford criteria (**Figure 4**). Aortic dissections are also categorized by chronicity which is another important management

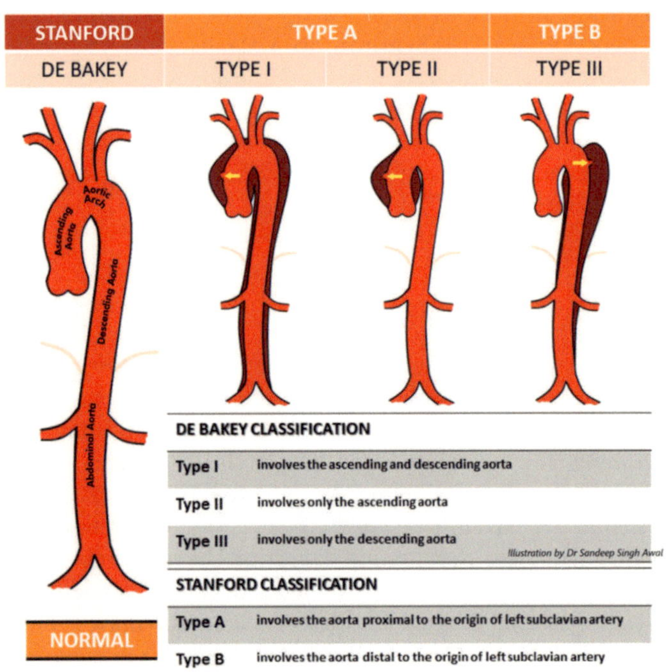

Figure 3.
Debakey and Stanford classification of aortic dissection [12]. (permission pending).

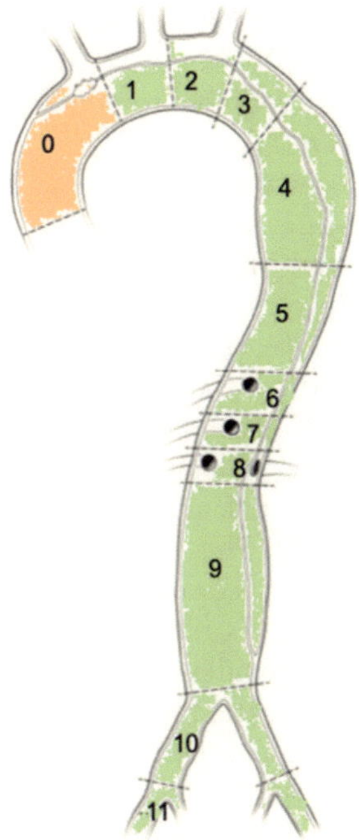

Type	Proximal Extent	Distal Extent
A	0	0
	1	1
	2	2
Entry tear in Zone 0	3	3
	4	4
B	5	5
Entry tear distal to Zone 0	6	6
	7	7
	8	8
I	9	9
	10	10
Unidentified tear	11	11
	12	12

Figure 4.
Society for vascular surgery and society of thoracic surgery aortic dissection classification scheme [14].

consideration reflecting morbidity, mortality, risk of endovascular intervention, and aortic remodeling. Acute dissections occur less than 14 days from symptom onset with a subcategory of hyperacute dissections occurring less than 24 hours from symptom onset. Subacute aortic dissections describe the period from 2 weeks to 3 months post-symptom onset, and finally chronic dissections include those older than 3 months from symptom onset [15]. New tears, including acute and, more specifically, hyperacute aortic dissections, have a thin septum that gradually thickens and becomes calcified and thus becomes less compliant with time. In the hyperacute and acute phase, the friability of the aortic wall leads to an increased risk of retrograde tearing with intervention.

6. Management

6.1 Nonoperative management

Type A aortic dissections are typically managed with emergent surgery and ascending aortic replacement with interposition grafting requiring hypothermic circulatory arrest and possible aortic valve repair or resuspension of which the details fall outside the scope of this chapter. Type B dissections without rupture or branch vessel malperfusion thus deemed uncomplicated are managed medically with blood pressure control, analgesia, and monitoring in the intensive care unit. In cases with rupture or compromised aortic branch vessel patency, intervention may be indicated to expand the true aortic lumen and re-establish branch perfusion. Initial management of uncomplicated type B aortic dissections involves blood pressure control which is commonly accomplished with intravenous beta blockade to decrease the pulse pressure with a target systolic blood pressure of 100–120 mmHg and heart rate of 60–80 beats per minute [16]. If additional agents are required to achieve control, parenteral calcium channel blockers and vasodilators may be added.

If presenting to a community hospital, transfer to a tertiary medical center with an intensive care unit and relevant surgical subspecialties should be initiated and strongly considered. Invasive blood pressure monitoring should be used and frequent laboratory testing to assess for chemical signs of malperfusion is recommended. Uncomplicated aortic dissection without signs of rupture, end-organ malperfusion and other high-risk features who undergo optimal medical management can often be safely transitioned to oral antihypertension medications and observed without surgery. Once beyond the acute phase, aortic remodeling is likely to occur if lifelong blood pressure control is maintained. Patients with high-risk aortic dissections which are not complicated, may warrant early intervention [17]. These include patients with maximal aortic diameter exceeding 4 cm, entry tears exceeding 1 cm, and false lumens exceeding 2.2 cm which have been shown to lead to aneurysmal degeneration [18]. Finally, patients with refractory pain, radiographic evidence of malperfusion, and hemorrhagic pleural effusion may also benefit from early intervention. To mitigate the risk of retrograde type A dissection, intervention in these cases is typically preferred in the subacute phase.

In the setting of end-organ ischemia or rupture, intervention is indicated. Malperfusion pathophysiology may be due to dynamic or static occlusion of branch vessels. In dynamic malperfusion, the highly mobile dissection flap temporarily occludes the branch vessel origin with hemodynamic changes during the cardiac cycle. In static obstruction, the dissection flap propagates into the branch vessel origin, causing true lumen to collapse with or without thrombosis. Malperfusion syndromes can affect any branch vessel but typically involve the renal arteries and visceral arteries but may also include the iliac arteries resulting in lower extremity ischemia, or the carotid and spinal arteries resulting in stroke or spinal cord ischemia, respectively. While more aggressive management is indicated in these scenarios, the principle of blood pressure control must still be applied.

6.2 Operative management

Repair should be done in an institution with an infrastructure in place to care for and manage these clinically complicated patients. This includes the availability of cardiothoracic surgical consultation in the event thoracotomy is indicated as well as the presence of a multidisciplinary team of experienced anesthesiologists, intensivists, nurses, and perfusionists and an intensive care unit familiar with the care of aortic dissection patients. Intravascular ultrasound and transesophageal echocardiogram capabilities may also be helpful. Preoperative considerations such as placement of a spinal drain to reduce the risk of spinal cord ischemia should be decided based on the acuity of the patient, the experience of the anesthesiologist and the anticipated length of aortic coverage. Since the goal is simply coverage of the entry tear to allow true lumen expansion, routine prophylactic lumbar drain placement usually is not necessary in the acute setting.

In 1999, Dake described the first TEVAR with a stent graft that is the current standard of care for the treatment of aortic dissections [19]. The advantages of TEVAR for type B aortic dissection repair include the ability to perform the procedure under local anesthesia with mild sedation, without requiring single lung ventilation as well as the decreased operative time and faster recovery of this minimally invasive procedure. Planning for TEVAR to repair type B aortic diameter includes consideration of the access vessels, intended aortic diameter, choice of available endografts, endograft diameter, and length of aortic coverage including proximal and distal seal zones with the potential need for proximal arch vessel coverage, as well as adjunctive techniques to assist with aortic remodeling.

The available FDA-approved endografts for the thoracic aorta include the Cook Zenith Alpha and Zenith TX2 (Cook Medical Incorporated, Bloomington, Indiana, USA); Gore c-TAG and TAG Thoracic Branch Endoprosthesis (W.L. Gore & Associates Incorporated, Newark, Delaware, USA); Medtronic Valiant (Medtronic PLC, Minneapolis, Minnesota, USA), and Terumo RelayPro and RelayPlus (Terumo Corporation, Shibuya City, Japan). The instructions for use of these devices vary and should be adhered to in order to achieve ideal results. Typically, 15–20 mm of healthy proximal and distal seal zones with a maximum aortic diameter of less than 42 mm are required for successful implantation. This may require coverage of one or more of the sura-aortic trunks, most frequently the left subclavian artery to achieve an adequate seal.

In the elective setting, subclavian revascularization with extra-anatomic bypass can be performed prior to TEVAR to reduce the risk of neurologic complications; however, in the emergent setting these patients are typically observed for signs of ischemia. A dominant left vertebral artery and a left internal mammary artery-based coronary artery bypass are obligatory indications for subclavian revascularization, typically *via* a left common carotid to left subclavian artery bypass.

The Gore TAG Thoracic Branch Endoprosthesis is a novel, off-the-shelf device with a built-in branch portal allowing for proximal seal in zone 2. Intravascular ultrasound is helpful to accurately measure aortic diameter and confirm true lumen positioning. The stent graft should be minimally oversized (<10%) to the native aorta to reduce the risk of retrograde dissection in a friable aorta [20]. The extent of graft coverage in the aorta should be limited to covering the entry tear with a single stent graft in the descending thoracic aorta which is often enough to allow for true lumen re-expansion without the increased risk of spinal cord ischemia that is associated with aortic coverage length [21].

The Cook Petticoat graft (Zenith® Dissection Endovascular System) represents a newer novel graft originally FDA-approved in 2019 and is a dissection-specific bare metal stent extension (Cook® Medical Incorporated, Bloomington, Indiana, USA) placed across the renovisceral segment. Known as the "Petticoat" technique in the case of more extensive dissections, has been shown to aid with positive aortic remodeling by reapposition of the dissection flap to the aortic wall over long-term follow-up [22].

In Patel's recent 2021 retrospective multicenter cohort of 120 patients from 10 European institutions with both complicated and uncomplicated type B aortic dissections treated with Zenith TX2 Dissection Endovascular Graft (ZDEG) and the Zenith Dissection Bare stent (ZDES) between 2011 and 2018, 30-day mortality was 5.8% post-surgery and 1.7% between 30 and 90 days of follow-up. Stroke and paraplegia occurred in 2.5% and 4.2% of patients, respectively. There was a 6.7% perioperative rate of type Ia endoleak and no instances of paraplegia, no permanent dialysis, and no requirement for adjunctive superior mesenteric stenting in the 33 patients (27.5%) who were treated by concurrent placement of ZDES distal to the ZDEG [23].

7. Complications

TEVAR for aortic dissection is not without its risk of serious complications. These include complications typical of endovascular access-based procedures such as femoral artery pseudoaneurysm, hematoma, vessel dissection, and thrombosis as well as potential problems specifically linked to instrumenting a damaged aorta such as aortic rupture, retrograde dissection propagation and stent graft induced new entry tears. Additional risks of inherent to TEVAR include stroke, spinal cord ischemia, myocardial infarction, acute kidney injury, bowel ischemia, and death.

8. Outcomes

TEVAR for aortic dissection has favorable long-term results compared with open surgical management. Results are also dependent on long-term optimal medical management of hypertension, wherein long-term mortality has been shown to be less than 10% at 1 year [24]. Short-term mortality is increased in patients presenting with hypotension, syncope, rupture, malperfusion syndromes including renal, mesenteric, limb and spinal ischemia, and advanced age [25]. With all aortic dissection patients treated with medical management, open surgery, and/or TEVAR, secondary interventions of the aorta are quite common and always necessitate long-term medical management and regular imaging surveillance in this patient population [26].

Regardless of surveillance, all-cause mortality at 1 year, 3 years, and 10 years was 15%, 24%, and 57%, respectively in this patient population and cumulative incidence of aortic-related mortality at 1 year, 3 years, and 10 years was 8.9%, 16.5%, and 27.2%, respectively. Nonaortic-related mortality was 2.7%, 7.2%, and 29%, respectively at 1 year, 3 years, and 10 years in this extremely ill cohort of patients [27].

9. Notes

The Terumo Thoraflex Hybrid, RelayPro, and RelayPlus (Terumo Aortic, Sunrise, Fl, USA) represent novel devices utilized in the therapies for thoracic aortic dissections and aneurysmal disease of the ascending and descending aorta, respectively.

The Thoraflex Hybrid graft is utilized in open repairs of the ascending aorta and arch for the frozen elephant trunk technique. The trial by Coselli [28] was published in 2024 and involved 12 US sites which included 65 patients without rupture in the primary study group and 9 patients recruited in the rupture group. Freedom from major adverse events was 81% at 1 year. Twenty-six patients underwent extension procedures including 22 endovascular procedures within a median of 122 days and freedom from MAE at 1 year was 71%.

The RelayPro represents the only on-label endovascular option to extend the Thoraflex Hybrid graft if the lesion requires extension after frozen elephant trunk. About 38% of patients need a downstream extension [29]. The RelayPro grafts offer 38% profile reduction in the graft with material tight woven polyester, a 24% profile reduction with new thin wall coiled primary introducer outer sheath and a 21% profile reduction of the inner sheath diameter. It is indicated for the treatment of thoracic aorta pathologies in adult patients such as aneurysms, pseudoaneurysms, dissections, and penetrating ulcers with intramural hematoma.

The study by Starnes et al. [30] published in 2024 was a prospective multicenter study assessing the low-profile RelayPro thoracic endograft in the treatment of traumatic aortic injury. The study enrolled 50 patients at 16 US centers from 2017 and 2021. Kaplan–Meier estimated freedom from major adverse events, all-cause mortality, paralysis, and stroke, was 98.0% at 30 days and 95.8% from 6 months to 4 years. RelayPro was deemed safe and effective and may provide an early survival benefit in the treatment of blunt traumatic aortic injury with long-term results still being followed.

In the study by Rossi [31], the RelayPro endograft was assessed for the treatment of acute complicated type B aortic dissection with initial primary end point of all-cause mortality at 30 days. The study consisted of 56 patients in 22 US centers and reported 7 major adverse events in 6 patients which consisted of paraplegia, paraparesis, disabling stroke, and renal failure. Estimated freedom from major adverse events was 89.1% at each interval from 30 days to 3 years.

The Relay Thoracic Stent-Graft with Plus Delivery System was specifically designed to accommodate the curvature and tortuosity of the thoracic aorta and originally approved by the FDA in 2012. Farber in 2017 looked at the RelayPlus in an investigational device exemption study with 3-year follow-up results with 100% technical success; 2.6% stroke rate; 0% Type I/III endoleak; 0% migration; 7.9% secondary interventions; and 0% fracture [32].

Malas in his post market approval study in 2021 [33] looked at thoracic aortic aneurysms and penetrating atherosclerotic ulcers undergoing thoracic endovascular aortic repair in novice and experienced users. There were 45 patients in the study with 2 deaths perioperatively. Three-year freedom from TEVAR-related mortality, all-cause mortality, and reinterventions was 95.6%, 84.0%, and 97.2%, respectively, with two type I endoleaks at 3 years: one type IB (distal) and one type IA (proximal). Early midterm results showed sustained freedom from TEVAR-related mortality. Follow-up continues to evaluate results of the low profile endograft.

Acknowledgements

Department of Cardiothoracic & Vascular Surgery, Montefiore Medical Center. The authors wish to thank Terumo Aortic for their generous support in publishing this manuscript.

Conflict of interest

The authors declare no conflict of interest.

Author details

Shuo Huang, James Hu, Matthew Carnevale and Paul Lajos*
Division of Vascular and Endovascular Surgery, Albert Einstein School of Medicine, Montefiore Medical Center, Bronx, New York, USA

*Address all correspondence to: plajos@montefiore.org

References

[1] Nicholls F. Observations concerning the body of his late Manistee, 26 October 1760. Philosophical Transactions. 1761;**52**(2):65-75

[2] Morgagni GB. De sedibus et causis morborum per anatomen indagatis (the seats and causes of diseases investigated by anatomy). Venice from the printing Remondiniana. Anatomo-Medical Letter. 1761;**713**(26):275

[3] Laennec RTMH. Traite de l'auscutation mediate, 2e. Paris: Tome II; 1826. pp. 695-704

[4] DeBakey ME, McCollum CH, Crawford ES, et al. Dissection and dissecting aneurysms of the aorta: Twenty-year follow-up of five hundred twenty-seven patients treated surgically. Surgery. 1982;**92**(6):1118-1134

[5] Nienaber CA, Fattori R, Lund G, Dieckmann C, Wolf W, von Kodolitsch Y, et al. Nonsurgical reconstruction of thoracic aortic dissection by stent-graft placement. The New England Journal of Medicine. 1999;**340**(20):1539-1545

[6] Dake MD, Kato N, Mitchell RS, Semba CP, Razavi MK, Shimono T, et al. Endovascular stent-graft placement for the treatment of acute aortic dissection. The New England Journal of Medicine. 1999;**340**(20):1546-1552

[7] Tsai T, Nienaber CA, Eagle KA. Acute aortic syndromes. Circulation. 2005;**112**(24):3802-3813

[8] Clouse WD, Hallett JW, Schaff HV, et al. Acute aortic dissection: Population-based incidence compared with degenerative aortic aneurysm rupture. Mayo Clinic Proceedings. 2004;**79**(2):176-180

[9] Al'Aref SJ, Girardi LN, Devereux R, et al. A contemporary review of acute aortic dissection. Emergency Medicine (Los Angel). 2015;**5**(274):2

[10] Cho JR, Shin S, Kim JS, et al. Clinical characteristics of acute aortic syndrome in Korean patients: From the Korean multi-center registry of acute aortic syndrome. Korean Circulation Journal. 2012;**42**(8):528-537

[11] Daily PO, Trueblood HW, Stinson EB, et al. Management of acute aortic dissections. The Annals of Thoracic Surgery. 1970;**10**(3):237-247

[12] Awal SS, Prasad N, Biswas S. CT evaluation of aortic dissection and other acute aortic syndromes: An update. International Journal of Radiology & Radiation Therapy. 2022;**9**(5):159-165

[13] DeBakey ME, Henly WS, Cooley DA, et al. Surgical management of dissecting aneurysms of the aorta. Journal of Thoracic and Cardiovascular Surgery. 1965;**49**(1):130-149

[14] Lombardi JV, Hughes GC, Appoo JJ, et al. Society for Vascular Surgery (SVS) and Society of Thoracic Surgeons (STS) reporting standards for type B aortic dissections. The Annals of Thoracic Surgery. 2020;**109**(3):959-981

[15] Hirst AE, Johns VJ, Kime SW. Dissecting aneurysm of the aorta: A review of 505 cases. Medicine (Baltimore). 1958;**37**:217-279

[16] Raymond CE, Aggarwal B, Schoenhagen P, et al. Prevalence and factors associated with false positive suspicion of acute aortic syndrome: Experience in a patient population transferred to a

specialized aortic treatment center. Cardiovascular Diagnosis and Therapy. 2013;**3**(4):196-204

[17] Acosta S, Blomstrand D, Gottsäter A. Epidemiology and long-term prognostic factors in acute type B aortic dissection. Annals of Vascular Surgery. 2007;**21**(4):415-422

[18] Trimarchi S, Eagle KA, Nienaber CA, et al. Importance of refractory pain and hypertension in acute type B aortic dissection: Insights from the international registry of acute aortic dissection (IRAD). Circulation. 2010;**122**:1283-1289

[19] Dake MD, Kato N, Mitchell RS, et al. Endovascular stent–graft placement for the treatment of acute aortic dissection. NEJM. 1999;**340**(20):1546-1552

[20] Baliga RR, Nienaber CA, Bossone E, et al. The role of imaging in aortic dissection and related syndromes. JACC: Cardiovascular Imaging. 2014;**7**(4):406-424

[21] Chiesa R, Melissano G, Marrocco-Trischitta MM, et al. Spinal cord ischemia after elective stent-graft repair of the thoracic aorta. Journal of Vascular Surgery. 2005;**42**:11-17

[22] Lombardi JV, Gleason TG, Panneton JM, et al. STABLE II investigators. STABLE II clinical trial on endovascular treatment of acute, complicated type B aortic dissection with a composite device design. Journal of Vascular Surgery. 2020;**71**(4):1077-1087

[23] Patel JJ, Kasprzak P, Pfister K, Tsilimparis N, et al. Early outcomes associated with use of the Zenith TX2 Dissection Endovascular Graft for the treatment of Stanford type B aortic dissection. Journal of Vascular Surgery. 2021;**74**(2):547-555

[24] White RA, Miller DC, Criado FJ, et al. Multidisciplinary society for vascular surgery outcomes committee. Report on the results of thoracic endovascular aortic repair for acute, complicated, type B aortic dissection at 30 days and 1 year from a multidisciplinary subcommittee of the society for vascular surgery outcomes committee. Journal of Vascular Surgery. 2011;**53**(4):1082-1090

[25] Tolenaar JL, Froehlich W, Jonker FH, et al. Predicting in-hospital mortality in acute type B aortic dissection: Evidence from international registry of acute aortic dissection. Circulation. 2014;**130**(11 suppl. 1):S45-S50

[26] Scali ST, Beck AW, Butler K, et al. Pathology-specific secondary aortic interventions after thoracic endovascular aortic repair. Journal of Vascular Surgery. 2014;**59**(3):599-607

[27] Hysa L, Khor S, Starnes B, et al. Cause-specific mortality of type B aortic dissection and assessment of competing risks of mortality. Journal of Vascular Surgery. 2021;**73**(1):48-60

[28] Coselli JS, Roselli EE, Preventza O, et al. Total aortic arch replacement using a frozen elephant trunk device: Results of a 1-year US multicenter trial. The Journal of Thoracic and Cardiovascular Surgery. 2024;**167**(5):1680-1692.e2

[29] Kandola S, Abdulsalam A, Field M, Fisher RK. Frozen elephant trunk repair of aortic aneurysms: How to reduce the incidence of endoleak and reintervention. JTCVS Techniques. 2020;**20**(3):13-20

[30] Starnes BW, Rajani RR, Rossi P, et al, Early survival benefit of a low-profile endograft in blunt traumatic aortic injury. Journal of Vascular Surgery. 2024;**80**(3):678-684.e1

[31] Rossi PJ, Desai ND, Malaisrie SC, et al. One-year results of a low-profile endograft in acute, complicated type B aortic dissection. Annals of Thoracic Surgery. 2024;**117**(2):336-343

[32] Farber MA, Lee WA, Szeto WY, et al. Initial and midterm results of the Bolton Relay Thoracic Aortic Endovascular Pivotal Trial. Journal of Vascular Surgery. 2017;**65**(6):1556-1566.e1

[33] Malas M, Locham S, Hughes C, et al. Midterm outcomes in patients undergoing endovascular repair of thoracic aortic aneurysms and penetrating atherosclerotic ulcers using the RelayPlus stent graft. Journal of Vascular Surgery. 2021;**73**(2):459-465

Chapter 2

Anatomic Completeness, Variations, Patency, and Functional Assessment of Circle of Willis: Implications for Chronic Aortic Dissection and Non-Emergent Arch Surgery

Antonio Nenna, Diletta Corrado, Francesco Loreni, Chiara Ferrisi, Gennaro Sorrentino, Omar Giacinto, Raffaele Barbato, Ciro Mastroianni, Mario Lusini and Massimo Chello

Abstract

Circle of Willis (CoW) variations are present in a significant number of patients. In patients undergoing non-emergent surgery for aortic dissection (e.g., chronic dissection or planned complex aortic arch surgery), an extensive preoperative examination is warranted as anatomic completeness, variation, patency, and functional assessment of CoW is crucial to optimize neuroprotection strategies. In non-emergent clinical presentations, unilateral or bilateral selective cerebral perfusion should be tailored to patient's anatomy to minimize intraoperative risk and improve outcomes. A new classification system provides a simple and comprehensive ontology of the described anatomical variations of the CoW. An accurate preoperative assessment might indicate the need for adjunctive perfusion in selected CoW configurations.

Keywords: circle of Willis, variants, variations, cerebral perfusion, cerebral protection, aortic arch surgery, dissection, aneurysm

1. Introduction

Circle of Willis (CoW) or cerebral arterial circle (CAC) is an arterial anastomotic network formed by a symmetrical polygonal-shaped connection between internal carotid arteries (ICAs) and vertebral arteries (VAs). It is located in the subarachnoid space on the base of the brain, around the optic chiasm and infundibulum of the pituitary stalk in the suprasellar cistern.

The anastomotic circle may be divided into 2 parts:

- Anterior circulation: formed by left and right internal carotid arteries (ICAs), horizontal segments (A1s) of the left and the right anterior cerebral arteries (ACAs), and a single anterior communicating artery (AcomA)

- Posterior circulation: consisting of left and right posterior communicating arteries (PcomAs), the horizontal segments (P1s) of left and right posterior cerebral arteries (PCAs), and a single basilar artery formed by the union of right and left VAs.

This anastomotic network allows an equal vascular supply between the two cerebral hemispheres and provides adequate perfusion in case of impaired or decreased blood flow through one or more of its segment arteries. However, other functions may be attributed to CoW, as demonstrated by Burlakoti et al. [1] through the measurement of cross-sectional area of incoming, communicating, and outgoing arteries of 51 cadaveric brains. The significant differences in the cross-sectional area of incoming and outgoing arteries, together with the area of communicating arteries, may be relevant for lowering the peak pressures of arterial blood perfusion of the brain, reducing hemodynamic stress, and proving a better distribution of pressure waves.

Four criteria are established to define the "normal" (non-variant) anatomy of the CoW [2]:

- All segments are present (AComA, A1s, PComAs, and P1s);

- All segments arise from their natural origins;

- No accessory arteries are present;

- All segments have an external diameter of >1 mm.

It is estimated that 68.22% of individuals in the neurologically healthy population have CoW variations, more frequent than the considered non-variant configuration. Commonly recorded variation types include hypoplasia, absence, and duplication. Hypoplasia is usually defined as a diameter <1 mm. Variations are a risk factor for cerebrovascular diseases, above all variations of CoW increase the risk of stroke, as analyzed by De Caro et al. [3] in a study where the prevalence of CoW variants increased in patients with ischemic stroke when compared to those who have other illnesses or symptoms besides stroke, due to a less efficient collateral flow. Another important cerebrovascular disease involved is arterial aneurysms, which may develop from the altered hemodynamics that characterize variations of CoW, as a result of high and low wall shear stress around the bifurcation sites [1]. Larger aneurysms have an increased risk of rupture, leading to subarachnoid hemorrhage and hemorrhagic ischemia. Variations of CoW are also involved in therapeutic options in preoperative assessment for vascular and heart surgery to choose the most appropriate method for cerebral perfusion and protection.

The purpose of this chapter is to give an overview of how variations influence the selection of cerebral perfusion techniques in aortic arch surgery.

2. Classification of variations

The considerable heterogeneity of variants of CoW leads to the need to create an anatomical and functional classification system, due to the relevance of variants in the preoperative assessment to decide the best surgical approach and the requirement of precautions. The study of CoW variants and adequate cerebral protection techniques reduce surgical errors and postoperative complications, improving the clinical outcome of patients after surgery. The aim is to prevent neurological sequelae after arch surgery during total or partial arch replacement through the classification of variations in risk categories which may help to use appropriate techniques of cerebral perfusion.

The elaborate embryological evolution of CoW and the shifting configurations that precede its definitive form predispose to abnormal development that may influence its capacity as a shunt mechanism. In 1961, Riggs and Rupp [4] classified the anomalous formation of CoW in four groups, based on the hypoplasia of communicating arteries (AcomAs and PcomAs), divisional branches of basilar artery (P1s), proximal anterior cerebral arteries (A1s) and both divisional branches of basilar and anterior cerebral. Although it is an admirable work where anatomical description encounters functional consequence, they described 21 anomalous configurations only considering hypoplastic segments, according to the configuration accepted as typical by Padget, without including absence or duplication of the cerebral arteries segments.

Later, in 1979, Lazorthes [5] described 22 different patterns of CoW, where type I is the typical CoW according to Padget's definition, and type II is the "fetal type", characterized by hypoplasia of all arterial segments. With regards to other configurations, they are based on the dependence or independence of the three main arterial axes (carotid arteries and basilar artery), but only segment hypoplasia is included and the lack of anatomical or functional distribution of variants in groups can generate confusion and misunderstanding about the functional consequence and the main feature of each variation. Moreover, the illustrations of CoW patterns are unclear and not exactly descriptive of hypoplasia.

In 1998, Krabbe-Hartkamp [6] outlined 18 variants using three-dimensional time-of-flight magnetic resonance angiography, dividing them into 2 groups based on the anatomical position, whether the hypoplasia or absence of segment is in the anterior or posterior circle. Hypoplasia was defined as a diameter smaller than 0.8 mm, therefore it may underestimate the frequency and the number of variations.

Afterward, Merkkola et al. [7] studied casts and angiographies made during forensic medicine autopsies to assess in theory weather perfusion through the right axillary artery is sufficient in providing uniform distribution of blood to both hemispheres of the brain (**Table 1**). They defined hypoplasia as a diameter below 0.5 mm but also repeated the analysis using 1 mm as threshold. In addition, they considered that critical arteries to examine are the AcomA and the left PcomA, because AcomA transports blood through the anterior circulation of CoW to the left cerebral hemisphere and PcomA establishes communication between the anterior and the posterior circulation. Then their absence is associated with hypoperfusion of the left hemisphere of the brain. They defined communicating arteries as normal, compromised, or missing depending on the diameter of the vessel, if >0.5 mm, <0.5 mm, or not present in either the permanent cast or the angiography. Then, they created four groups: the first one was referred to as excellent because both communicating arteries were normal; the second group called "good" was characterized by only one normal communicating

Study (year)	Patients	CoW variants, details, and outcomes
Merkkola et al. [7]	87	Exellent: AcomA+AcomPsn N 35% Good: AcomA N+ AcomPsnM 32%, AcomA M+ AcomPsn N 8%, AcomA C + AcomPsn N 8% Compromised: AcomA m + AcomPsn C 1%, AcomA C + AcomPsn M 2% Bad: AcomA M+ AcomPsn M 14%
Papantchev et al. [8]	99	CoW type Ia Left PCoA or both PCoA Left MCA 27.3% (27/99) 26.6% (22/83) CoW type Ib AcoA Left ACA 0% (0/99) 2.4% (2/83) CoW type IIa ACoA and left PCoA Left ACA; left MCA 3.1% (3/99) 3.6% (3/83) CoW type IIb Right VA or left PCA (P1 segment) Left MCA; left PCA 9.1% (9/99) 7.2% (6/83) CoW type III Right ACA (A1 segment) Right ACA; left ACA; left MCA 3.1% (3/99) 7.2% (6/83) CoW type IV Right VA and right ACA (A1 segment) Right ACA; left ACA; left MCA; left PCA 0% (0/99) 1.2% (1/83) Total 42.4% (42/99) 48.2% (40/83)
Papantchev et al. [9]	500	Type IA Left PComA Left middle cerebral artery 35.6% (178/500) Type IB AComA Left anterior cerebral artery 2% (10/500) Type IIA Left PComA + AComA Left anterior cerebral artery + left middle cerebral artery 4.8% (24/500) Type IIB Left P1 or right VA Left middle cerebral artery + left posterior cerebral artery 9.2% (46/500) Type IIIA Right A1 + right anterior cerebral artery + left anterior cerebral artery + left middle cerebral artery 6% (30/500) Type IIIB AcomA + right VA Left anterior cerebral artery + left middle cerebral artery + left posterior cerebral artery 0.2% (1/500) Type IV Right A1 + right VA or right A1 + left P1 Right anterior cerebral artery + left anterior cerebral artery + left MCA + left PCA 0.8% (4/500) Total: 58.6% (293/500)

Table 1.
Studies describing anatomic variances of CoW during autopsies after sudden cardiac/cerebrovascular death.

artery; the patients who belonged to the compromised group, the third one, had both arteries compromised or one compromised and the other one missing; the last group was characterized by the absence of both the communicating arteries. This classification is limited because only considers two segments of CoW and does not look at vertebral arteries, right A1 and left P1 abnormalities. The proposed classification included in the same group a missing and a hypoplastic segment, which may generate confusion and may not represent an accurate analysis of the hypoperfusion risk of unilateral cerebral perfusion technique.

As we discussed, the incompleteness of these classification systems brought Ayre et al. [2] to propose a comprehensive classification system through the distribution of 82 distinct anatomical variations into five groups, based on the type of abnormalities (hypoplastic or absent segment), which can provide a clear and complete vision about all the patterns we may detect in patients. In this classification, the absence of segments is included, both hypoplastic and absent segments, and the presence of accessory segments. This system allows us to clearly distinguish every potential variation, but it is only based on an anatomical examination without information about functional implications. In addition, to identify the specific variants which may be observed in patients and attribute them to the corresponding group, it is necessary to consult the illustrated table of Ayre's classification. This approach may be impractical and time-consuming, especially in an emergent or urgent situation. Another disadvantage in using this classification as a reference for cerebral perfusion in cardiac surgery is the absence of vertebral artery abnormalities, not taken into consideration either by classification previously seen. However, it may be helpful and more convenient for the attribution to each group and subgroup of an ideal perfusion technique to warrant blood flow for each cerebral hemisphere, based on a primary empirical evaluation, to enhance the identification and categorization of CoW variants.

Coulier et al. [10] described the frequencies of variations of CoW, identifying 27 types of variations in 511 patients with Computed Tomographic Angiographic 3D Volume Rendering reconstruction of the cerebral arterial circle (CAC). They classify variants into 3 groups: complete CACs (22.5%) with seven robust segments (6.1%) or with hypoplastic segments, nearly complete CAC (30.72%) with only one segment absent and incomplete CAC. They found that the posterior arch (73.18%) is much more frequently incomplete than the anterior arch (18.4%), due to the lack of PComAs, unilaterally or bilaterally.

Above all, it is important to highlight variations characterized by some very precarious vascular supplies, such as complete isolation of the MCA (iMCA), found in 1.8% of patients and detected in seven different types of configurations. The MCA is isolated when it is not connected to the contralateral ICA through the anterior circulation for the absence of ipsilateral or contralateral A1 segment of ACA or AcomA and, at the same time, it is not connected to vertebral arteries through the posterior circulation, due to the absence of PcomA or ipsilateral P1 segment of PCA. The most common configuration is the absence of both communicating arteries, anterior and posterior, followed by the absence of ipsilateral A1 and PcomA. Banga et al. [11] found that iMCA is an independent predictor of immediate neurological events after CEA using cross-clamping technique without shunt protection. Fortunately, in 545 patients who underwent CEA, the iMCA was found in 6.3%, so it's a rare CoW variation.

Other situations of anomalous CoW are complete separation of the 2 hemispheres (2.15%), complete separation of basilar and carotid territories (40.1%, frequently missing both PComAs), complete separation of the three main arterial axis of CAC (both ICAs and VB trunk, 8.6%, frequently missing all the communicating arteries).

As seen, the posterior arch is most involved in CoW variations, specifically for the PcomA-P1-P2 complex, involving a particular variant named "Fetal Posterior Cerebral Artery" (FPCA) in which the distal posterior carotid artery territory is dependent on the ipsilateral ICA. All the posterior arch variations can be divided into 5 groups:

- Agenesis of the PcomA (30.52% unilateral, 35% bilateral)
- Hypoplasia of the PcomA (25.24% unilateral, 19% bilateral)
- "Intermediate" type of FPCA, in which the caliber of P1 is quite similar to PcomA
- "Partial" type of FPCA, where the caliber of PcomA is greater than P1
- "Full" FPCA type, characterized by the absence of P1 and a robust PcomA.

Those variants may influence the extension of an ischemic stroke, hence the prognosis of patients, which can be worse or better than patients without variations. For instance, in patients with unilateral full FPCA type, a basilar artery occlusion may result in a smaller lesion, although an ICA obstruction may result in a wider ischemia compared to patients without CoW variation [3].

Rangus et al. [12] demonstrated that more than one-third of patients with CoW variations suffer ischemic stroke, especially in the posterior circulation rather than the anterior. A higher frequency of right-sided FPCA was registered among patients with CoW variants affected by stroke. All the patients affected by this condition were reclassified into having one territory lesion stroke pattern from an initial categorization as more than one territory pattern after performing MRI examinations. Initially, vertebrobasilar territory stroke was re-classified as ICA territory stroke, re-assigning the stroke from the posterior to the anterior territory. These patients are more prone to misclassification of stroke patterns, which could affect care, not only in the acute phase but may also compromise the choosing of the appropriate secondary prevention protocol.

It appears clear that some classifications do not include types of variations that may be fundamental in the preoperative evaluation, such as iMCA and the absence of vertebral arteries, probably due to the different aims and methods of each classification, as well as the different types of population involved and different threshold to define hypoplasia. For example, the Krabbe-Hartkamp classification is functional in understanding the role of CoW variations in patients with various degrees of carotid stenosis, and since it involved healthy subjects, it is focused on the diameter variations of segments. On the other hand, the Riggs and Rupp classification was obtained by patients with clinical signs of neurological dysfunction and it is centered on the hypoplasia of the segments without even a mention of segment absence, pursuing the aim to reconstruct the embryological derivation and subsequently the defects. It may underestimate the presence of CoW variants in healthy population.

Another difference is the type of method utilized to study CoW variations, such as imaging techniques (CTA, MRA) or anatomic dissection at autopsy. Each method has a different sensibility and specificity, so it may lead to miss variations that play an important role in cardiac and vascular surgery.

Despite the numerous attempts to create a complete and comprehensive classification system, it is indispensable to study a new categorization of CoW variants that allows easier and faster identification of the ideal perfusion technique for each variation when aortic arch surgery is performed.

Therefore, the important incidence of variations of CoW and the multitude types of configurations, despite the different implications of each configuration in neurological outcomes after vascular and cardiac surgery, support the use of Computer Tomography Angiography (CTA). This examination, adopted as a complementary high-quality evaluation for the preoperative assessment of non-emergent pathologies, such as chronic aortic dissection, reduces postoperative neurological complications.

3. Techniques of cerebral protection and neuromonitoring

Aortic arch surgery performed with the open distal anastomosis technique requires a blood-free operating field and it may be ensured through a period of circulatory arrest (CA). This strategy requires the interruption of all body circulation, including cerebral perfusion, and several studies demonstrated that it is indispensable to provide an adequate cerebral protection technique during CA, to reduce the risk of neurological postoperative complications.

After cardiac surgery, neurological injuries may occur. Roach classifies them into two categories: Type 1, which includes transient ischemic attack (TIA), fatal and non-fatal stroke, stupor, coma and hypoxic encephalopathy; Type 2, which includes epilepsy without focal deficit, memory loss, cognitive decline and delirium. Later, Ergin introduced a new classification to distinguish the characteristics of neurological damage on the basis of clinical expression, describing Transient Neurologic Deficit (TND) and Permanent Neurologic Dysfunction (PND), a useful system to compare the outcome of each cerebral protection strategy. TND is defined as a global ischemic injury, which is the result of inadequate or interrupted cerebral protection but is considered a benign self-limiting condition with complete resolution before the discharge. It manifests clinically as delirium, agitation, obtundation, postoperative confusion, or transient Parkinson's without evidence in cerebral imaging such as CT. PND is represented by ischemic stroke, due to an embolic event and it is not correlated with the strategy used for brain protection. MR shows cerebral lesions in the first 12–18 hours after the event, while CT after 24–48 hours. Symptoms and clinical manifestation depend on the site and the extension of the ischemic insult.

The deep hypothermic circulatory arrest (DHCA) was used in the 70s as a substitute for cardiopulmonary bypass (CPB) and, later, used for cerebral protection during arch surgery in aortic aneurism. The aim is to reduce metabolism and oxygen use for cerebral tissue. Deep or profound hypothermia is defined as a temperature below 20° C, which makes it possible to reduce the oxygen consumption of the human brain from 2.9 mL/g/min at 37°C to 0.2 mL/g/min at 20°C. A retrospective review [13] analyzed DHCA performed at a main temperature of 16.5°C versus DCHA with RCP at 20.5°C in patients who underwent aortic hemiarch reconstruction for elective aortic aneurysm or acute type A aortic dissection. This study demonstrated the operative mortality and postoperative stroke rate were comparable and there was no significant difference in long-term prognosis, in both elective and acute ascending aortic pathologies. CA time was shorter in the DCHA group (9 vs. 15 mins), according to the STS database study of type A dissection, which suggested that isolated DHCA less than 20 minutes might be safe during hemiarch replacement for aortic dissection. Unfortunately, it is difficult to predict the exact limit in terms of safe time to warrant cerebral protection and the temperature threshold to avoid deleterious systemic effects of deep hypothermia, although it is considered to be 18°C. A period >40 and >65 minutes of circulatory arrest is predictive of ischemic stroke and mortality respectively. Another disadvantage of DHCA is the prolonged CPB time, due to the longer period to cool down and to warm up the patient.

Englum et al. demonstrated the importance of combining deep hypothermia with a cerebral perfusion technique to reduce the incidence of postoperative stroke and neurological complications, without any differences in terms of operative mortality and neurological outcomes between retrograde and anterograde cerebral perfusion [14]. They also compared different grades of hypothermia and found no differences among various grades of hypothermia when a cerebral perfusion technique was included. The different grades of hypothermia experimented on in this study were defined and divided into three groups: high-moderate (24.1–28°C), low-moderate (20.1–24°C), and deep or profound (<20°C).

Ueda et al. described, for the first time, the use of retrograde cerebral perfusion (RCP) in aortic arch surgery. This technique consists of perfusing the brain through the superior vena cava with a retrograde blood flow. The main perfusion pressure is maintained between 20 and 25 mmHg but there is no possibility for direct monitoring. This type of perfusion may eliminate toxic metabolites and cerebral air and embolic debris from the arterial side, but the effectiveness remains uncertain. It may be disadvantageous for prolonged CPB time, as over 80 minutes, and if pressure is maintained over 30 mmHg because it may cause cerebral edema, worsening cerebral damage. Moreover, the veno-venous shunting of blood flow from the cerebral to the systemic venous circulation may occur, which could reduce the perfusion of brain capillary and, therefore, the efficacy and benefits of RCP in cerebral protection. However, meta-analysis demonstrates that RCP is associated with lower postoperative stroke and operative mortality compared with DHCA, with no difference in any outcome when comparing ASCP, even if DHCA is performed principally but not exclusively at a main temperature of 20°C. If executed at low-moderate temperature, RCP has no differences with ASCP in terms of neurological complications and post-operative stroke, so it allows for lowering the grade of hypothermia. Thus, this cerebral protection technique is least utilized when performing elephant trunk surgery, preferring bilateral or unilateral ASCP, probably due to the prolonged CPB time.

The anterograde selective cerebral perfusion (ASCP) remains the most used technique for cerebral protection. It was first used by De Bakey in 1957, and later, by Kazui in 1995 and Pacini in 2010, who demonstrated the efficacy in terms of postoperative morbidity and mortality. ASCP is based on cerebral perfusion directly through the epiaortic vessels and it may be unilateral or bilateral, in relation to the cannulation of one or both carotid arteries, even if the preferred cannulation site is the right axillary artery or both the right and left axillary artery in the case of bilateral ASCP to avoid manipulation of the supra-aortic vessels and the risk of atherosclerotic plaques dislocation. The main blood flow is regulated at 8–16 ml/Kg/min to maintain a radial blood pressure between 40 and 70 mmHg, with higher flows in warmer temperature strategies but below 16 mL/Kg/min in order to avoid an increased cerebral pressure. The core temperature is kept between 20 and 30°C, while perfusate temperature is kept between 20 and 26°C, and the left subclavian artery is clamped to avoid the subclavian steal syndrome. The use of this cerebral protection offers the advantage of prolonging the safe time of circulatory arrest, which is very useful when a more complex and longer surgery technique is performed. It also allows the use of bilateral perfusion if both anterior and posterior communicating arteries are absent, to reduce the risk of hypoperfusion of the left cerebral hemisphere. This procedure is not without its risks, such as embolic events and vascular injury of cannulated vessels.

Multiple factors contribute to the final neurological outcome after aortic arch surgery: temperature management, blood flow, pharmacologic protection, aortic cross-clamping, and duration of CA. The type of perfusion strategy adopted is the most deciding factor for the neurological outcome, as the cannulation site is for ASCP, providing the following options: the femoral artery, the right or left axillary artery, the carotid arteries, the innominate or subclavian artery and the ascending aorta in the true lumen. The right axillary artery is the preferred cannulation site, due to the lack of sandblast effect of turbulent flow, which may cause the disaggregation of atheromatous plaques and calcifications, with a reduced risk of cerebral embolization. Another advantage is the continuous backflow in all aortic arch vessels which minimizes the risk of cerebral air embolization. In contrast, the left axillary artery exploits posterior cerebral circle anterograde perfusion through the left vertebral artery. However, this may not ensure a complete cerebral perfusion in the case of CoW variants, as in the case of iMCA where there is no connection from the contralateral internal carotid artery and at the same time there is no connection from the vertebral arteries. In an emergent situation, when isolating the axillary artery is time-consuming, direct innominate artery (IA) cannulation may be used as an alternative, which is non-inferior to axillary artery with regard to neurological outcomes in elective aortic arch surgery, as demonstrated by a randomized trial comparing axillary and innominate artery as cannulation sites [15]. In addition, IA cannulation reduces procedural and CPB times, particularly in obese patients, and warrants lower flow resistance, decreasing blood loss in the operative field and/or kinking of the cannula. In case of shortness or dissection of IA, the right subclavian artery cannulation without infraclavicular incision may be used as a cannulation site. Left common carotid artery is a feasible and fast approach, used for an emergency option, mostly in obese patients, due to the high compliance of the vessel which allows high CPB flow. On the other hand, in case of small lumen, it will not support high CPB flows. Ascending aorta as a cannulation site is usually avoided due to the high risk of false lumen perfusion and rupture or dissection of the aortic wall while the femoral artery has long been the standard site for peripheral cannulation in non-elective cases permitting the cerebral blood flow through retrograde aortic perfusion, but a diseased abdominal and descending thoracic aorta increases the risk of cerebral emboli and malperfusion. The absence of obstructive clamps or cannulas within the field and direct aortic manipulation in femoral artery cannulation is advantageous for the surgical technique. However, the disadvantages of retrograde perfusion are the possible development of new re-entry tears and the perfusion of re-entry tears. In these circumstances, there is an important risk of epiaortic vessels and visceral malperfusion and, then, an increased risk of neurological damage. On those grounds, in the last 10 years, the cannulation of femoral artery gradually diminished.

In most centers, unilateral ASCP is performed with the axillary artery as a cannulation site, while bilateral ASCP may be performed using the right axillary artery and the left common carotid artery or the so-called "Kazui technique" [16] based on the direct cannulation of both the right and left carotid arteries.

Consensus regarding optimal cerebral protection strategy in aortic arch surgery is lacking, so the ideal method of cerebral perfusion remains undefined and is still a matter of debate. A systematic review and meta-analysis [17] assess the difference between cerebral protection strategies in terms of postoperative mortality and disabling stroke, by comparing different types of aortic arch surgery and pathologies: degenerative aortic aneurysm, acute type A aortic dissection, and post-dissection chronic aneurysm. The group of patients with unilateral ASCP had the lowest rate of operative mortality and disabling stroke. This was observed despite the unilateral ASCP group having the highest proportion of acute aortic dissections, especially relative to the bilateral group. The longest CPB, aortic cross-clamp, hypothermic circulatory arrest, and selective cerebral perfusion times were noted in the bilateral ASCP group, whereas bilateral ASCP was mainly used for total arch replacement. Even if it seems advantageous to prefer unilateral ASCP in case of a short period of circulatory arrest, not all patients may be suitable for this cerebral perfusion technique because of their cerebral vascular anatomy and physiology.

Even if some studies demonstrate the importance of collateral vessels like ophthalmic arteries, leptomeningeal vessels, and external carotid arteries which may permit the use of unilateral ASCP in patients with CoW variations, it is not considered protective when the duration of circulatory arrest is more than 50 minutes. For these reasons, De Paulis et al. recommend using bilateral ASCP if the duration is estimated to exceed 30–40 minutes [18]. Patel et al. support the use of bilateral ASCP, especially when the duration of circulatory arrest time is estimated to be greater than 30 minutes, due to the complexity of the procedure, as a total arch replacement, since 6–17% of adult population has an incomplete CoW, even if unilateral ASCP is a simple and reproducible technique [19].

In relation to CoW variations, the current expert consensus document of EACTS and ESVS recommends preoperative imaging studies to assess the patency and the morphology of CoW where treatment involves the aortic arch. Furthermore, it may not be feasible in an acute setting, as acute type A aortic dissection (ATAAD), which has a mortality rate of 50% in the first 48 hours after the onset of symptoms if surgery is not timely. Overall, the mortality rate of non-surgical treated patients is 58% while among surgically treated patients is 26%, with an incidence of postoperative neurological deficit of about 10–30%.

A systematic review and meta-analysis [20] show the difference between ASCP and RCP, also comparing bilateral with unilateral ASCP in patients affected by ATAAD who underwent emergent surgery. TND risk did not differ between RCP and ASCP, even if ACP increases the risk of embolic events and neurologic deficit while RCP theoretically decreases the risk of emboli formation but cannot provide physiological brain perfusion with a greater risk of hypoperfusion. However, the pooled risk ratio for TND demonstrates that unilateral ASCP is superior to bilateral in preventing neurological deficit, even if the ICU stay is longer in the unilateral group than in the bilateral one. No significant differences were shown between RCP and ASCP, either bilateral or unilateral, in terms of mortality and PND. Hence, circulatory arrest times were longer in the ASCP group than the RCP group, according to other studies where ASCP is preferred over other brain perfusion strategies, mainly bilateral, for longer periods of circulatory arrest. Furthermore, the core temperature was elevated in the ASCP group, resulting in reduced durations for cooling and rewarming, even if no significant difference in the CPB duration was seen.

In conclusion, for acute pathologies and emergency aortic arch surgery, bilateral ASCP is suggested for longer circulatory arrest durations; unilateral ASCP is safe for shorter durations but is a superior strategy for preventing TND and may be encouraged in case of augmented neurological deficit risk as poor preoperative mental status, diabetes, and peripheral arterial disease if it is allowed by surgeon expertise and resources; RCP is the less complicated method and can be performed in more centers and by most surgeons but requires a greater grade of hypothermia.

ASCP is the preferred strategy both in acute type A aortic dissection and in elective aortic arch surgery because the physiological blood flow pattern direct to the brain is associated with improved neurological protection with a lower risk for embolization into the right-sided cerebral vessels.

For chronic pathologies and non-emergent aortic arch surgery, in addition to circulatory arrest duration and co-morbidities, preoperative imaging of CoW may contribute to the selection of the most appropriate cerebral perfusion strategy, because the presence of any CoW variation could be decisional. Elective surgery allows to improve the preoperative study of patients with chronic pathologies, such as aortic arch aneurysm or type B aortic dissection, who may have a CoW variant, because of the important prevalence in the neurologically healthy population (62,22%) and who may benefit from a specific cerebral protection technique rather than another one, with the aim to reduce TND and postoperative stroke. Even if neurological events are less frequent in elective surgery (3.4%) than the emergent one (12%), the efficacy of cerebral protection strategy is still the most important determinant of favorable postoperative neurological outcomes both in elective and emergent aortic arch surgery. It is important to underline that neurological complications are associated with increased mortality, longer hospitalization, healthcare resources utilization, and impaired quality of life.

Therefore, it is appropriate to perform CTA in non-acute pathologies and non-emergent surgery involving aortic arch to identify patients who may require a bilateral ASCP, in addition to intraoperative monitoring.

As concerns neuromonitoring, it may guide the decision of the cerebral brain protection strategy, because bilateral monitoring assures the achievement of a sufficient amount of arterial blood and, then, an adequate supply of oxygen in both cerebral hemispheres. According to many studies, a longer duration of DHCA is associated with neurocognitive impairment, but TND is consistent with ASCP as well. The question of an effective distribution and ideal quantity of cerebral blood flow, particularly in the left hemisphere in presence of CoW variants, is one of the main issues about unilateral ASCP.

Intraoperative neurological monitoring may prevent negative consequences of a suboptimal cerebral perfusion. Different techniques are available for neuromonitoring [21], such as near-infrared spectroscopy (NIRS), which is a non-invasive method used to determine the regional oxygen saturation of hemoglobin (rSO2) regarding blood in the brain, based on the different absorption capacity of unsaturated and saturated hemoglobin in the near-infrared spectrum. This method employs disposable sensors placed on each side of the patient's forehead which allows the detection of rSO2 of the cortical brain tissue (3–4 cm of depth) perfused by anterior and middle cerebral arteries, but it only detects rSO2 reduction in the frontal lobes. It permits to continuously monitor changes in the local brain oxygen imbalance to recognize early hypoperfusion through prolonged rSO2 desaturation. The cut-off to define a high risk of neurological injury varies among available NIRS devices, and may be defined as a drop of $\geq$10% from the baseline with the ForeSight method or $\geq$20% with the INVOS system, due to the different grades of depth detection, 20 mm below the skin for INVOS and 25 mm for ForeSight [22]. The disadvantage is the lack of monitoring of the parietal and occipital lobes which are part of the posterior arterial territory, useful in CoW variants with absence of anastomosis between the anterior and the posterior circle. Moreover, it does not detect the perfusion of deeper brain regions, as required in elderly patients in which cortical atrophy gets the cortex away from the skull, and the signal may be influenced by ambient light and skin or muscle blood flow. Hemoglobin, total bilirubin, end-tidal carbon dioxide concentration, blood pressure, and inspired oxygen fraction are known factors influencing rSO2 measurement. In emergent surgery, when CTA is not performed to detect CoW variants, an impaired rSO2 may be caused by interrupted CoW if the cannula is not displaced or the arterial line is not obstructed. In this case, a switch from unilateral ASCP to bilateral should be considered. NIRS can be helpful in detecting the opposite situation: persistent hyperemia caused by hyperperfusion and hyperoxia induces vasogenic edema, the major determinant of cerebral hyperperfusion syndrome characterized by migraine symptoms, delirium, focal neurologic deficit, seizures, and coma.

Choi et al. [23] observed that, during CEA, a significant predictor for shunt insertion is the fractional reduction of rSO2 from the preclamping reference point recorded with NIRS system. A fractional decrease of 25.8% considered as cut-off value was not influenced by the patency of the CoW. In case of not patent anterior circulation of CoW, in patients with shunt placement, the maximum fractional decrease of rSO2 and the degree of stenosis in their contralateral carotid artery are significantly higher. Anyway, the drop in the cerebral oxygen saturation registered with NIRS system during the period of uASCP, may be the result of hypoperfusion of left cerebral hemisphere if selected CoW variations are present. Switching to bASCP may lead to restoration of perfusion in the left cerebral hemisphere with a significant increase in cerebral oxygen saturation. Despite its high false positive rate, cerebral oximetry may be properly sensitive to predict cerebral ischemia during CEA as suggested by these findings. While the positive predictive value was lower, cerebral oximetry could be an advantageous intraoperative device during aortic arch surgery owing to its high negative predictive value.

The latest evolution in terms of optical techniques are Diffuse Correlation Spectroscopy (DCS) and Frequency-Domain NIRS (FDNIRS). These techniques are based on the evaluation of the optical properties of tissues correlated to blood flow and hemoglobin concentration, respectively. Further to cerebral oxygen saturation, they also offer quantitative measures of cerebral blood volume and perfusion, useful for the calculation of a quantitative index of cerebral oxygen consumption (iCBF). However, the role of these techniques in cardiac anesthesia is still to be defined.

Transcranial Doppler (TCD) is a non-invasive method useful for the evaluation of blood flow in large intracranial vessels (i.e., middle cerebral artery) and the detection of micro- and macro-emboli. In particular, for patients with an incomplete CoW, when an inadequate cross-filling is detected and there is no perfusion in one of the middle cerebral arteries (i.e., due to iMCA), a shift from uASCP to bilateral could be quickly performed. When the decrease of middle cerebral artery velocity is ≥50% from the baseline during cerebral perfusion, it may guide the decision to change cerebral protection strategy. The TCD, differently from NIRS, allows real-time detection of cerebral blood flow, possibly optimizing the perfusion strategy earlier. Unfortunately, TCD is not applicable in approximately 20% of patients because of poor acoustic transcranial window [24]. It is not a recommended technique to detect CoW variants in an intraoperatory setting because a percentage of patients, estimated to be 15%, do not tolerate carotid compression for the assessment of CoW function. Even under the carotid compression test, the exact hemodynamic condition of cerebral perfusion is not accurately simulated, so the effective perfusion pressure during brain perfusion could be underestimated. Patients with severe carotid atherosclerosis who undergo aortic arch repair, estimated to be 3% of all patients, should avoid carotid compression. Thus, hemodynamics between preoperative and intraoperative evaluation with TCD is very different, because of the effects of non-pulsatile blood flow, lower mean pressures, hypothermia, and anesthesia which are not considered during the initial functional evaluation of CoW. Lastly, TCD is largely reliant on the operator and has not been commonly employed in cardiac surgery. These findings encourage the preoperative assessment of CoW with CTA whenever possible and the limitation of TCD as an integrative approach for NIRS in intraoperative monitoring in selected cases.

Electroencephalogram (EEG) has been widely used as an intraoperative monitoring tool to detect cerebral ischemia. Variations in EEG, such as diffuse or focal attenuation of the high and the middle frequencies, asymmetric changes in frequency and amplitude of the recording, and persistent increase of slow waves, are considered signs of cerebral ischemia. However, this method is susceptible to influences by anesthetic effects, leading to potential false negatives, especially in the case of micro-embolism. It cannot detect subcortical lobe ischemia or silent brain stroke caused by micro-embolisms. In this regard, the Bispectral index (BIS) is a processed EEG parameter introduced to indicate the depth of anesthesia and cerebral ischemia. A certain decrease in BIS may be indicative of cerebral ischemia, but the exact threshold has not been yet identified and it has a limited positive predictive value, so false positives may occur.

Somatosensory evoked potential (SSEP) is the electrical activity response measured at the skin's surface following controlled peripheral nerve stimulation and may indicate cerebral ischemia if it changes ≥50% from the baseline. Unlike EEG and NIRS, SSEP analyzes not only the cortex but also the deepest structure of the brain, but it demands expertise and may not properly evaluate all aspects of cerebral perfusion. Thus, EEG and SSEP measurements are affected by hypnotic agents and electrosurgical devices, including electrocautery.

As demonstrated by various studies, the intraoperative neuromonitoring technique cannot replace CTA as preoperative technique for the evaluation of CoW variants and they are characterized by different limitations and positive or negative predictive values. In conclusion, neuromonitoring is useful to shift cerebral perfusion technique for emergent surgery, when CTA is not performed and is reasonable to suspect CoW variants, and in elective surgery to evaluate technical intraoperative problems with CPB or cerebral protection strategy, such as cannula malposition or arterial line obstructions.

4. Systematization of CoW variants and cerebral perfusion techniques

As discussed, a new and specific classification is needed when performing non-emergent and elective aortic arch surgery in patients affected by CoW variants, in order to choose the best approach to cerebral perfusion.

The normal anatomy of CoW protects patients from ischemia because it warrants the perfusion of all cerebral areas, even when an internal carotid artery is clamped and even when the contralateral internal carotid artery is occluded, despite the brain being perfused only *via* the basilar artery. However, during cardiac and vascular surgery, in presence of anomalies of the CoW, the perfusion of some cerebral areas can become insufficient and produce clinical neurological deficits. Besides the variable presence of connections in leptomeningeal and extracranial networks, collateral flow in the brain (which includes the brain stem, the cerebellum, and both cerebral hemispheres) is primarily dependent on the CoW. For these reasons, unilateral ASCP is not always suitable and in selected cases, it is indispensable to perform a bilateral ASCP, while RCP is always suitable but is CPB-time limited and it is impossible to determine whether the brain is really perfused with oxygenated blood or it is shunted with cerebral oedema as a major complication. In addition, DHCA, if performed for 20 minutes is considered safe, but this period is too short for complex arch reconstruction. A recent European survey [18] showed that approximately two-thirds of centers prefer bASCP, whereas one-third of them deliver the cerebral perfusate in an unilateral manner; DHCA and RCP are rarely used in Europe.

The aim is to develop a systematic classification of CoW variants which are likely to have an increased neurological deficit risk if aortic arch surgery is performed with unilateral ASCP. The preoperative prediction of bilateral ASCP reduces cerebral hypoperfusion and, consequently, TND and neurological complications.

Evidence are summarized from studies in patients undergoing carotid artery surgery (**Tables 2** and **3**) and non-emergent arch surgery (**Tables 4** and **5**).

Urbanski et al. [32] divided CoW variations into three groups: in the first group, there is only one hypoplastic or absent segment; both sides of the second group had abnormalities in the posterior pre-communicating (2a) or communicating arteries (2b); in the third group, the abnormalities are in both anterior and posterior segments of the CoW on one or even on both sides. This last group is the only one that might benefit from bASCP and, in some cases (missing posterior communicating segments on the left and anterior communicating segments on the right, as iMCA, or above two

Study (year)	Patients	Age	Clinical presentation / neurological comorbidities	Intervention	CoW preoperative assessment (method)	Functionally complete CoW (%)	Intraoperative cerebral protection strategy	Intraoperative cerebral protection monitoring	In-hospital mortality	Stroke (minor, transient, major, global brain ischemia)
Banga et al. [11]	545	Patients without Immediate Neurologic Events (INE): 68 ± 8.2) Patients with INE: 71.6 ± 8.9	38% with previous neurological symptoms	CEA	CT angiography	60.3%	Selective shunt	N/A	0.2%	3.7% (8 patients with permanent stroke, 12 patients with transient stroke)
Choi et al. [23]	310 (273 shunt, 37 no shunt)	Group shunting (GS), 66.6 ± 10.4 Group no shunting (GNS), 67.3 ± 8	N/A	CEA	MR angiography	N/A	Selective shunt	Clinical evaluation in awake patient	0	1.0% (dysarthria, disorientation, and headaches at territories of the middle cerebral artery and anterior communicating artery)
Gibello et al. [25]	503	73.34 ± 7.43	33.7% with previous neurological symptoms	CEA	CT angiography	N/A	Pruitt-Inahara selective shunt	N/A	N/A	Previous neurological symptoms, diabetes and female sex are correlated with a lower tolerance to carotid cross-clamping. Chronic obstructive pulmonary

Study (year)	Patients	Age	Clinical presentation / neurological comorbidities	Intervention	CoW preoperative assessment (method)	Functionally complete CoW (%)	Intraoperative cerebral protection strategy	Intraoperative cerebral protection monitoring	In-hospital mortality	Stroke (minor, transient, major, global brain ischemia)
										disease is correlated to higher tolerance to carotid cross-clamping.
Montisci et al. [26]	71	Group “Complete CoW” (35 patients), 71.8 ± 7.2). Group “one agenesia/ obstruction in the CoW” (21 patients), 71.6 ± 9.6. Group “2+ agenesias / obstructions in the CoW” (15 patients), 73.1 ± 5.2	29.5% preoperative neurological symptoms	CEA	MR angiography	78.9%	Pruitt-Inahara shunt (11 patients)	Clinical evaluation in awake patient	0	0
Pennekamp et al. [27]	431	69 ± 9	Neurological symptoms: 88% (TIA 65%, stroke 23%)	CEA	CT angiography (33%); MR angiography (67%)	83.8% of patients studied with MR angiography	Selective shunt	TCD + EEG	0.7%	3% stroke

Study (year)	Patients	Age	Clinical presentation / neurological comorbidities	Intervention	CoW preoperative assessment (method)	Functionally complete CoW (%)	Intraoperative cerebral protection strategy	Intraoperative cerebral protection monitoring	In-hospital mortality	Stroke (minor, transient, major, global brain ischemia)
Soares et al. [28]	98 (54 with complete CoW, 44 incomplete CoW)	72.8 ± 3.0	Previous neurological symptoms (53.1%)	CEA	CT angiography, MR angiography	55%	Selective shunt	EEG	2%	3.1%
Zhou et al. [29]	482	61.2 ± 10.4	Hypertension in subjects with incomplete CoW was significantly greater vs. complete CoW (72.2% vs. 55.7%; P = 0.011)	/	MR angiography	12.7%	/	/	/	/

Table 2.
Studies describing completeness of CoW in patients undergoing carotid endarterectomy: Details and methods.

Study (year)	CoW variants, details and outcomes	Comments
Banga et al. [11]	Complete CoW: 1 INE Isolated anomaly in anterior semicircle (72 patients): 1 INE Isolated anomaly in posterior semicircle (196 patients): 2 INEs No differences in INEs between complete CoW and single/isolated anomaly ($P = 0.57$) Abnormalities in both semicircles (215 patients): 16 INEs. Significant differences compared to other groups in terms of INEs ($P = 0.001$). Among these patients, 8 out of 34 patients with iMCA (isolated middle cerebral artery) had INEs (23.5%). iMCA is a strong predictor of INEs (OR 11.1, 95%CI 3.6–35.9, $P < 0.01$)	An iMCA (isolated middle cerebral artery) carries more than a 10-fold higher risk of INEs after CEA with cross-clamping without shunt protection. In these patients, routine shunting is recommended to prevent INEs.
Choi et al. [23]	Absence of the anterior circulation in CoW is the most important factor for shunt insertion, assuming no stenosis in the contralateral carotid artery during CEA. rSO_2 can be applied in predicting shunt insertion, irrespective of the patency of the circle of Willis, although the positive predictive value was low. The cut-off value was 25.8%.	When the anterior circulation was non-patent, the probability of shunt insertion increased as the contralateral carotid arteries were more severely stenosed.
Gibello et al. [25]	The most common anomaly is the ipsilateral or contralateral hypoplasia/occlusion of the posterior communicating artery. Significant correlation between the number of CoW anatomic anomalies and neurological tolerance to cross-clamping: two or more hypoplasic or occluded segments of the circle are positively correlated to worse cerebral compensation.	A proposed score (PTOT) is the summary of patency of CoW and the supraortic trunk. PTOT is a strong predictor of cerebral tolerance to carotid cross-clamping.
Montisci et al. [26]	Strong association between intolerance to carotid cross-clamping and two or more agenesiae / obstructions in the CoW (OR 51, 95% CI 5–480, $P < 0.001$). No significant difference in the risk of developing carotid cross-clamp intolerance between the presence of one agenesia/obstruction in the CoW versus complete CoW (OR 1.7, 95% CI 0.1–28.7, $P = 0.71$). Probability of having two agenesiae / obstructions in the CoW in patients with carotid cross-clamp intolerance: 82% Probability of having zero or one agenesia / obstruction in patients without carotid cross-clamp intolerance: 90% Probability of a patient having carotid cross-clamp intolerance when the CoW has two agenesiae / obstructions: 60% Probability of a patient not having carotid cross-clamp intolerance when the CoW has zero or one agenesia / obstruction: 96%	Two or more agenesia / obstructions of the CoW were associated with a high risk of intolerance to carotid cross-clamp.
Pennekamp et al. [27]	Posteriorly, the most observed abnormality was a not-visible P-coms (47% and 45% for the ipsilateral	In the MRA group, any not-visible anterior (OR 4.96, 95% CI 1.95–

Study (year)	CoW variants, details and outcomes	Comments
	and contralateral P-com respectively) 1. Circle of Willis morphology with MR (284 patients) 1A) Not visible anterior segment (any) (48 patients); among them, shunt used in 14 patients ($P < 0.01$) 1B) Not visible posterior segment ipsilateral (any) (136 patients); among them, shunt used in 34 patients ($P < 0.01$) 2. CoW morphology with MRA / CTA (431 patients) 2A) Absent anterior segment (any) (77 patients); among them, shunt used in 21 patients ($P < 0.01$) 2A1) Absent A-com (49 patients); among them, shunt used in 12 patients ($P = 0.05$) 2A2) Ipsilateral A1 segment hypoplastic (61 patients); among them, shunt used in 1 patient ($P < 0.01$) 2B) Absent ipsilateral post segment (241 patients); among them, shunt used in 49 patients ($P = 0.01$) 2B1) P-com not-visible (201 patients); among them, shunt used in 38 patients ($P = 0.04$) 2B2) P-com < P1 (121 patients); among them, shunt used in 9 patients ($P < 0.01$) 2C) Absent contralateral post segment (194 patients); among them, shunt used in 25 patients ($P = 0.75$)	12.58) or ipsilateral posterior segment of the CoW (OR 5.08, 95% CI 2.10–12.32) was independently related to the need of shunt use during CEA In the CT group none of the factors were independently related to the need for shunt use during CEA. Therefore, only predictors describing morphology of CoW derived from MRA findings were included in this model. Imaging with MR seems superior compared to TC in terms of image quality and clinical / prognostic implications.
Soares et al. [28]	During CEA 4 patients required selective shunt (2 with complete CoW, 2 with incomplete CoW; $P = 0.15$). The incidence of postoperative stroke was 3.1% (asymptomatic 2%, symptomatic 1.1%), with no differences among CoW complete and incomplete groups (3.7 vs. 2.3%, $P = 0.68$).	The completeness of the CoW might not influence the outcomes of carotid interventions. Anatomy of the CoW is not a strong enough predictive factor for the prognosis of cross-clamping intolerance during CEA
Zhou et al. [29]	The prevalence of incomplete CoW was significantly higher in Posterior-COW than that of anterior CoW (79.7% [384/482] versus 40.7% [196/482], $P < 0.001$). The prevalence of an incomplete A-COW was significantly higher in patients with presence of carotid intraplaque hemorrhage than those with a complete CoW (52.7 versus 38.5%; $P = 0.022$) especially with the absence of ACoA (69.2%; $P = 0.001$) Incomplete A-COW significantly associated with the presence of intra-plaque hemorrhage before (OR, 1.781; 95% CI, 1.083–2.931; $P = 0.023$) and after adjusted for clinical risk factors including age, sex, body mass index, smoking, diabetes mellitus, pulse pressure, and hyperlipidemia (OR, 1.945; 95% CI, 1.139–3.321; $P = 0.015$)	An incomplete CoW is independently associated with intraplaque hemorrhage of carotid atherosclerotic plaques.

Table 3.
Studies describing completeness of CoW in patients undergoing carotid endarterectomy: Outcomes and clinical implications.

Study (year)	Patients	Age	Clinical presentation / comorbidities	Intervention	CoW preoperative assessment (method)	Functionally complete CoW (%)	Cannulation strategy and hypotermic arrest	Intraoperative cerebral protection monitoring	In-hospital mortality	Stroke (minor, transient, major, global brain ischemia)
Mariscalco et al. [30]	76 (61 m, 15 f)	65.4 ± 16.8	atherosclerotic descending thoracic aortic aneurysms (35, ruptured 3), chronic type B dissecting aneurysm or complicated acute type B dissection (16), penetrating ulcers (14, ruptured 2), traumatic pseudoaneurysms (11, chronic 3).	TEVAR	CT angiography	70	not applicable	—	12	0 hemorrhagic stroke, 7 ischemic (embolic) stroke, 1 low-flow ischemic stroke
Smith et al. [31]	391	62 ± 12 years, 61% male (n. 237)	—	aortic arch replacement	CT angiography	27% complete Cow (107)	temperature of 25° two 15-French perfusion cannulas into the ostia of the innominate and left common carotid arteries	—	—	—
Urbanski et al. [32]	99 (67 m, 32 f)	65 years (range 25–84 years)	—	aortic arch replacement	CT angiography	—	the left (93) or right (1) carotid artery was prepared in 94 patients. moderate hypothermia with rectal temperature of 30°C.	trans-cranial doppler	1	—

Study (year)	Patients	Age	Clinical presentation / comorbidities	Intervention	CoW preoperative assessment (method)	Functionally complete CoW (%)	Cannulation strategy and hypotermic arrest	Intraoperative cerebral protection monitoring	In-hospital mortality	Stroke (minor, transient, major, global brain ischemia)
							circulatory arrest and unilateral cerebral perfusion time: 18 ± 10 min (range 7–70).			

Table 4.
Studies describing completeness of CoW in patients undergoing cardiac / arch surgery: Details and methods.

Study (year)	CoW variants, details, and outcomes	Comments
Mariscalco et al. [30]	CVA Willis anomal vs. CVA normal Willis 37.5% vs. 4.4%, p < 0.01).	incompleteness of the Willis circle (OR 17.19, 95% CI 2.10 to 140.66; p = 0.008) and presence of coronary artery disease (OR 6.86, 95 CI% 1.18 to 40.05; p = 0.032) predicted neurological events
Smith et al. [31]	Moderately safe group, Total moderately safe group 70 (18) Left fetal variant 12 (3) ACoA dysfunction 9 (2) Bilateral fetal variant 30 (8) ACoA and right PCoA dysfunction 7 (2) ACoA dysfunction and right fetal variant 6 (2) Right PCoA dysfunction and left fetal variant 6 (2) Unsafe group, Total unsafe group 40 (10) ACoA and left PCoA dysfunction 6 (2) ACoA dysfunction and left fetal variant 0 (0) ACoA dysfunction and bilateral fetal variant 5 (1) ACoA and bilateral PCoA dysfunction 15 (4) ACoA and right PCoA dysfunction and left fetal variant 1 (<1) ACoA and left PCoA dysfunction and right fetal variant 1 (<1) Right VA dysfunction 12 (3)	ischemic brain damage during right u-ASCP (28%) is greater than during bi-ASCP (<1%) 62% functional CoW safe for uSCP 10% PCoAr disfunction (41) 13% PCoAl disfunction (50) 17% bilateral PCoA disfunction (65)
Urbanski et al. [32]	59 variants, 3 groups, 18 patients group I: abnormality anterior or posterior part group II: hypoplastic or missing posterior communicating arteries on both sides group III: abnormalities within the anterior and posterior communicating arteries	—

Table 5.
Studies describing completeness of CoW in patients undergoing cardiac / arch surgery: Outcomes and clinical implications.

anomalous positions within the CoW) even a bASCP could not warrant a sufficient cerebral perfusion. In this study, 99 patients affected by different CoW variants underwent elective aortic arch surgery, with hemiarch, subtotal, or total arch replacement. uASCP was performed through the left carotid artery as a cannulation site and, when required, the right carotid artery was used as adjunctive perfusion cerebral artery for bASCP. Unexpectedly, during the carotid artery occlusion test with TCD, no significant decrease of flow velocity in the MCA was observed and for patients in whom the use of TCD has not been possible, no signs of cerebral ischemia were observed at EEG and SSEP. Even the measurement of blood pressure in the radial arteries, which reflects the blood pressure in subclavian and, then, in vertebral arteries, demonstrated that there aren't differences in cerebral blood supply during uASCP in patients with complete and incomplete CoW. Urbanski supports that incompleteness of CoW does not correlate with insufficient cerebral protection during uASCP and, for this reason, does not recommend CTA as a standard procedure before elective aortic arch surgery, only functional carotid occlusion test and intraoperative neurovascular monitoring are considered essential. These conclusions are probably influenced by very short duration of ASCP, optimal pharmacological cerebral protection, and the etiopathology of degenerative or atherosclerotic aneurysm. Since atherosclerosis is a generalized disease, in this particular patient's cohort, there is a possibility for pathological expansion of secondary collaterals (as leptomeningeal and ophthalmic arteries). Moreover, the old-generation CT scan used in this study might misclassified segments with a diameter over 1 mm as aplastic or hypoplastic, because of the low spatial resolution of this equipment.

Mariscalco et al. [30] demonstrated that patients affected by atherosclerotic descending thoracic aortic aneurysm, chronic type B dissecting aneurysm or complicated acute type B dissection, penetrating ulcers and traumatic pseudoaneurysm who underwent thoracic endovascular aortic repair (TEVAR) intervention, were prone to cerebrovascular accidents after the procedure if they had incompleteness of CoW. This study, then, proves that anomalies of CoW are independent cerebrovascular accident predictors after TEVAR procedure.

Smith et al. [31] assumed that a Cow variant may be considered functionally safe as long as the collateral flow when performing uASCP did not have to reach a vessel beyond the left MCA. An example is the isolated variation of PcomA because the blood flow of the left MCA and the left A1 is possible through the AcomA, while the basilar and the right vertebral arteries can perfuse the left PCA. In this case, uASCP is considered safe. When the cerebral areas were inaccessible to the CoW-dependent collateral blood flow during right uASCP, the functional variation is defined as unsafe, such as right vertebral artery dysfunction, combined with either bilateral PcomA dysfunction or combined with fetal type variant. Finally, right uASCP was defined as moderately safe if right-to-left posterior-to-anterior collateral perfusion had to arrive at a vessel outside the left MCA. On this basis, they propose a clinical traffic light algorithm (red light, amber, and green light) categorizing different functional anatomical variants as unsafe, moderately safe, and safe for uASCP. They also consider vertebral arteries hypoplasia or absence, differently from other studies. This classification is based not on the morphology but on the functional anatomy of CoW as is to be expected during uASCP, lie on preoperative transcranial color-coded duplex (TCCD) examination of bilateral common, internal and external carotid artery, and both vertebral arteries, performing carotid compression test whenever possible. As emphasized by Etz and Borger [24], a significant number of patients are not eligible for the proposed TCD assessment of CoW functionality, and its clinical significance for the majority of patients remains unclear. Therefore, a preoperative CTA-based classification is needed.

Papantchev et al. [9] studied 500 CoW with two different methods: 250 were obtained from cadavers via routine dissection, while the others were visualized with CTA imaging technique. Otherwise, other classifications that are not considered relevant whether the variation is on the right or left side of the circle, the left–right lateralization in uASCP is of crucial importance, since in uASCP with the cannulation of the right axillary artery or brachiocephalic trunk, the brain receives blood only via the right common carotid artery and right vertebral artery (VA). Therefore, the protective effect of uASCP is entirely based on the CoW which maintains adequate perfusion of the contralateral left cerebral hemisphere through A1s, P1s, AcomA, and PcomAs segments. Variations of the circle exist in at least 50% of the people, so it is a not inconsiderable factor to take into account in the selection of the adequate cerebral perfusion strategy. Moreover, the classifications seen before do not consider vertebral arteries variations because they are not part of the CoW, but variations in those arteries could have crucial importance during uASCP. For these reasons, Papantchev defines five segments of CoW as critical for uASCP: right A1, AcomA, left PcomA, left P1, and right VA. A diameter of 1 mm was used as the threshold for hypoplasia, in order to be consistent with other major morphological studies of the CoW reported in the literature. Nine circle configurations were identified and they were subdivided into seven groups, according to the number of major cerebral vessels (ACAs, MCAs, PCAs) at risk of hypoperfusion during uASCP:

- Type IA includes all circles with hypo- or aplasia of left PcomA. With this variation, the territories supplied by the left MCA are at risk of hypoperfusion during uASCP. This is the most frequent variant (35.6%), according to data reported in literature where PcomAs is the most variable part of the circle;

- Type IB includes all circles with AcomA variations. The territories supplied by the left ACA are at risk of hypoperfusion;

- Type IIA includes all circles with hypo- or aplasia of both left PcomA and AcomA. The left cerebral territories supplied by ACA and MCA are at risk of hypoperfusion;

- Type IIB includes all circles with left P1 or right VA variations, which leads to hypoperfusion risk of brain territories perfused by both left MCA and left PCA;

- Type IIIA includes all circles hypo- or aplasia of right A1, with high hypoperfusion risk of brain territories supplied by left MCA, right and left ACA

- Type IIIB includes all circles hypo- or aplasia of both AcomA and right VA. If this circle type is present, the entire left hemisphere is at risk of hypoperfusion during uASCP. This is the rarest variation (0.2%);

- Type IV includes all circles with hypo- or aplasia of both right A1 and right VA or both right A1 and left P1. This is the most severe variation because it leads to the risk of hypoperfusion of territories perfused by right ACA, left ACA, left MCA, and left PCA.

Hence, if the CoW variation leads to the risk of hypoperfusion of only one major cerebral vessel, it is classified in group I and so on. All types were present in 58.6% of all examined CoW, according to the high frequency of CoW variants in healthy people found by other studies. Papantchev's classification is simple and straightforward, dividing a large number of complex CoW variations into only seven types, which is a small number if compared to other classifications. It is focused on high-risk variations that may benefit from bASCP when the preoperative neurological examination with CTA method is possible.

The study of Papantchev may be integrated with vascular surgery studies, comparing patients with CoW variants who needed shunting during CEA, to be able to predict, in the preoperative assessment, when the use of bilateral ASCP is recommended to prevent neurological sequelae.

Patients who underwent CEA intervention, affected by CoW variants, are estimated to be 50%, the same frequency encountered in cardiac surgery. When performing CEA during vascular surgery, the carotid cross-clamping (CC) intolerance and the demand for shunting in patients affected by some specific types of CoW variants, can be helpful in creating a complete classification of high-risk variants because CC is based on the same principle of unilateral ASCP, where cerebral blood flow is provided by only one carotid artery. The identification of high-risk variants simplifies the choice between unilateral and bilateral ASCP in elective aortic arch surgery, because patients with some specific CoW variants may require a bilateral ASCP instead of unilateral to ensure adequate cerebral perfusion in both brain hemispheres, even when CPB time is short.

Bagan et al. [33] found that configurations type number 5, 14, and 15 according to Lazorthes' classification are likely to have CC intolerance. Type 5 is characterized by the absence of AcomA and PcomA ipsilateral, while in type 14 A1 segment contralateral and PcomA ipsilateral are absent and in type 15 AcomA and P1 segment contralateral are absent. The common peculiarity of these configurations is the absence of 2 segments and, except for type 15, the isolation of the middle cerebral artery from the contralateral carotid artery and vertebral arteries. Later, Montisci et al. [26] demonstrated that the number of absent segments in the CoW is significantly associated with intolerance to CC, independent of the CoW configurations. When two or more segments are absent, a cerebral perfusion deficit is highly probable, whereas other factors such as ipsilateral, contralateral carotid stenosis, and preoperative symptoms are not statistically associated with CC intolerance. The absence of only one segment does not appear to be correlated with CC intolerance if not associated with contralateral carotid occlusion or low blood pressure. The location of the absent segments can influence the extension of hypoperfused cerebral area and consequent clinical signs. In those patients with the absence of two or more segments without CC intolerance, it is likely that a very small area or a neurologically irrelevant area was hypoperfused. Also, TCD investigation showed correlation between undetectable CoW segments and decreased flow velocity in MCA with ischemic EEG abnormalities. Even if the patients of this report were studied using magnetic resonance angiography (MRA), it is recommended to prefer CTA for the preoperative assessment of CoW because CTA is not flow-dependent and allows for image reformation along any plane. Gibello et al. [25] found a strong association between the insertion of shunt during CEA and the number of obstructed or hypoplastic CoW vessels. The results revealed that there is no one specific CoW configuration that is more susceptible to carotid CC intolerance, but the increased number of hypoplastic or occluded CoW segments leads to a higher likelihood of neurological deficits following carotid CC. Hence, it is reasonable to adopt bilateral ASCP as a preferred cerebral perfusion strategy in patients with two or more absent segments of CoW to prevent hypoperfusion of cerebral areas.

Banga et al. [11] studied the impact of iMCA on immediate neurological events, such as transient ischemic attack and stroke, diagnosed immediately after CEA. They divided CoW into two semicircles: the anterior, formed by the contralateral anterior cerebral artery (A1), anterior communicating artery (AcomA) and ipsilateral A1; the posterior, composed by the ipsilateral carotid artery (P1) and posterior communicating ipsilateral artery (PcomA). Among the patients with normal CoW, only one had a stroke and among patients with one hypoplastic or absent segment in the anterior or the posterior semicircle, three had immediate neurological events. Statistical data

Papantchev's group	Variation	Incidence	Proposed strategy of cerebral perfusion
Group I Group I-A Group I-B	Left PComA AComA	30–35% 2–5%	Monolateral (RS/RIA) Monolateral (RS/RIA)
Group II Group II-A Group II-B iMCA	Left PComA + AComA Left P1 or right vertebral artery Isolated middle cerebral artery	3–8% 7–10% 2–5%	Bilateral (RS/RIA + LCC) Monolateral (RS/RIA) Bilateral (RS/RIA + LCC)
Group III Group III-A Group III-B	Right A1 AComA + right vertebral artery	4–8% 1–2%	Trilateral (RS/RIA + LCC + LS) Bilateral (RS/RIA + LCC)
Group IV	Right A1 + right vertebral artery / left P1	1–2%	Trilateral (RS/RIA + LCC + LS)

PComA: posterior communicating artery; AComA: anterior communicating artery; RS: right subclavian / axillary artery; RIA: right innominate artery; LCC: left common carotid artery; LS: left subclavian artery.

Table 6.
Proposed management strategy of antegrade cerebral perfusion during non-emergent arch surgery based on CoW variants. In group I, there is only one location of an anatomical variation (hypoplasia, aplasia) within the CoW. In this group, an adequate collateral supply of the entire CoW could generally have been expected, even if it had been supplied through only one artery (i.e., the right carotid artery). In group II, the abnormalities existed within the posterior pre-communicating (group II-A) or communicating arteries (group II-B) on both sides. In cases belonging to group II-A, a sufficient supply of the posterior cerebral region could have been expected, regardless of whether the CoW had been supplied from the left side (left carotid artery) or from the right side (right carotid and right vertebral arteries). However, in cases belonging to group II-B, a perfusion only from the right side would offer a sufficient collateral flow. In group III, the pathologies were found in both anterior and posterior components of the CoW on one or even on both sides so that an insufficient cerebral supply could have occurred during the perfusion of the left side and in some cases (e.g., missing anterior communicating components on the right and posterior communicating components on the left or in cases with more than two abnormal locations within the CoW) even during perfusion from the anterior part of the right side; therefore a 3-way perfusion (right innominate artery + left carotid + left subclavian) would have been advised. In group IV, functional incompleteness of CoW is total and a 3-way perfusion appears mandatory.

confirms that there is no difference in terms of neurological deficits between patients with complete CoW and patients with only one semicircle affected. The difference becomes significant when both semicircles (the anterior and the ipsilateral posterior) have at least one hypoplasia or absent segment at the same time. This evaluation allows us to consider hypoplasia as absent when both semicircles are involved in anomalous CoW, confirming the hypothesis of augmented neurological risk when two or more segments are absent or, in addition, hypoplastic. Among the patients with at least one absent or hypoplastic segment in both semicircles, those with iMCA carried more than a 10-fold higher risk of immediate neurological events after CEA with CC without shunt protection. This means that, on the side of the clamped ICA, the MCA flow is not supported by contralateral carotid nor from the vertebral artery, due to the absence of communication between the two semicircles.

Thus, iMCA may be considered a particularly high-risk variant in the group of two absent segments who are susceptible to bilateral ASCP. Therefore, all CoW variants characterized by at least two absent segments, in addition to Papantchev's types IIA, IIIB, and IV, may benefit from bASCP.

Other vascular surgery studies [23] in patients who underwent CEA procedure demonstrated that the absence of anterior circulation was the primary factor in the insertion of a shunt, given that there was no stenosis in the contralateral carotid artery. In this case, the evaluation of contralateral carotid stenosis became important because it increases about 27% the probability of shunt insertion. Previous studies documented that the collateral flow rates in AcomA rose with the increases of the degree of stenosis of ICA and this is particularly true when AcomA is absent because an augmented blood flow and pressure is registered in patients with ICA stenosis, probably due to a physiological increased blood flow through leptomeningeal collaterals if a patient has poor CoW integrity. This is also the reason why an incomplete CoW is a risk factor for intraplaque hemorrhage and atherosclerotic plaque rupture [29]. Hence, the second risk group may be constituted of patients with CoW variants involving absent segments in the anterior circle who may need an evaluation of contralateral carotid stenosis with carotid ultrasound, in addition to the first risk group formed by the absence of at least two segments and the iMCA subgroup. The cut-off of contralateral carotid stenosis which allows patients with anterior segments absence to benefit the bilateral ASCP instead of unilateral, is estimated to be above 50% (**Table 6**).

5. Conclusions

Neurological injuries, stroke, and paraplegia are the most devastating complications of aortic arch surgery. The non-emergent surgery and chronic diseases of aortic arch permit to notably reduce neurological deficits by the given opportunity to study in a preoperative assessment with CTA the patients' CoW which may be affected by various abnormalities, such as hypoplasia or absence of one or more segments.

A simple systematic classification may provide decisional criteria to prefer bASCP over uASCP in selected CoW variations to easily identify, among 82 variants, the ones which have a high risk of hypoperfusion during uASCP. Papantchev's classification may be integrated by carotid cross-clamping studies during CEA, which allows to identify other two high-risk groups: the first one, which includes CoW variants with the absence of at least two segments (which includes types IIA, IIIB, and IV), characterized by a subgroup identified as iMCA; the second group, which includes at least one absent segment in the anterior circle and the contralateral carotid stenosis over 50%.

The intraoperative monitoring of cerebral blood perfusion is essential but cannot replace preoperative CTA because the evaluation of CoW incompleteness is decisional in preferring a determinate cerebral perfusion strategy, due to an augmented risk of stroke and TND if aortic arch surgery is performed with uASCP. bASCP is recommended over uASCP in high-risk groups to warrant an adequate cerebral perfusion and the reduction of postoperative neurological complications. The use of uASCP when the CoW proves to have an adequate and sufficient collateral capacity, and bASCP only when necessary and in emergent situations, may minimize surgical manipulation of supraortic vessels, and subsequently decrease the rate of embolic stroke.

Acknowledgements

Authors would like to acknowledge the efforts of Marco Piastra for their help in English language.

Conflict of interest

The authors declare no conflict of interest.

Appendices

ACAs	anterior cerebral arteries
AcomA	anterior communicating artery
ASCP	anterograde selective cerebral perfusion
bASCP	bilateral anterograde selective cerebral perfusion
CA	circulatory arrest
CC	carotid cross-clamping
CEA	carotid endarterectomy
CoW	circle of Willis
CPB	cardio-pulmonary bypass
CTA	computed tomography angiography
DHCA	deep hypothermic circulatory arrest
EEG	electroencephalogram
ICAs	internal carotid arteries
iMCA	isolated middle cerebral artery
MCAs	middle cerebral arteries
MRA	magnetic resonance angiography
NIRS	near-infrared spectroscopy
PCAs	posterior cerebral arteries
PcomAs	posterior communicating arteries
PND	permanent neurological deficit
RCP	retrograde cerebral perfusion
SSEP	somatosensory evoked potential
TCD	transcranial Doppler
TEVAR	thoracic endovascular aortic repair
TND	transient neurological deficit
VAs	vertebral arteries

Author details

Antonio Nenna*, Diletta Corrado, Francesco Loreni, Chiara Ferrisi, Gennaro Sorrentino, Omar Giacinto, Raffaele Barbato, Ciro Mastroianni, Mario Lusini and Massimo Chello
Unit of Cardiac Surgery, Fondazione Policlinico Universitario Campus Bio-Medico di Roma, Rome, Italy

*Address all correspondence to: a.nenna@policlinicocampus.it

References

[1] Burlakoti A, Kumaratilake J, Taylor J, Massy-Westropp N, Henneberg M. The cerebral basal arterial network: Morphometry of inflow and outflow components. Journal of Anatomy. 2017; **230**(6):833-841

[2] Ayre J, Bazira P, Abumattar M, Makwana H, Sanders K. A new classification system for the anatomical variations of the human circle of Willis: A systematic review. Journal of Anatomy. 2022;**240**(6):1187-1204

[3] De Caro J, Ciacciarelli A, Tessitore A, et al. Variants of the circle of Willis in schemic stroke patients. Journal of Neurology. 2021;**268**(10):3799-3807

[4] Riggs H, Rupp C. Variation in form of circle of Willis—The relation of the variations to collateral circulation: Anatomic analysis. Archives of Neurology. 1963;**8**:8-14

[5] Lazorthes G, Gouazé A, Santini J, Georges S. Le cercle artériel du cerveau (circulus arteriosus cerebri). Anatomia Clinica. 1979;**1**(3):241-257

[6] Krabbe-Hartkamp M, Van der Grond J, De Leeuw F, De Groot J, Algra A, Hillen B, et al. Morphologic variation on three-dimensional time-of-flight MR angiograms. Radiology. 1998;**207**(1): 241-257

[7] Merkkola P, Tulla H, Ronkainen A, et al. Incomplete circle of Willis nad right axillary artery perfusion. The Annals of Thoracic Surgery. 2006;**82**(1):74-79

[8] Papantchev V, Hristov S, Todorova D, Naydenov E, Paloff A, Nikolov D, et al. Some variations of the circle of Willis, important for cerebral protection in aortic surgery–A study in eastern Europeans. European Journal of Cardio-Thoracic Surgery. 2007;**31**(6):982-989. DOI: 10.1016/j.ejcts.2007.03.020

[9] Papantchev V, Stoinova V, Aleksandrov A, et al. The role of Willis circle variations during unilateral selective cerebral perfusion: A study of 500 circles. European Journal of Cardio-Thoracic Surgery. 2013;**44**(4):743-753

[10] Coulier B. Morphological variants of the cerebral arterial circle on computed tomographic angiography (CTA): A large restrospective study. Surgical and Radiologic Anatomy. 2021;**43**(3):417-426

[11] Banga P, Varga A, Csobay-Novàk C, et al. Incomplete circle of Willisi is associated with higher incidence of neurologic events during carotid eversion endarterectomy without shunting. Journal of Vascular Surgery. 2018;**68**(6):1764-1771

[12] Rangus I, Milles L, Galinovic I, et al. Reclassifications of ischemic stroke patterns due to variants of the circle of Willis. International Journal of Stroke. 2022;**17**(7):770-776

[13] Arnaoutakis G, Ogami T, Bobba C, et al. Cerebral protection using deep hypothermic circulatory arrest versus retrograde cerebral perfusion for aortic hemiarch reconstruction. Journal of Cardiac Surgery. 2022;**37**(10):3279-3286

[14] Englum B, He X, Gulack B, et al. Hypothermia and cerebral protection strategies in aortic arch surgery: A comparative effectiveness analysis from the STS adult cardiac surgery database. European Journal of Cardio-Thoracic Surgery. 2017;**52**(3):492-498

[15] Peterson M, Garg V, Mazer C, Chu M, Bozinovski J, Dagenais F, et al. A

randomized trial comparing axillary versus innominate artery cannulation in aortic surgery. The Journal of Thoracic and Cardiovascular Surgery. 2020;**164** (5):1426-1438-e2

[16] Kazui T. Total arch replacement with separated graft technique and selective antegrade cerebral perfusion. Annals of Cardiothoracic Surgery. 2013;**2**(3):353-357

[17] Abjigitova D, Veen K, Van Tussenbroek G, et al. Carebral protection in aortic arch surgery: Systematic review and meta-analysis. Interactive Cardiovascular and Thoracic Surgery. 2022;**35**(3):ivac128

[18] De Paulis R, Czerny M, Weltert L, et al. Current trend in cannulation and neuroprotection during surgery of aortic arch in Europe. European Journal of Cardio-Thoracic Surgery. 2015;**47**(5): 917-923

[19] Patel V, Orozco-Sevilla V, Coselli J. Cerebral protection in aortic arch surgery: A systematic review and meta-analysis. Interactive Cardiovascular and Thoracic Surgery. 2022;**35**(6):ivac270

[20] Rahimi M, Sahrai H, Norouzi A, et al. Cerebral protection in acute type a aortic dissection surgery: A systematic review and meta-analysis. Journal of Thoracic Disease. 2024;**16**(2):1289-1312

[21] Montisci A, Maj G, Cavozza C, Audo A, Benussi S, Rosati F, et al. Cerebral perfusion and neuromonitoring during complex aortic arch surgery: A narrative review. Journal of Clinical Medicine. 2023;**12**:3470

[22] Stilo F, Montelione N, Paolini J, Strumia A, Cuccarelli M, Nenna A, et al. Current status of brain monitoring during carotid endarterectomy. JVS Vascular Insights. 2024 (in press). ISSN 2949-9127. DOI: 10.1016/j.jvsvi.2024.100060

[23] Choi B, Park S, Shin S, et al. Neurological derangement and regional cerebral oxygen desaturation associated with patency of the circle of Willis during carotid endarterectomy. Journal of Cardiothoracic and Vascular Anesthesia. 2015;**29**(5):1200-1205

[24] Etz C, Borger M. Commentary—Functional assessment of circle of Willis: Interesting observation or critical consideration? The Journal of Thoracic and Cardiovascular Surgery. 2019;**158**: 1305-1306

[25] Gibello L, Varetto G, Spalla F, et al. Impact of the supra-aortic trunks and circle of Willis patency on the neurological compensation during carotid endarterectomy. Annals of Vascular Surgery. 2019;**60**:229-235

[26] Montisci R, Sanfilippo R, Bura R, Branca C, Piga M, Saba L. Status of the circle of Willis and intolerance to carotid cross-clamping during carotid endarterectomy. European Journal of Vascular and Endovascular Surgery. 2013;**45**(2):107-112

[27] Pennekamp CW, van Laar PJ, Hendrikse J, den Ruijter HM, Bots ML, van der Worp HB, et al. Incompleteness of the circle of Willis is related to EEG-based shunting during carotid endarterectomy. European Journal of Vascular and Endovascular Surgery. 2013;**46**(6):631-637. DOI: 10.1016/j.ejvs.2013.09.007

[28] de Athayde Soares R, Câmara Costa Ferreira ZM, Viana Portela MV, Valentim M, Matielo MF, Nakamura ET, et al. The importance of the circle of Willis in carotid interventions outcomes: A real-life study. Annals of Vascular

Surgery. 2024;**101**:127-133. DOI: 10.1016/j.avsg.2023.11.026

[29] Zhou C, Yuan C, Li R, et al. Association between incomplete circle of Willis and carotid vulnerable atherosclerotic plaques. Arteriosclerosis, Thrombosis, and Vascular Biology. 2018; **38**(11):2744-2749

[30] Mariscalco G, Piffaretti G, Tozzi M, et al. Predictive factors for cerebrovascular accidents after thoracic endovascular aortic repair. The Annals of Thoracic Surgery. 2009;**88**(6):187-1881

[31] Smith T, Jafrancesco G, Surace G, Morshuis WJ, Tromp SC, Heijmen RH. A functional assessment of the circle of Willis before aortic arch surgery using transcranial Doppler. The Journal of Thoracic and Cardiovascular Surgery. Nov 2019;**158**(5):1298-1304. DOI: 10.1016/j.jtcvs.2019.01.007

[32] Urbanski P, Lenos A, Blume J, et al. Does anatomical completeness of the circle of Willis correlate with sufficient cross-perfusion during unilateral cerebral perfusion? European Journal of Cardio-Thoracic Surgery. 2008;**33**(3): 402-408

[33] Began P, Vidal R, Martinod E, et al. Cerebral ischemia during carotid artery cross-clamping: Predictive value of phase contrast magnetic resonance imaging. Annals of Vascular Surgery. 2006;**20**(6):747-752

Chapter 3

History and Evolution of the Management of Acute Type-A Aortic Dissection

Nikhil Chandra, David Tang, Kamaraj Radhakrishnan and Sean D. Galvin

Abstract

Acute type A aortic dissection (ATAAD) is a condition associated with high morbidity and mortality. The first known classification system came from DeBakey and team in the 1960s. In 1970 the Stanford group proposed that dissections involving the ascending and/or proximal arch warranted urgent surgical repair and those that only involved the descending aorta to be managed medically. Globally there remains a debate with regards to the operative extent at the index presentation. Since then, there has been significant evolution of the understanding of the disease process, its classification systems, diagnostic tools, operative/canulation strategies, cerebral protection, extent of replacement and development of surveillance programs and multi-disciplinary aortic meetings. This has improved post operative and long-term survival. We look at the history and evolution of the diagnosis and management of acute type A aortic dissection.

Keywords: type A aortic dissection, dissection classification, malperfusion, true lumen, false lumen, AV resuspension, root replacement, arch reconstruction, FET, TEVAR, deep hypothermic circulatory arrest, peripheral cannulation

1. Introduction

1.1 Evolution of surgery for aortic dissection

Dr. Nicholls, physician to King George II in the 1760s, provided the first documented description of acute aortic dissection in western literature during a postmortem examination [1]. Over the next two centuries with the development of increasingly sophisticated imaging techniques our understanding of both acute and chronic aortic syndromes has significantly expanded. Yet, despite these advancements, there remains challenges in timely diagnosis, performing surgery with low morbidity and mortality whilst optimizing long term survival and deducting the requirement for aortic reintervention and late mortality from secondary aortic complications.

The surgical management of acute type A aortic dissection has gone through various phases of evolution. Early surgical techniques focused on limited repair of the ascending with a clamped anastomosis to prevent intra-pericardial rupture, correct aortic regurgitation and prevent coronary ischaemia. The next phase evolved to focus on open distal aortic anastomosis and hemiarch replacement. Improved imaging has now allowed the understanding of the complex physiology and anatomy of both acute and chronic dissections. There has been a transition in the mindset and surgical approach away from a purely central aortic operation to surgical techniques that allow subsequent management of the entire "aortic organ". Current surgical techniques recognize the importance of aortic valve function, malperfusion, false lumen (FL) patency and the potential for future complex aneurysm development. This current holistic phase of surgical therapy has evolved to include aortic arch repair, sophisticated techniques of cerebral protection, frozen elephant trunks (FET). FET is a specially designed stent graft that is deployed within the proximal descending thoracic aorta. It allows simultaneous repair of the aortic arch and the proximal DTA in a single operation. It acts as a landing zone for potential future endovascular interventions in the distal aorta.

We will discuss the evolution of aortic dissection surgery focusing on changing techniques and outcomes and touch on what the future might hold.

2. Aortic dissection and evolution of classification systems

Aortic dissection primarily involves an intimal tear that extends into the aortic media. This tear typically occurs at points where the aortic wall experiences the highest tension (entry tear). The separation of the aortic media from the intima results in the formation of a multi channeled aorta, where an aortic dissection flap divides the aortic lumen into parts known as the true and false lumens. Re-entry tears typically occur in the intima, creating additional connections between the true and false lumens in the lower or distal part of the aorta. The true lumen tends to be narrow with high-velocity blood, while the false lumen is often larger and experiences slower, turbulent blood flow [2].

Early diagnoses were previously limited, with only 40–50% of cases identified pre-mortem [3]. Before the advent of cardiopulmonary bypass (CPB), safe surgical interventions were unavailable.

The DeBakey classification categorizes aortic dissections into three types based on the extent of the dissection along the aorta [4].

Type I – involves ascending and descending aorta.

Type II – involves only the ascending aorta.

Type III – involves the ascending and descending aorta.

Daily and Shumway at Stanford highlighted from their case series from 1964 to1969 that there are substantial differences in both treatment and prognosis between aortic dissections affecting the ascending aorta and those limited to the descending aorta. Patients with dissection involving the ascending aorta had a much-improved survival with surgical intervention compared to medical management in contrast to dissections involving just the descending thoracic aorta who had comparable outcomes with medical and surgical treatment [5]. This observation formed the basis of the Stanford classification for aortic dissection which groups dissections into 2 categories.

Type A – involves the ascending aorta proximal to the left subclavian artery (LSCA).

Type B – involves the aorta distal to the LSCA.

Whilst the Stanford classification underscores of the descriptions of aortic dissection into contemporary surgical literature the growth of endovascular therapies and our understanding of malperfusion syndromes have led to the ongoing development of classifications that describe both the radiological appearances of the dissection and clinical consequences. Some of the newer classification systems include:

DISSECT: A mnemonic based system [6].

D - duration of disease, *I* - intimal tear location, *S* - size of the dissected aorta, *S* - segmental *E*xtent of aortic involvement, *C* – clinical complications of the dissection and *T*hrombus within the aortic false lumen.

TEM classification [7]. This was an extension of the Stanford classification (A and B) by adding **T**ype non-A and non-B, primary **E**ntry tear and *M*alperfusion.

A 0 was added if the primary entry tear was not visible; 1, if it was in the ascending aorta; 2, if it was in the arch; and 3, if it was in the descending aorta (E0, E1, E2, E3).

A 0 if malperfusion was absent; 1, if coronary arteries; 2, if supra-aortic vessels; and 3, if visceral/renal and/or a lower extremity was affected (M0, M1, M2, M3).

Plus (+) was added if malperfusion was clinically present and minus (−) if it was a radiological finding.

The Penn Classification [8].

A - Hemodynamically stable without signs or symptoms of ischaemia.

B – Haemodynamically stable but with evidence of branch vessel malperfusion with signs or symptoms of ischaemia (eg: stroke, ST segment changes, abdominal pain, limb ischaemia).

C – Global malperfusion from circulatory collapse (with or without cardiac involvement).

B-C – Global malperfusion from circulatory collapse plus evidence of local ischaemia.

Recognizing not only the radiological aspects of dissections, but these newer classification systems also focus on the importance of clinical malperfsuion and ischaemia and may allow for more sophisticated tools to plan the extent of surgery at the index operation.

3. Phase 1: Pioneering surgery on the aorta and cardiopulmonary bypass

Initially, the main challenge with ATAAD was diagnosing it correctly. Once diagnosed, there was no safe method to manage it before the advent of CPB, often leading to the condition being identified postmortem. The difficulty in accurately diagnosing these patients was just one aspect of the problem. Surgical treatment was unexplored, and early medical approaches such as sedation and bed rest were largely ineffective. Consequently, the natural course of acute aortic dissection, whether involving the ascending, arch or descending, was fatal.

Initial experience in aortic surgery was garnered from procedures on peripheral arterial aneurysms which later translated to abdominal and thoracic aortic aneurysms. From the late eighteenth century onwards, many techniques were described to address aortic aneurysms. This ranged from inserting hot needles into the aneurysmal sac to stimulate thrombosis, inserting wires or coils to stimulate fibrous tissue growth within the sac, ligature of the vessel proximal to the aneurysm, endoaneurysmorrhaphy and in the early 1900s, polyethylene wrapping (cellophane wrapping) [9–13]. Aortic rupture was not always prevented with these techniques and a more robust and definite strategy was necessary.

3.1 Flap fenestration and early aortic graft replacement

In 1935, the first surgical method for addressing an acute aortic dissection was described by performing an iliac fenestration to treat an ischemic leg resulting from acute aortic dissection by Gurin et al. The fenestration helped to decompress a non-re-entering false lumen [14]. Over the subsequent 5 decades, advancements in the treatment of aortic dissection have primarily concentrated on managing the tear in the aorta and preventing proximal aortic rupture, which is the leading cause of mortality.

DeBakey et al. at Houston in 1955 managed an ATAAD by creating a re-entry tear in the proximal descending thoracic aorta to decompress the false lumen in the ascending aorta and aortic arch with suture obliteration of the distal false lumen [15]. Shaw et al. at Massachusetts General Hospital also performed flap fenestration of the abdominal aorta for an ATAAD around the same time [16]. This procedure had a high operative mortality rate close to 50%. Flap fenestration was soon acknowledged as palliative because it did not restore the structural integrity of the ascending aorta and arch [4]. However, interventions on the ascending aorta and arch without cardiopulmonary bypass either necessitated complex extra-anatomic bypasses or involved ineffective circumferential aortic wrapping.

Suture obliteration of the proximal and distal false lumen followed by primary anastomosis of the native aorta was soon replaced by graft replacement of the diseased aorta. This was initially reserved for chronic dissections, however, with favorable results from DeBakey's series between 1961 and 1965, more acute dissections were managed with emergency surgery at other centres. The Stanford group were instrumental in advocating for replacement of the ascending aorta in ATAAD [5]. Replacement of the ascending or arch of aorta was more challenging using the clamp and sew technique as there was no safe way to protect the brain and distal body from ischaemic injury during the period of no flow.

In the 1950's, Michael DeBakey, Denton Cooley, and Oscar Creech Jr. described a series of patients who had their dissected aneurysmal part resected and in suitable cases, end-to-end anastomosis was attempted. In others, freeze-dried homografts were used to bridge the aortic defect. It is worth noting that these repairs were performed in the descending thoracic or the thoracoabdominal aorta prior to the availability of conventional cardiopulmonary bypass (CPB) machines. However, these experiences led to the development of several important universal principles in the surgical repair of aortic dissection. In that paper, the authors described the goal of surgical therapy is directed towards prevention of propagation of intramural dissection and terminal rupture through the outer adventitial layer and restoration of blood flow in the true lumen [15]. The understanding of the pathophysiology of aortic dissection then was of incredible accuracy despite the lack of readily available imaging technology. Some proposed concepts like cystic media necrosis, mechanical shear stress on the aorta, and the association with hypertension still hold true today. During the 1950s, the search for an ideal aortic replacement conduit intensified. Initially, homografts were used by most surgeons as conduits to replace diseased regions of the aorta [17]. However, the drawbacks of homografts, such as calcification and deterioration, became increasingly evident. The need for durable, synthetic material that could be manufactured at scale grew dire. The eventual discovery of Dacron as a vascular conduit almost happened by accident. When DeBakey was experimenting with materials for vascular grafts, he went to a department store in Houston, Texas to look for Nylon. The clerk informed him that they had run out of Nylon but they had a "new fabric" called Dacron. DeBakey purchased a yard of the material and was working on them at home using his wife's sewing machine [18]. He first implanted the Dacron graft at the VA Hospital in Houston and by the mid 1960's, his team had performed over 250 cases of aortic dissection repair, and the Dacron graft is still widely used in cardiovascular surgeries today and Dr. DeBakey would go on to do more than 60,000 cardiovascular surgeries until his retirement [18–20].

The advent of the CPB machine ushered in a new era of surgical intervention for ATAAD that was previously unimaginable. Several pivotal milestones in scientific discoveries paved the way to the modern CPB machine. In 1813, Le Gallois first conceptualized the idea of extracorporeal circulation, but his vision was far ahead of its time. The limited understanding of blood biology made the clinical application of CPB a distant reality [21]. It was not until the end of the century that transfusion medicine emerged as a field, with the discovery of blood types, storage methods, and transfusion techniques [22]. Interestingly, heparin was first isolated in 1916 by McLean, a medical student from Johns Hopkins University, who was initially searching for a novel procoagulant. Heparin later became the mainstream anticoagulant in cardiovascular surgery and is still used today. Its reversal agent, protamine, was later discovered by Chargraff and Olson in 1937 [23].

The next critical development was the vertical screen oxygenator by John Gibbon, in collaboration with the International Business Machines Corporation (IBM). This breakthrough culminated over two decades of Gibbon's work on the CPB machine. His initial experiments on feline subjects achieved long-term survival following 10-20 minutes of CPB. However, his first clinical attempts to correct cardiac anomalies in patients were discouraging, compounded by misdiagnoses, technical failures, and air embolism [24, 25]. The concept of the cardiac surgery team arose from these mishaps, underscoring the need to elevate the standards and competencies of every team member involved.

In the spring of 1955, Dr. John Kirklin et al. at the Mayo Clinic reported their first successful series of intracardiac surgeries using a modified version of the original Gibbon-IBM model [26]. This success was later mirrored by Lillehei and DeWall with their bubble oxygenation system featuring a defoaming coil [27]. These luminary figures revolutionized cardiovascular surgery, creating the specialty as we know it today.

In the mid 1960's, Michael DeBakey and associates in Houston amassed significant experience operating on 179 patients with aortic dissections of which 37 of whom had ATAAD. Remarkably, they achieved an operative survival rate of over 70% in the ATAAD group [4]. In retrospective analysis of their data, there may have been some Type B dissections included in the 70% survival rate. They also devised the DeBakey Classification for aortic dissection and outlined the recommended operative approach for each type.

Operative repairs of DeBakey Type I and II aortic dissection became feasible after the advent of the CPB machine. For Type I, DeBakey advocated for the transection of the ascending aorta a few centimeters above the aortic valve, obliterating the false lumen by approximation of the intimal layer and the outer wall by means of continuous suture of both the proximal and distal cut ends, and subsequent end-to-end anastomosis of the transected aorta with the goal to restore mural integrity and perfusion into the true lumen. This technique, though not employed in modern repair, principally prevented further retrograde extension of the dissection into the aortic root, which could result in fatal coronary obstruction or torrential acute aortic insufficiency.

In Type II dissections, DeBakey described resecting and replacing the entire ascending aorta on occluding clamps. The aorta was divided between occluding clamps placed proximal to the innominate artery whilst a Dacron graft is sewn to the distal cut end. At that time, it was believed then that acceptable cardiac function was maintained via continuous pulmonary ventilation and retrograde perfusion from the coronary sinus return and bronchial arterial flow. This technique has now been superseded by cardioplegic arrest which provides more superior myocardial protection. The proximal anastomosis was achieved by trimming the dissected aorta down to the aortic annulus with myocardial protection achieved via direct coronary perfusion catheters. In both types, valvular insufficiency was common, and the aortic valve was resuspended via fixation of the leaflet attachments, or in some cases of significantly dilated annulus, bicuspidisation annuloplasty or aortic valve replacement with a prosthesis would be performed [4].

4. Phase 2: Future proofing the aorta

Historically, many centres have taken a conservative approach to the aortic valve and root during surgical repair of ATAAD in the absence of significant aortic regurgitation or massively dilated root. Typically opting to preserve them using supra-coronary aortic grafts, commissural resuspension of the aortic valve, and various methods to repair the sinus of Valsalva. The concern with this strategy is the potential need for further interventions due to late-onset aortic valve insufficiency. One of the more common and globally accepted technique is to perform complete resection of the intimal tear and replacing the ascending aorta with or without hemiarch replacement. An open distal anastomosis without aortic clamping is usually preferred as it allows more accurate re approximation of the dissected layers and a better haemostatic anastomosis [28–32]. Aortic clamping could induce false lumen pressurization. This could lead to propagation of the dissection downstream and further malperfusion.

4.1 Aortic valve and root

Acute aortic regurgitation in ATAAD can arise from several mechanisms: (I) rapid enlargement of the aortic root due to expansion of the false lumen, leading to inadequate closure of the aortic valve; (II) extension of the dissection into the aortic root, disrupting the attachments of the aortic valve commissures and causing prolapse of the valve leaflets; and (III) prolapse of a portion of the dissection flap through the aortic valve during diastole, preventing proper closure of the valve leaflets. Because the morphology of the valve leaflets remains intact, preservation of the native valve is often feasible for most patients.

When the aortic root is partially dissected, repair can involve resuspension of the aortic valve. However, extensive dissection of the aortic root typically necessitates more definitive interventions such as aortic root replacement using a composite valve graft or a valve-sparing root replacement where appropriate and in experienced hands. Techniques that retain the sinuses and conserve the valve may not be suitable for patients with underlying root pathologies like Marfan syndrome or annulo-aortic ectasia. In such cases, aortic root replacement with a composite prosthesis or valve-sparing root replacement is recommended to address both the dissection and the underlying structural issues of the aortic root.

In cases of ATAAD preserving the native aortic valve is preferred if the cusps are relatively normal, given the absence of an ideal prosthetic valve. Both preoperative clinical assessment, radiological features, intraoperative transesophageal echocardiography and operative assessment, play critical roles in determining the suitability of preserving the valve and/or the root [33].

When abnormal cusp pathology or traumatic dissection make preserving the native valve impractical, replacement becomes necessary. Bioprosthetic valves have shown durability in older patients (over 65 years old), but younger patients undergoing aortic valve replacement (AVR) with bio prostheses, whether alone or as part of a composite valve graft (CVG) root replacement, face a significantly higher risk of structural valve deterioration within 15 years [34].

Mechanical prosthetic AVR requires lifelong anticoagulation, carrying risks of bleeding and embolic complications, yet offers a lower risk of reoperation and potentially improved survival for patients aged 50–69 years [35]. Typically, mechanical valves are recommended for AVR in patients under 60–65, barring contraindications to anticoagulation, while bioprosthetic valves are favored for patients over 65–70. Decisions for those aged 60–70 should weigh factors such as life expectancy and comorbidities [36].

Even when root replacement becomes necessary, there are cases where a conservative approach towards preserving the valve can still be maintained, particularly under the care of experienced surgeons. The Tirone David re-implantation technique for valve-sparing root replacement (VSRR) has shown promising mid-term outcomes in carefully chosen younger patients with ATAAD who are not in critical condition [37].

Several methods have been proposed to preserve the aortic valve and reinforce proximal anastomosis and commissural resuspension. Originally, Teflon felt was used both internally and externally at proximal and distal anastomoses to strengthen the fragile native aorta [38]. Additionally, Teflon was applied externally (within the adventitia) to fortify the aorta and fill the false lumen [28]. Starting in the 1980s, biological glue has been infused between the dissected layers of the aorta as part of this remodeling technique [39, 40]. The "French" gelatin-resorcinol-formaldehyde (GRF) glue gained popularity for reinforcing delicate sinuses of Valsalva tissue and assisting in sewing the proximal anastomosis, resulting in reasonable mid-term outcomes [41]. However, concerns about tissue toxicity and the occurrence of false aneurysms in glued aortic segments dampened enthusiasm, particularly with GRF French glue due to formalin toxicity concerns. Despite advancements in newer biological glue formulations like bovine serum albumin with glutaraldehyde (BioGlue), designed to mitigate formalin-related issues, concerns remain about tissue necrosis and the potential for false aneurysms [42, 43].

Preserving the aortic valve and root could lead to re-operations in future for either. This was the rationale for some groups that urged for a more aggressive approach at the index operation, arguing that a re-do in such cases would be added morbidity and mortality for something that could have been tackled prior. Since the 1970s there were two schools of thought with one group advocating for root replacement and another urging for an aortic valve replacement for anyone with an ATAAD and aortic regurgitation [44–47].

In patients ATAAD, the native valve often remains functional despite extensive root dissection and aortic regurgitation [48]. For patients with intact valves but severe sinus damage, supra-coronary replacement of the ascending aorta with valve resuspension is usually acceptable. There are techniques that involve reconstructing the aortic root with Teflon felt strips (external only or sandwich) or a circular cuff of dacron graft [49, 50]. In experienced hands and in high volume centres, techniques such as valve sparing root replacements have demonstrated favorable long-term outcomes, particularly among Marfan patients [51]. The choice between root replacement strategies depends on the likelihood of preserving the valve long-term. Conversely, patients at higher risk of re-intervention due to pre-existing root issues (dilated root), connective tissue disorders or extensive dissection may benefit from more aggressive root replacement approaches at the index operation.

Performing an aortic root replacement during an ATAAD repair prolongs the aortic cross clamp and cardiopulmonary bypass times. It adds a level of complexity dealing with dissected aortic tissue when mobilizing the coronary buttons. While mortality risks may not significantly differ in experienced hands and at high volume centres, caution is advised in universally recommending root replacement for ATAAD patients as many centres would have relatively low numbers of acute or elective proximal aortic surgeries [52, 53]. At our institution around 25% of the ATAAD would receive an aortic root replacement.

In a nutshell, surgically managing the proximal aorta in ATAAD involves weighing the risks and benefits of preserving versus replacing the aortic valve and root. Clinical judgment and patient-specific factors play crucial roles in determining the optimal surgical strategy, aiming for durable outcomes and minimizing the need for re-intervention.

4.2 Conquering the arch

Aortic arch replacement surgery involves a range of techniques and materials tailored to the individual patient's condition and the surgeon's expertise. The goal is to effectively restore blood flow through the aortic arch while minimizing risks and complications associated with the surgery.

- *Types of grafts*: Aortic arch replacements typically use knitted or woven Dacron prostheses. These are synthetic materials that are durable and biocompatible. The grafts are often coated with substances like albumin, gelatin, or bovine collagen to make them impervious and reduce the risk of clot formation or infection.

- *Types of graft configurations:*

    - *Straight grafts*: These are simple tubular grafts used to replace the diseased segment of the aortic arch.

    - *Anteflow grafts*: These grafts have a side arm that functions as a perfusion port. This is useful for maintaining arterial inflow during CPB. Once the distal anastomosis of the aortic graft is performed, the dacron graft is clamped and the arterial inflow (distal to the clamp) is through this side arm.

    - *Variations with branches*: Some grafts are designed with three or four branches (usually about 8-10 mm in diameter). These branches are used to debranch the arch vessels (such as the innominate artery, left common carotid artery, and left subclavian artery). This allows the surgeon to perform selective antegrade cerebral perfusion (SACP) and maintain blood flow to the brain during surgery.

- *Use of Teflon felt strips*: Teflon felt strips are often used to reinforce the anastomoses (surgical connections) between the graft and the remaining native aorta. This reinforcement helps to prevent bleeding and ensures a secure seal at the graft-to-aorta junction.

- *Technique variability*: The choice of specific techniques and materials can vary based on several factors:

    - *Location of intimal tear*: The exact location of the primary intimal tear or the extent of the aortic pathology can influence the choice of graft and technique.

    - *Size of aortic arch*: The size and shape of the aortic arch also play a role in determining which type of graft and configuration is most suitable.

    - *Surgeon's preference and experience*: Surgeons may have preferences based on their training and experience with certain techniques and graft types.

When the primary initial tear is located within the aortic arch, an approach to replace the arch is considered. In the past, surgeries involving the arch carried substantial risks due to insufficient protection for the brain, leading to mortality rates as high as 42% [54]. The traditional approach for replacing the transverse aortic arch refers to performing the distal anastomosis first. Cooley et al. recommended routinely performing open distal anastomosis with profound hypothermic circulatory arrest (PHCA) to improve visibility, assess the intima of the arch, and ensure the continuity of the true lumen while closing off the false lumen [55].

Performing the distal aortic anastomosis with aortic clamping avoids the need for profound hypothermia and circulatory arrest and is faster. However, this approach may compromise the technical quality of the anastomosis, increasing the risks of issues such as bleeding, graft dehiscence, pressurization of the distal aorta, further propagation of the dissection, and late false aneurysm formation, which could necessitate reoperation [56]. At our institution we practice open distal anastomosis with SACP and avoid clamping dissected aortas.

As experience with PHCA increased, surgeons began extending operations for ATAAD involving the arch. This extension of the surgery to involve the arch was fraught with complications and did not readily attain widespread uptake among all centres. The primary concern was adequate cerebral protection, this led to the development of cerebral protection strategies such as antegrade and retrograde cerebral perfusion.

Kazui introduced selective antegrade cerebral perfusion (SACP) at 10 mL/kg/min during PHCA, demonstrating comparable neurological outcomes to PHCA alone in total aortic arch replacement cases, and suggesting enhanced safety during extended circulatory arrest periods [57]. This approach gained popularity with the development of axillary artery cannulation techniques pioneered by Sabik and Baribeau, facilitating SACP with direct or small caliber graft cannulation. Despite the additional procedural time required for axillary artery dissection and graft placement, this method has been successfully employed globally in emergency ATAAD settings [58, 59].

Ueda et al. innovated the use of RCP for neuroprotection, demonstrating effective arch repair without head vessel clamping. Its simplicity and minimal impact on cannulation strategy allowed for rapid deployment in both elective and emergency scenarios [60]. However, limitations such as internal jugular vein valve competency and veno-venous shunting have constrained its effectiveness, resulting in reduced cerebral blood delivery compared to other methods. Animal studies indicated potential risks of cerebral oedema with RCP, albeit effective for particulate emboli clearance when combined with inferior vena cava occlusion. Further studies and retrospective reviews put forward the opinion that RCP is an adjunct for cooling and does not contribute much towards oxygenation. The authors are careful to mention that the conversion from SACP to RCP is not advocated and ACP is still the preferred cerebral protection strategy for extensive and complex arch surgery [60–62].

Recognizing the critical need for optimal neuroprotection strategies, Svensson et al. conducted a randomized trial comparing intermittent antegrade brain perfusion with RCP in elective arch operations, revealing no statistically significant difference between the two approaches. However, the trial's short circulatory arrest periods may have limited the ability to discern subtle differences in brain protection efficacy [63].

Many centres globally perform unilateral SACP using right axillary perfusion by sewing on an 8 mm dacron graft and clamping of the arch vessels to prevent back flow into the operative field. Direct cannulation of the arch vessels is another strategy utilized. At our institution we perform branch first arch replacement and commence the procedure by sequentially debranching the arch vessels. All these strategies deliver approximately 10 ml/kg/min of blood flow to the brain with moderate to deep hypothermia.

There is a 5–10% stroke risk in aortic arch surgery despite the advancements in cerebral protection strategies. Abjigitova et al. performed the largest meta-analysis on this matter. It included 222 studies and 43,720 patients [64]. The data is largely based on observational studies and makes it very difficult to make a direct comparison between Unilateral antegrade cerebral perfusion, bilateral antegrade cerebral perfusion, retrograde cerebral perfusion and DHCA with no cerebral perfusion, given the significant change in practice with minimal standardization. The procedures included hemiarch or total arch replacement, emergency and elective cases and the experience of the operating centre all varied. The selection of one technique over the other or the lowest temperature attained was not uniform. These could have been influenced pre-existing stroke, complexity of the procedure, experience of the surgeon. The authors concluded that unilateral ACP had lower mortality (6.6%) and stroke rate (4.8%), whereas bilateral ACP (9.1% mortality and 7.3% stroke), retrograde (7.8 and 6.4%) and DHCA without cerebral perfusion (9.2, 6.3%). In our centre a single surgeon experience of branch first aortic arch replacement over the last 10 years had a mortality rate of 5.3% in emergency type A dissections with no elective mortality. Stroke rate of 2.1% in emergency type A dissections in patients with pre-operative cerebral malperfusion and no elective strokes.

Our current practice emphasizes an aggressive approach to proximal arch replacement in all ATAAD patients with involvement extending into the arch. We employ SACP via the branch first arch replacement technique described by Matalanis et al. [65]. We use the modified trifurcation dacron graft (**Figure 1**) with a perfusing side arm port that allows to set up a separate head circuit on our CPB machine. The arch vessels are sequentially disconnected and debranched onto the trifurcation graft with

DOI: http://dx.doi.org/10.5772/intechopen.1009147

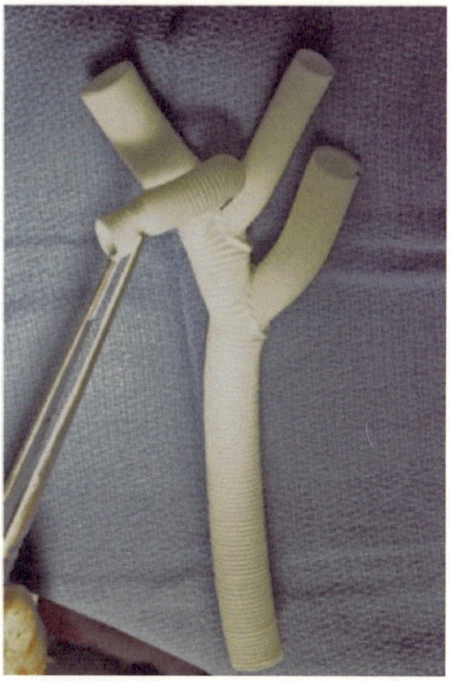

Figure 1.
Intra-operative image of the modified 3-branched Dacron graft (TAPP graft). This graft has the advantage of having an additional limb (held by forceps) which allows for antegrade cerebral perfusion following completion of each branch anastomosis and removes the need for separate axillary cannulation to supply inflow to the graft.

the heart ejecting (**Figure 2**). During the debranching process the patient is cooled. This approach aims for thorough distal reconstruction while minimizing the period of hypothermia and cardiopulmonary bypass durations (**Figures 3–5**).

Moderate systemic hypothermia (Nasopharyngeal ~20–22°C, bladder temperature 24–26°C) is typically sufficient for acute type A aortic dissection (ATAAD) and routine ascending aortic and arch procedures with continuous cerebral perfusion. For more complex cases involving arch rupture, extensive dissection, or young patients with connective tissue disorders, total arch replacement with or without a frozen elephant trunk is performed with deep hypothermia at nasopharyngeal temperature of 20°C. After completion of the open distal anastomosis, body flow is reinstated using the anteflow limb of the dacron graft and the patient is rewarmed as we address the proximal aorta. We routinely perform femoral artery cannulation for ATAAD. Occasionally we perform direct cannulation of the true lumen of the distal ascending aorta or arch using seldinger technique under TOE guidance and epiaortic ultrasound [66].

The choice of arterial cannulation and perfusion strategy is crucial for ensuring safe cerebral protection during aortic arch surgeries. The more common peripheral cannulation techniques include femoral, axillary, carotid, subclavian. Femoral artery cannulation ensures a rapid and reproducible setup, however, there are concerns about pressurization of the false lumen and malperfusion. Centres that routinely perform other peripheral arterial cannulation techniques reserve the use of femoral artery cannulation during situations of haemodynamic distress or when there is extensive axillary artery dissection [67].

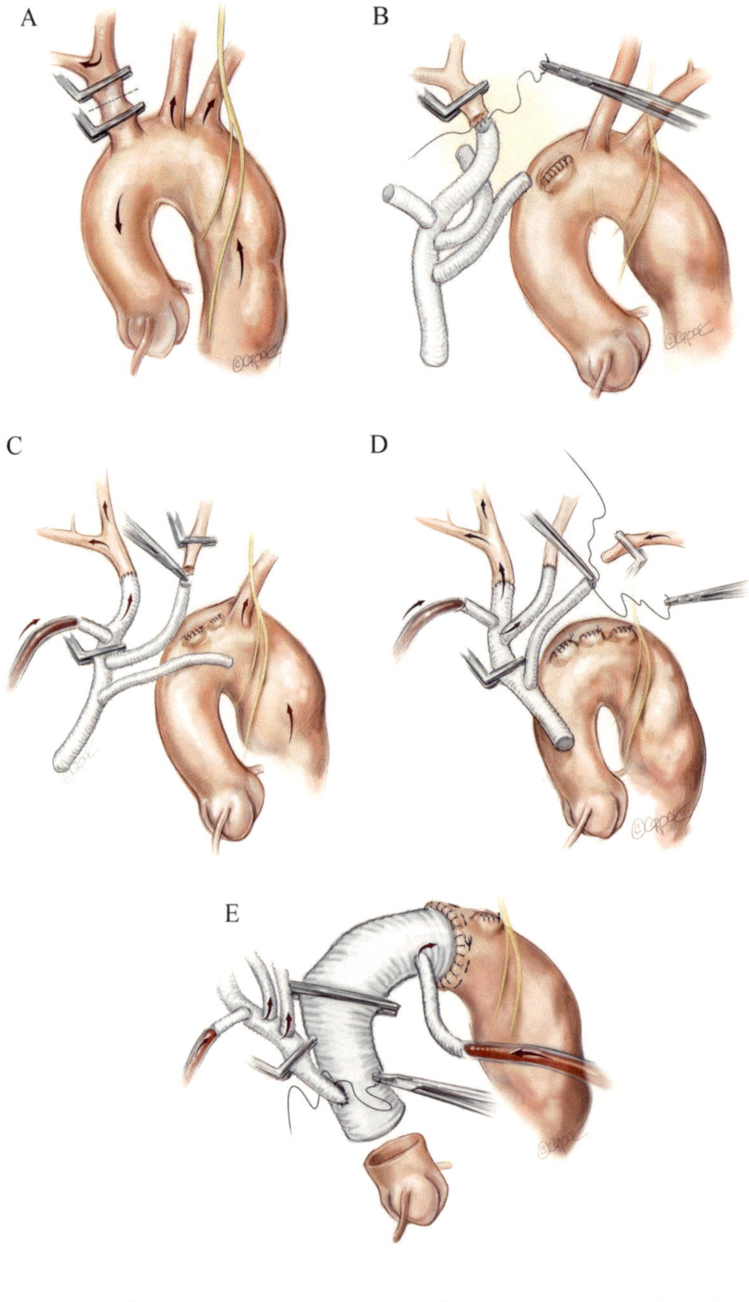

Figure 2.
Sequence of the "branch-first" aortic arch reconstruction. A. The innominate artery is clamped proximal to its bifurcation and distal to its origin from the arch. Right hemispheric cerebral perfusion is maintained through the left common carotid and left subclavian arteries via collateral channels, B. The innominate stump is ligated and the anastomosis to the branched graft completed; C. Antegrade right hemispheric cerebral perfusion is resumed via perfusion side arm. Left hemispheric cerebral perfusion during construction of the left common carotid anastomosis is maintained via the same collaterals; D. Left Subclavian anastomosis is completed; E. The distal aortic anastomosis is completed under hypothermic body circulatory arrest. After completion of the root anastomosis, connection of the trifurcation graft to the ascending graft proceeds without interruption of cerebral perfusion.

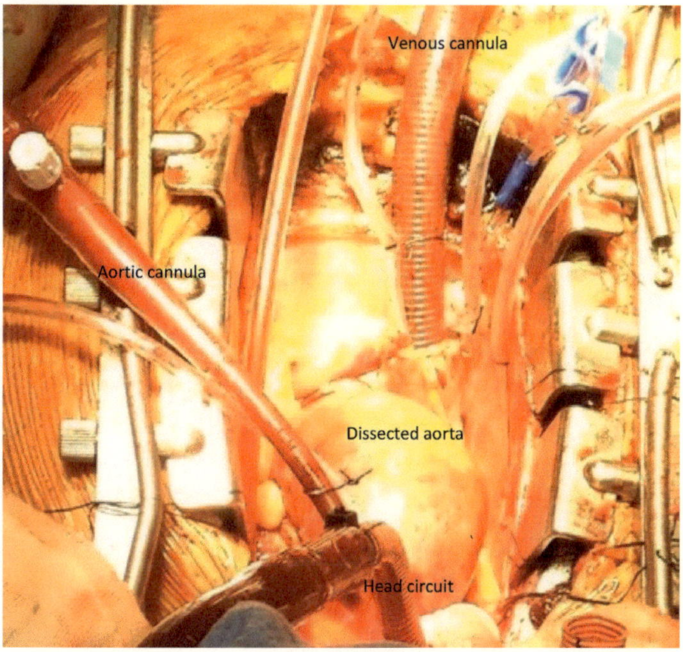

Figure 3.
Intraoperative view of a dissected aorta. In this instance, direct aortic cannulation into arch under TOE guidance using seldinger technique. Venous cannula into right atrium (RA). Head circuit is an extra pump set up in the CPB circuit that allows antegrade cerebral perfusion as the arch vessels are debranched using the trifurcation graft.

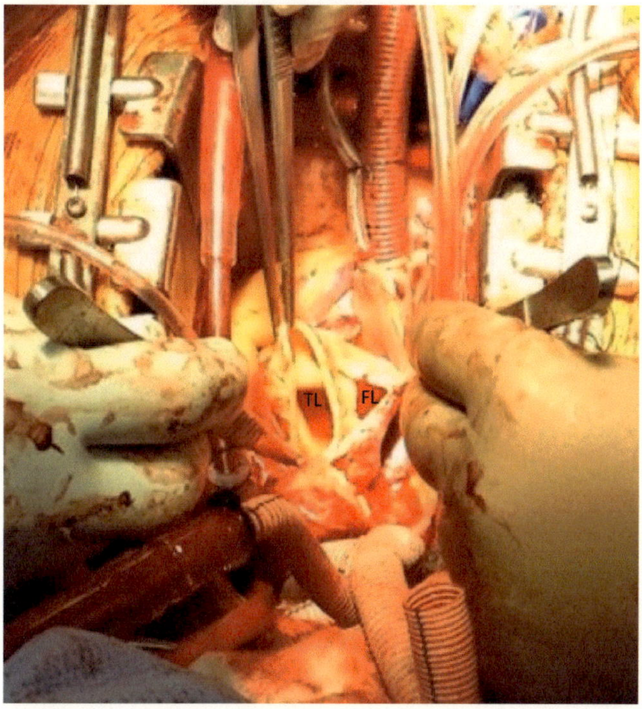

Figure 4.
Intra-operative view of a dissected aorta post transection. True Lumen (TL) and Fale Lumen (FL) in view.

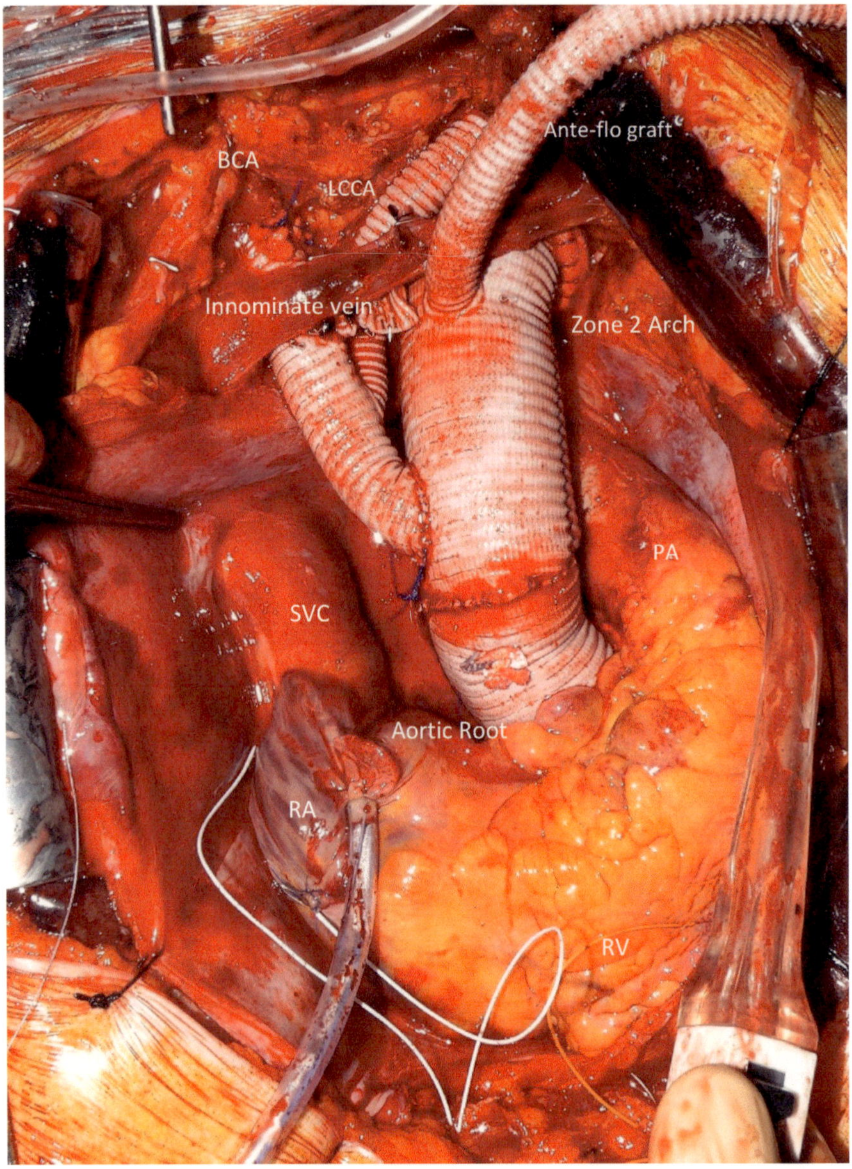

Figure 5.
Intraoperative view of a replaced ascending aorta with an Ante-flo graft. Brachiocephalic artery (BCA) and left common carotid artery (LCCA) debranched onto a trifurcation graft. Common stem of trifurcation graft proximalised onto ascending aorta, allowing greater landing zone for future TEVAR procedures.

Numerous studies have sought to determine the optimal surgical approach for repairing acute aortic dissection. The debate over whether a more conservative or more aggressive procedure is preferable in the acute phase remains unresolved and should be considered alongside careful evaluation of both short-term and long-term outcomes and patient's age and comorbidities.

Malvindi et al. from Europe suggested three key aspects that can be definitively examined. The first is survival following the initial repair. An approach involving more extensive surgery may reduce the need for reoperation, but it comes with a potenital risk of perioperative complications. Therefore, more aggressive proximal procedures should be reserved for cases with significant root involvement or dilation. Complete or partial arch replacement should be considered if the primary entry tear is located distal to the ascending aorta. The second aspect is the progress after the initial repair. It is always advised to maintain routine, lifelong imaging and clinical follow-ups to detect complications and assess the growth of untreated aortic segments. The third aspect is the outcome of reoperation. Reoperation after an acute dissection repair can be safely performed, offering a favorable long-term prognosis. A redo procedure does not necessarily reflect a less extensive repair in the initial surgery [68].

Kato introduced the frozen elephant trunk in 1996 as a modification of the conventional elephant trunk. This allows to safely address multi segment aortic disease. It provides safe proximal anastomosis within proximal descending thoracic repair. It also serves as an excellent landing zone for a future thoracic endovascular repair (TEVAR) graft. The essence of this device is that the stent graft is delivered into the open aorta under circulatory arrest and sutured into position [69–71]. The branch first debranching and arch replacement technique we utilize provides more of a landing zone for a 2nd stage TEVAR by relocating the arch vessels.

Ultimately, decisions regarding the extent of surgical intervention must prioritize patient survival, with concerns about downstream aortic reoperation secondary in importance.

We recommend managing these patients in a multi-disciplinary aortic MDM that allows for robust discussion on the best way forward for patients with residual aortic disease. Close surveillance is important to pick up complications of aortic dissection such as aneurysmal degeneration, visceral malperfusion or persistent false lumen. In select cases where there is residual thoracoabdominal aortic disease, we implement the branch first technique to replace the descending aorta via a thoracolaparotomy [72]. This is usually performed as a combined procedure with our vascular surgery colleagues at our institution.

5. Phase 3: The endovascular era

The next generation of evolution in the surgical management of ATAAD is primarily on endovascular techniques. At the cusp of the twenty-first century, two landmark papers published in the New England Journal of Medicine described the earliest clinical experiences with managing aortic dissection with entry tear beyond the left subclavian artery using endovascular stenting, with compelling clinical data TEVAR might surmount the gold-standard open surgical approach that has been established since the 1950's [73, 74]. The first experience in treating ATAAD via endovascular techniques was in cases with the primary intimal tear in the descending aorta and retrograde extension into the arch and ascending aortic. The primary tears were occluded by stent-graft placement which led to thrombosis of the false lumen, restoration of distal perfusion, and lower early procedural mortality compared to open repair [74].

In contrast, stent deployment in the ascending aorta on the other hand poses significant technical anatomical challenge. In 2000, Gerald Dorros and his team in

Wisconsin described the first stent deployment in the proximal ascending aorta for ATAAD. The team were presented with a patient post emergency coronary bypass operation which was complicated with ATAAD and was surgically repaired with a prosthetic graft. Five months later, the patient remained symptomatic, and imaging showed that she had a residual entry tear proximal to the innominate artery. A balloon expandable covered stent was deployed with a transseptal guidewire stabilization which resulted in resolution of the patient's symptom. Unfortunately, she passed away three weeks after the procedure; however, postmortem found that the stent was expanded and in good opposition to the aortic wall [75].

Subsequent use of TEVAR in the ascending aorta, particularly in cases of ATAAD, remained largely experimental and was limited to a select group of patients with favorable anatomy [76]. The largest single-centre experience till date was reported by Caisheng Ye et al. from Guangzhou. A total of 45 patients were managed with TEVAR from the year 2001 to 2009. In their series, the patients were categorized based on the anatomical locations of the entry tears: ten (22.2%) in the ascending aorta, 14 (31.1%) in the aortic arch, and 21 (46.7%) in the distal aortic arch or proximal descending aorta. The latter groups all had retrograde extension involving the ascending aorta. Ye's paper described different endovascular approaches based on the anatomical location of the entry tears. For those located in the ascending aorta, stents were introduced via either the left common carotid artery (LCCA) or the right common femoral artery. The former necessitates a preceding left subclavian artery (LSA)-LCCA bypass whilst in the latter, only patients with "at-risk" anatomy underwent LSA-LCCA-right common carotid artery (RCCA) bypass procedure. For entry tears in the arch, it is technically challenging to achieve adequate landing zone without compromising blood flow to the arch vessels. Resultantly, a hybrid approach with arch vessel debranching was necessary to facilitate safe deployment of TEVAR grafts across the arch. For entry tears in the distal arch or the descending aorta, most patients were treated with TEVAR alone, except for those with a non-dominant right vertebral artery or non-intact Circle of Willis, who required an LSA-LCCA bypass. The overall surgical success rate was 97.8%, with a 30-day mortality was 6.7%. Despite the heterogeneity of the patient group, comprising 30 (66.6%) ATAAD cases (onset up to 14 days) and 15 patients presenting beyond 14 days since symptom onset, the study sets a strong precedent with optimistic results demonstrated in a high-volume specialized center [77].

For half a century, the dogma of surgical treatment of ATAAD was to resect the dissected ascending aorta and to reestablish aortic continuity with a graft conduit to prevent immediately fatal sequalae of the disease itself. The procedure improves the prognosis of the patient and is ultimately lifesaving. It is however a palliative procedure in principle. As operative techniques evolved, the focus has shifted to improving late survival rate and freedom from reoperation from subsequent aneurysmal changes of the residual dissection in the aortic arch and descending aorta.

In 2002, the birth of the first hybrid procedure for the treatment of ATAAD was described by Masaaki Kato and associates in Osaka attempted to address the shortcoming of the conventional ascending aortic replacement. They described a less invasive total arch graft implantation aimed to achieve complete closure of intrathoracic entry sites for ATAAD compared to the conventional total arch replacement. In the procedure, the aortic arch is transected and a 30F curved catheter sheath is advanced under transesophageal echocardiography guidance to the target landing zone, which was described as a point of tight contact between stent graft and vascular wall. The deployment of an open-style self-expandable stent obviates the need for a distal anastomotic suture which is technically less challenging, whilst providing non-inferior survival outcomes [78].

The hybrid arch repair and later the invention of the frozen elephant trunk technique is an attractive option that provides a comprehensive single-stage repair in patients with extensive dissection involving both the aortic arch and the descending thoracic aorta. However, extensive preoperative comorbidities and limited physiological reserve in certain patient subgroups preclude an invasive surgical approach. The ascending aorta and aortic arch pose unique challenges for the endovascular surgeon, often considered the final frontier in the treatment armamentarium of the entire aortic organ. The curvature of the aortic arch is challenging to navigate and in the case of dissection, aggressive oversizing would result in radial tension exerted on the true lumen, resulting in stent graft-induced new entry (SINE) or catastrophic aortic rupture. The proximity to the aortic valve and the coronary ostia presents significant challenges in planning endovascular therapies for the ascending aorta. In 2014, Bartosz Rylski and associates from the University of Pennsylvania introduced a novel composite endovascular valved graft. It involves a single piece of device with three distinct portions: (1) a prosthetic aortic valve, (2) an uncovered graft portion which allows for unobstructed diastolic coronary perfusion, and (3) a covered graft portion. Compared to converntional TEVAR, this composite graft has three landing zones: the aortic annulus, the sino-tubular junction and the distal ascending aorta or the proximal arch [79].

Although the composite graft was initially designed for patients with concomittant aortic stenosis and post-stenotic ascending aortic anerusym, in 2023, Mehrdad Ghoreishi et al. at the University of Maryland adapted this concept for repairing ATAAD. They developed the "Endo-Bentall" device, which incorporates a self-expanding transcatheter aortic valve (TAVR) sewn circumferentially to a TEVAR graft. This graft includes two nitinol-reinforced fenestrations for coronary artery stenting, all contained within a modified TEVAR delivery system. In cases where endoleak is detected, the coronary ostia can be accessed through the fenestrations and stented using a covered balloon-expandable stent. This system was deployed in two patients with prohibitive surgical risks, yielding satisfactory medium-term outcomes with complete false lumen thrombosis and adequate coronary perfusion [80]. However, the long-term patency of the stented coronary ostia remains uncertain. Additionally, the transapical deployment of composite graft in ATAAD has also been proposed in setting of haemopericardium, as cardiac tamponade could be rapidly relieved whilst it circumvents the steep aortic curvate at the arch and facilitate wire placement into the true lumen. [80]

The evolution of endovascular techniques represents a significant advancement in the management ATAAD. The transition from traditional open surgical approaches to innovative hybrid and endovascular solutions highlights the ongoing quest to improve patient outcomes, reduce procedural mortality, improve freedom from reintervention and enhance long-term survival.

Imaging review of a 74 year old female with acute type a aortic dissection and left leg pain with compressed true lumen and obstruction of left common iliac artery. Previous CABG x 3 in 2001 (LIMA – LAD, RIMA y graft to diag and OM) (**Figures 6-13**).

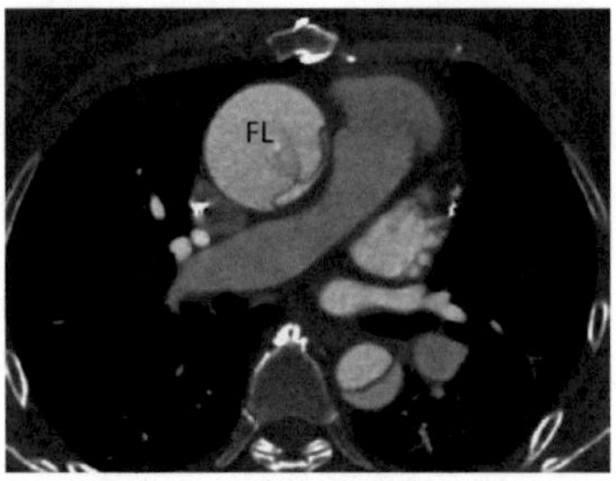

Figure 6.
Large false lumen in ascending aorta.

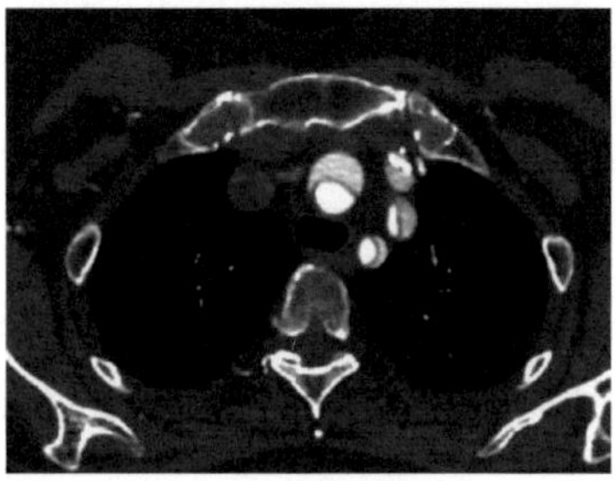

Figure 7.
All 3 arch vessels dissected.

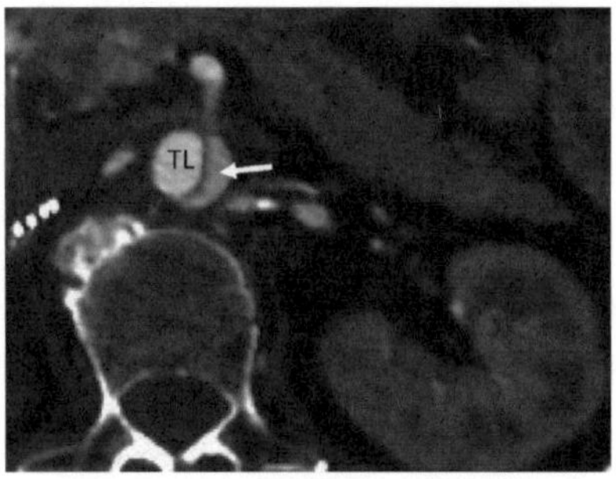

Figure 8.
Renal artery off false lumen.

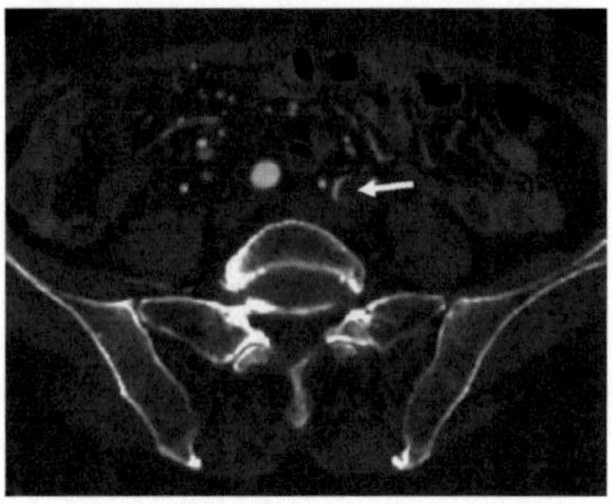

Figure 9.
Occluded left common iliac artery.

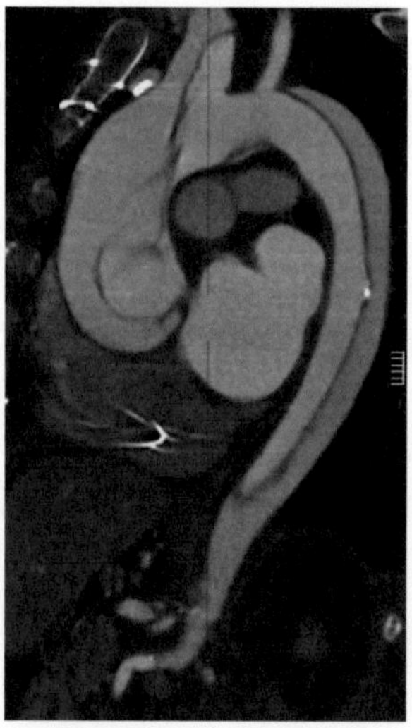

Figure 10.
Sagittal view showing Type A and Type B dissection.

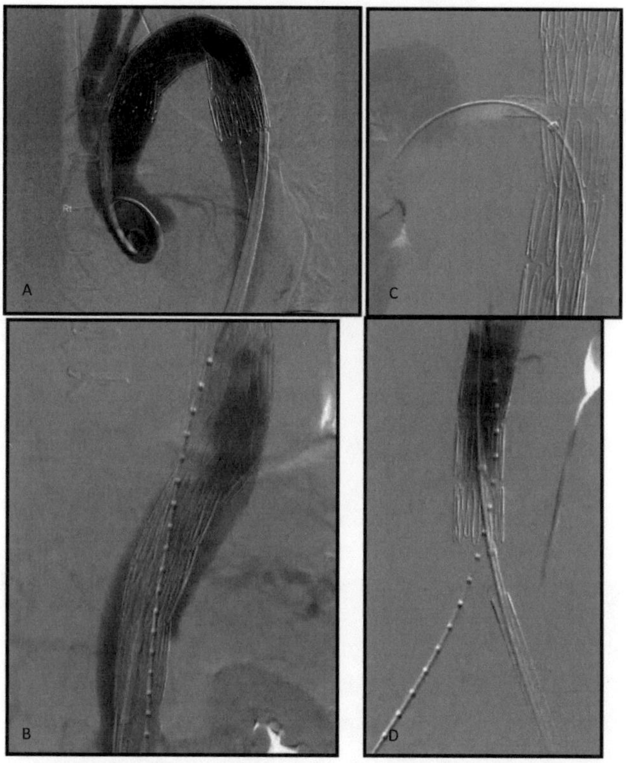

Figure 11.
Patient presenting with true lumen collapse following acute Type A Aortic Dissection and persistent occlusion of left common iliac artery - managed with Brach First Total Arch Replacement. Imaging shows completion STABILIZE technique. As the common stem of the trifurcation graft is now located proximal on the ascending aortic graft second stage endovascular treatment is simplified in even the most complex of cases, including dissections. A: Covered stent graft in arch, B: Uncovered stent graft in descending thoracic aorta down to aortic bifurcation, C: Left renal artery – covered stent, D: 2 uncovered stents in right common and right external iliac artery.

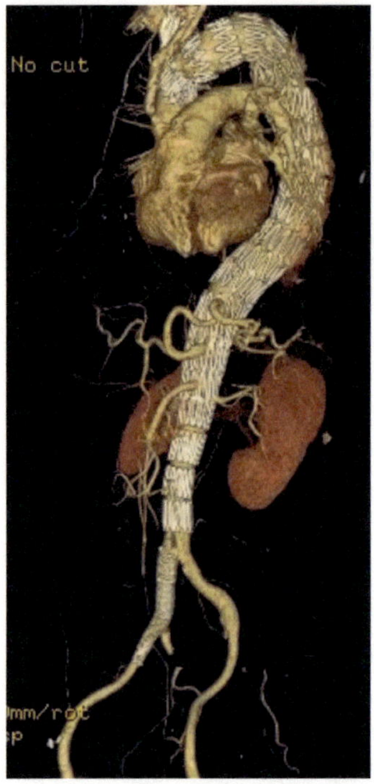

Figure 12.
Ct aortogram 12 months following branch first arch replacement followed by STABILIZE TEVAR with full expansion of the residual trye lumen and complete remodeling of the residual dissected thoracoabdominal aorta.

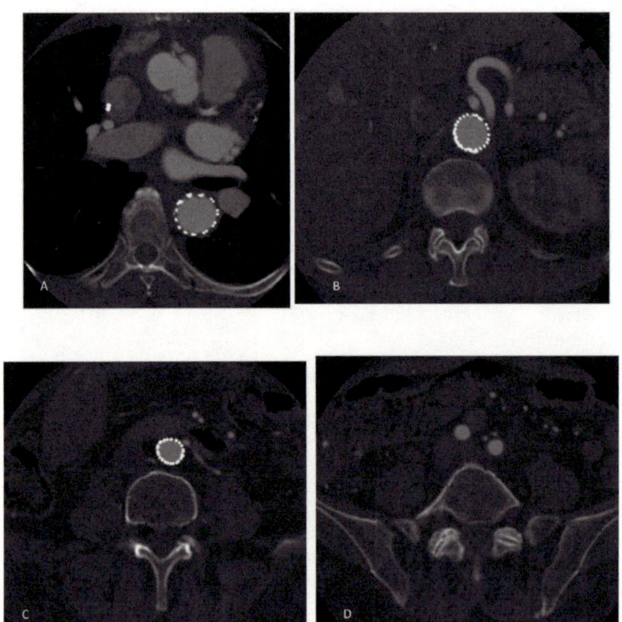

Figure 13.
A–D: Ct aortogram 12 months following branch first arch replacement followed by STABILIZE TEVAR with full expansion of the residual true lumen and complete remodeling of the residual dissected thoracoabdominal aorta.

6. Conclusions

The evolution of aortic dissection surgery has seen a shift from high-mortality open surgeries to more effective, refined and occasionally less invasive methods with the advent of endovascular techniques. There have been newer classification systems to help diagnose and manage aortic dissections better. This evolution has significantly improved survival rates, reduced complications, and enhanced long-term recovery. As surgical and diagnostic technologies continue to advance, the outlook for patients with aortic dissection continues to improve. The extent of replacement at the index operation remains up for debate and is mostly decided based on the institution's experience and patient factors. We believe having a dedicated aortic team with robust aortic MDMs would immensely improve outcomes for these patients.

Conflict of interest

The authors declare no conflict of interest.

Author details

Nikhil Chandra*, David Tang, Kamaraj Radhakrishnan and Sean D. Galvin
Wellington Hospital, Wellington, New Zealand

*Address all correspondence to: nikhil.chandra@ccdhb.org.nz

References

[1] Nicholls F. Observations concerning the body of his late majesty, October 26, 1760. Philosophical Transactions of the Royal Society B. 1761;**52**:265-275

[2] Macura KJ, Corl FM, Fishman EK, Bluemke DA. Pathogenesis in acute aortic syndromes: Aortic dissection, intramural hematoma, and penetrating atherosclerotic aortic ulcer. AJR. American Journal of Roentgenology. 2003;**181**(2):309-316. DOI: 10.2214/ajr.181.2.1810309

[3] Hirst AE, Johns VJ, Kime SW. Dissecting aneurysm of the aorta: A review of 505 cases. Medicine (Baltimore). 1958;**37**:217-279

[4] DeBakey ME, Henly WS, Cooley DA, Morris GC Jr, Crawford ES, Beall AC Jr. Surgical management of dissecting aneurysms of the aorta. The Journal of Thoracic and Cardiovascular Surgery. 1965;**49**:130-149

[5] Daily PO, Trueblood HW, Stinson EB, et al. Management of acute aortic dissections. The Annals of Thoracic Surgery. 1970;**10**:237-247. DOI: 10.1016/S0003-4975(10)65594-4

[6] Dake MD, Thompson M, van Sambeek M, et al. Dissect: A new mnemonic-based approach to the categorization of aortic dissection. European Journal of Vascular and Endovascular Surgery. 2013;**46**:175-190. DOI: 10.1016/j.ejvs.2013.04.029

[7] Sievers HH, Rylski B, Czerny M, Baier ALM, Kreibich M, Siepe M, et al. Aortic dissection reconsidered: Type, entry site, malperfusion classification adding clarity and enabling outcome prediction. Interactive Cardiovascular and Thoracic Surgery. 2020;**30**(3):451-457. DOI: 10.1093/icvts/ivz281

[8] Augoustides JG, Geirsson A, Szeto WY, Walsh EK, Cornelius B, Pochettino A, et al. Observational study of mortality risk stratification by ischemic presentation in patients with acute type a aortic dissection: The Penn classification. Nature Clinical Practice. Cardiovascular Medicine. 2009;**6**(2):140-146. DOI: 10.1038/ncpcardio1417. Epub 2008 Dec 9

[9] Siddique K, Alvernia J, Fraser K, Lanzino G. Treatment of aneurysms with wires and electricity: A historical overview. Journal of Neurosurgery. 2003;**99**(6):1102-1107. DOI: 10.3171/jns.2003.99.6.1102

[10] Brock RC. The life and work of sir Astley Cooper. Annals of the Royal College of Surgeons of England. 1969;**44**(1):1-18

[11] Tuffier T. *Intervention chirurgicale directe pour* un *anévrysme* de la *crosse* de l'*aorte*: Ligature du sac. Presse méd. 1902;**1**:267

[12] Lozano-Sanchez FS, García-Cenador MB. The first aortic endoaneurysmorrhaphy: Ricardo Lozano Monzón (1872-1934). Annals of Surgery Open. 2021;**2**(3):e086. DOI: 10.1097/AS9.0000000000000086

[13] Harrison PW, Chandy J. A subclavian aneurysm cured by cellophane fibrosis. Annals of Surgery. 1943;**118**(3):478-481. DOI: 10.1097/00000658-194309000-00017

[14] Gurin D, Bulmer JW, Derby R. Dissecting aneurysm of the aorta: Diagnosis and operative relief of acute

arterial obstruction due to this cause. New York State Journal of Medicine. 1935;**35**:1200-1202

[15] De Bakey ME, Cooley DA, Creech O Jr. Surgical considerations of dissecting aneurysm of the aorta. Annals of Surgery. 1955;**142**:586-610; discussion, 611-582.

[16] Shaw RS. Acute dissecting aortic aneurysm; treatment by fenestration of the internal wall of the aneurysm. The New England Journal of Medicine. 1955;**253**(8):331-333. DOI: 10.1056/NEJM195508252530807

[17] Schafer PW, Hardin CA. The use of temporary polythene shunts to permit occlusion, resection and frozen homologous graft replacement of vital vessel segments. Surgery. 1952;**31**:186-193

[18] Oransky I, Micheal EDB. Orbit. 2008;**732**(9638):530

[19] DeBakey ME, Cooley DA, Crawford ES, Morris GC Jr. Clinical application of a new flexible knitted Dacron arterial substitute. The American Surgeon. 1958;**24**:862-869

[20] DeBakey ME, McCollum CH, Crawford ES, Morris GC Jr, Howell J, Noon GP, et al. Dissection and dissecting aneurysms of the aorta: Twenty-year follow-up of five hundred twenty-seven patients treated surgically. Surgery. 1982;**92**(6):1118-1134

[21] Galletti PM, Brecher GA. Heart-Lung Bypass: Principles and Techniques of Extracorporeal Circulation. Philadelphia, PA: Grune & Stratton; 1962

[22] Galletti PM, Mora CT. Cardiopulmonary bypass: The historical foundation, the future promise. In: Mora CT, editor. Cardiopulmonary Bypass. Berlin, Germany: Springer-Verlag; 1995. pp. 3-21

[23] Bechtel L. Commentary: 1916-1940—Brief history of heparin. In: History and Heritage of Cardiovascular Surgery, Perfusion and the American Society of ExtraCorporeal Technology. 1885-2011. Richmond, VA: American Society of ExtraCorporeal Technology; 2012. p. 17

[24] Bull BS, Huse WM, Brauer FS, Korpman RA. Heparin therapy during extracorporeal circulation. II. The use of a dose-response curve to individualize heparin and protamine dosage. The Journal of Thoracic and Cardiovascular Surgery. 1975;**69**:685-689

[25] Romaine-Davis A. John Gibbon and his Heart-Lung Machine. Philadelphia, PA: University of Pennsylvania Press; 1991

[26] Kirklin JW. The middle 1950s and C. Walton Lillehei. The Journal of Thoracic and Cardiovascular Surgery. 1989;**98**(8):822-824

[27] DeWall RA. The evolution of the helical reservoir pumpoxygenator system at the University of Minnesota. The Annals of Thoracic Surgery. 2003;**76**:S2210-S2215

[28] Yun KL, Miller DC. Technique of aortic valve preservation in acute type a aortic dissection. Operative Techniques in Thoracic and Cardiovascular Surgery. 1996;**1**:68. DOI: 10.1016/S1085-5637(07)70082-7

[29] Lai DT, Miller DC, Mitchell RS, et al. Acute type a aortic dissection complicated by aortic regurgitation: Composite valve graft versus separate valve graft versus conservative valve repair. The Journal of Thoracic and Cardiovascular Surgery.

2003;**126**:1978-1986. DOI: 10.1016/S0022-5223(03)01279-0

[30] Svensson LG, Crawford ES, Hess KR, et al. Dissection of the aorta and dissecting aortic aneurysms. Improving early and long-term surgical results. Circulation. 1990;**82**:IV24-IV38

[31] Elefteriades JA. What operation for acute type A dissection? The Journal of Thoracic and Cardiovascular Surgery. 2002;**123**:201-203. DOI: 10.1067/mtc.2002.120330

[32] Strauch JT, Spielvogel D, Lansman SL, et al. Long-term integrity of teflon felt-supported suture lines in aortic surgery. The Annals of Thoracic Surgery. 2005;**79**:796-800. DOI: 10.1016/j.athoracsur.2004.08.028

[33] Movsowitz HD, Levine RA, Hilgenberg AD, et al. Transesophageal echocardiographic description of the mechanisms of aortic regurgitation in acute type A aortic dissection: Implications for aortic valve repair. Journal of the American College of Cardiology. 2000;**36**:884-890. DOI: 10.1016/S0735-1097(00)00766-X

[34] Johnston DR, Soltesz EG, Vakil N, et al. Long-term durability of bioprosthetic aortic valves: Implications from 12,569 implants. The Annals of Thoracic Surgery. 2015;**99**:1239-1247. DOI: 10.1016/j.athoracsur.2014.10.070

[35] Chiang YP, Chikwe J, Moskowitz AJ, et al. Survival and long-term outcomes following bioprosthetic vs mechanical aortic valve replacement in patients aged 50 to 69 years. JAMA. 2014;**312**:1323-1329. DOI: 10.1001/jama.2014.12679

[36] Svensson LG, Crawford ES, Hess KR, et al. Composite valve graft replacement of the proximal aorta: Comparison of techniques in 348 patients. The Annals of Thoracic Surgery. 1992;**54**:427-437; discussion 438-9. DOI: 10.1016/0003-4975(92)90432-4

[37] Leshnower BG, Myung RJ, McPherson L, et al. Midterm results of David v valve-sparing aortic root replacement in acute type a aortic dissection. The Annals of Thoracic Surgery. 2015;**99**:795-800; discussion 800-1. DOI: 10.1016/j.athoracsur.2014.08.079

[38] Pessotto R, Santini F, Pugliese P, Montalbano G, Luciani GB, Faggian G, et al. Preservation of the aortic valve in acute type a dissection complicated by aortic regurgitation. The Annals of Thoracic Surgery. 1999;**67**(6):2010-2013; discussion 2014-9. DOI: 10.1016/s0003-4975(99)00417-8

[39] Fabiani JN, Jebara VA, Deloche A, Stephan Y, Carpentier A. Use of surgical glue without replacement in the treatment of type A aortic dissection. Circulation. 1989;**80**(Suppl 1):264-268

[40] Bachet J, Gigou F, Laurian C, et al. Four-year clinical experience with the gelatin-resorcine-formol biological glue in acute aortic dissection. The Journal of Thoracic and Cardiovascular Surgery. 1982;**83**:212-217

[41] Hata M, Shiono M, Sezai A, et al. Type a acute aortic dissection: Immediate and mid-term results of emergency aortic replacement with the aid of gelatin resorcin formalin glue. The Annals of Thoracic Surgery. 2004;**78**:853-857; discussion 857. DOI: 10.1016/j.athoracsur.2004.03.061

[42] Hata H, Takano H, Matsumiya G, et al. Late complications of gelatin-resorcin-formalin glue in the repair of acute type A aortic dissection. The Annals of Thoracic Surgery. 2007;**83**:1621-1626. DOI: 10.1016/j.athoracsur.2007.01.025

[43] Ngaage DL, Edwards WD, Bell MR, et al. A cautionary note regarding long-term sequelae of biologic glue. The Journal of Thoracic and Cardiovascular Surgery. 2005;**129**:937-938. DOI: 10.1016/j.jtcvs.2004.07.046

[44] Halstead JC, Spielvogel D, Meier DM, et al. Composite aortic root replacement in acute type a dissection: Time to rethink the indications? European Journal of Cardio-Thoracic Surgery. 2005;**27**:626-632; discussion 632-3. DOI: 10.1016/j.ejcts.2004.12.059

[45] Appelbaum A, Karp RB, Kirklin JW. Ascending vs descending aortic dissections. Annals of Surgery. 1976;**183**:296-300. DOI: 10.1097/00000658-197603000-00015

[46] Kouchoukos NT, Karp RB, Blackstone EH, et al. Replacement of the ascending aorta and aortic valve with a composite graft. Results in 86 patients. Annals of Surgery. 1980;**192**:403-413. DOI: 10.1097/00000658-198009000-00016

[47] Kidd JN, Ruel GJ Jr, Cooley DA, et al. Surgical treatment of aneurysms of the ascending aorta. Circulation. 1976;**54**:III118-III122

[48] Rylski B, Bavaria JE, Milewski RK, Vallabhajosyula P, Moser W, Kremens E, et al. Long-term results of neomedia sinus valsalva repair in 489 patients with type a aortic dissection. The Annals of Thoracic Surgery. 2014;**98**(2):582-588; discussion 588-9. DOI: 10.1016/j.athoracsur.2014.04.050. Epub 2014 Jun 10

[49] Cohen RG, Hackmann AE, Fleischman F, Baker CJ, Cunningham MJ, Starnes VA, et al. Type a aortic dissection repair: How I teach it. The Annals Thoracic Surgery. 2017;**103**(1):P14-P17

[50] Xue Y, Zhou Q, Pan J, Cao H, Fan F, Zhu X, et al. Root reconstruction for proximal repair in acute type A aortic dissection. Journal of Thoracic Disease. 2019;**11**(11):4708-4716. DOI: 10.21037/jtd.2019.10.62

[51] David TE, David CM, Manlhiot C, et al. Outcomes of aortic valve-sparing operations in marfan syndrome. Journal of the American College of Cardiology. 2015;**66**:1445-1453. DOI: 10.1016/j.jacc.2015.07.041

[52] Yang B, Norton EL, Hobbs R, Farhat L, Wu X, Hornsby WE, et al. Short- and long-term outcomes of aortic root repair and replacement in patients undergoing acute type A aortic dissection repair: Twenty-year experience. The Journal of Thoracic and Cardiovascular Surgery. 2019;**157**(6):2125-2136. DOI: 10.1016/j.jtcvs.2018.09.129. Epub 2018 Dec 21

[53] Brown JA, Zhu J, Navid F, Serna-Gallegos D, Sehra R, Warraich N, et al. Preservation versus replacement of the aortic root for acute type A aortic dissection. The Journal of Thoracic and Cardiovascular Surgery. 2024;**167**(6):2037-2046.e2. DOI: 10.1016/j.jtcvs.2022.04.053. Epub 2022 Jul 14

[54] Debakey ME, Henly WS, Cooley DA, et al. Aneurysms of the aortic arch: Factors influencing operative risk. The Surgical Clinics of North America. 1962;**42**:1543-1554

[55] Cooley DA, Livesay JJ. Technique of "open" distal anastomosis for ascending and transverse arch resection. Cardiovascular Diseases. 1981;**8**:421-426

[56] Geirsson A, Shioda K, Olsson C, Ahlsson A, Gunn J, Hansson EC, et al. Differential outcomes of open and clamp-on distal anastomosis techniques in acute type A aortic dissection. The Journal of Thoracic and Cardiovascular

Surgery. 2019;**157**(5):1750-1758. DOI: 10.1016/j.jtcvs.2018.09.020. Epub 2018 Sep 29

[57] Kazui T, Washiyama N, Muhammad BAH, Terada H, Yamashita K. M Takinmi improved results of atherosclerotic aneurysm surgery using a refined technique. The Journal of Thoracic and Cardiovascular Surgery. 2000;**121**:491-499

[58] Sabik Joseph F et al. Axillary artery: An alternative site of arterial cannulation for patients with extensive aortic and peripheral vascular disease. The Journal of Thoracic and Cardiovascular Surgery. 1995;**109**(5):885-891

[59] Baribeau YR, Westbrook BM, Charlesworth DC. Axillary cannulation: First choice for extra-aortic cannulation and brain protection. The Journal of Thoracic and Cardiovascular Surgery. 1999;**118**(6):1153-1154. DOI: 10.1016/S0022-5223(99)70124-8

[60] Ueda Y, Miki S, Kusuhara K, Okita Y, Tahata T, Yamanaka K. Surgical treatment of aneurysm or dissection involving the ascending aorta and aortic arch, utilizing circulatory arrest and retrograde cerebral perfusion. The Journal of Cardiovascular Surgery. 1990;**31**(5):553-558

[61] Griepp RB, Griepp EB. Perfusion and cannulation strategies for neurological protection in aortic arch surgery. Annals of Cardiothoracic Surgery. 2013;**2**(2):159-162. DOI: 10.3978/j.issn.2225-319X.2013.03.12

[62] Ueda Y. A reappraisal of retrograde cerebral perfusion. Annals of Cardiothoracic Surgery. 2013;**2**(3):316-325. DOI: 10.3978/j.issn.2225-319X.2013.01.02

[63] Svensson LG, Blackstone EH, Apperson-Hansen C, Ruggieri PM, Ainkaran P, Naugle RI, et al. Implications from neurologic assessment of brain protection for total arch replacement from a randomized trial. The Journal of Thoracic and Cardiovascular Surgery. 2015;**150**(5):1140-7.e11. DOI: 10.1016/j.jtcvs.2015.07.054. Epub 2015 Jul 26

[64] Abjigitova D, Veen KM, van Tussenbroek G, Mokhles MM, Bekkers JA, Takkenberg JJM, et al. Cerebral protection in aortic arch surgery: Systematic review and meta-analysis. Interactive Cardiovascular and Thoracic Surgery. 2022;**35**(3):ivac128. DOI: 10.1093/icvts/ivac128

[65] Matalanis G, Perera NK, Galvin SD. Aortic arch replacement without circulatory arrest or deep hypothermia: The "branch-first" technique. The Journal of Thoracic and Cardiovascular Surgery. 2015;**149**(2 Suppl):S76-S82. DOI: 10.1016/j.jtcvs.2014.07.100. Epub 2014 Aug 10

[66] Khaladj N, Shrestha M, Peterss S, Strueber M, Karck M, Pichlmaier M, et al. Ascending aortic cannulation in acute aortic dissection type A: The Hannover experience. European Journal of Cardio-Thoracic Surgery. 2008;**34**(4):792-796. DOI: 10.1016/j.ejcts.2008.05.014; disussion 796. Epub 2008 Jun 25

[67] Benedetto U, Raja SG, Amrani M, et al. The impact of arterial cannulation strategy on operative outcomes in aortic surgery: Evidence from a comprehensive meta-analysis of comparative studies on 4476 patients. The Journal of Thoracic and Cardiovascular Surgery. 2014;**148**:2936-43.e1-4

[68] Malvindi Pietro G et al. Reoperation after acute type a aortic dissection repair: A series of 104 patients. The Annals of Thoracic Surgery. 2012;**95**(3):922-927

[69] Kato M, Ohnishi K, Kaneko M, Ueda T, Kishi D, Mizushima T, et al. New graft-implanting method for thoracic aortic aneurysm or dissection with a stented graft. Circulation. 1996;**94**(9 Suppl):II188-II193

[70] Roselli EE, Subramanian S, Sun Z, Idrees J, Nowicki E, Blackstone EH, et al. Endovascular versus open elephant trunk completion for extensive aortic disease. The Journal of Thoracic and Cardiovascular Surgery. 2013;**146**(6):1408-1416. DOI: 10.1016/j.jtcvs.2013.07.070; discussion 1416-7. Epub 2013 Sep 24. Erratum in: J Thorac Cardiovasc Surg. 2016 Jul;152(1):291. doi: 10.1016/j.jtcvs.2016.04.005. Idrees, Jahanzaib J [corrected to Idrees, Jay J]

[71] Chiu P, Miller DC. Evolution of surgical therapy for stanford acute type A aortic dissection. Annals of Cardiothoracic Surgery. 2016;**5**(4):275-295. DOI: 10.21037/acs.2016.05.05

[72] Matalanis G, Ch'ng SL. Thoracoabdominal aortic aneurysm - The branch first technique. Seminars in Thoracic and Cardiovascular Surgery. 2019;**31**(4):708-712. DOI: 10.1053/j.semtcvs.2019.03.013. Epub 2019 Apr 11

[73] Nienaber CA, Fattori R, Lund G, Dieckmann C, Wolf W, von Kodolitsch Y, et al. Nonsurgical reconstruction of thoracic aortic dissection by stent-graft placement. The New England Journal of Medicine. 1999;**340**(20):1539-1545

[74] Dake MD, Kato N, Mitchell RS, Semba CP, Razavi MK, Shimono T, et al. Endovascular stent-graft placement for the treatment of acute aortic dissection. The New England Journal of Medicine. 1999;**340**(20):1546-1552

[75] Dorros G, Dorros AM, Planton S, et al. Transseptal guidewire stabilization facilitates stent-graft deployment for persistent proximal ascending aortic dissection. Journal of Endovascular Therapy. 2000;**7**:506-512. DOI: 10.1177/15266028

[76] Horton JD, Kolbel T, Haulon S, et al. Endovascular repair of type a aortic dissection: Current experience and technical considerations. Seminars in Thoracic and Cardiovascular Surgery. 2016;**28**:312-317. DOI: 10.1053/j.semtcvs.2015.12.004

[77] Ye C, Chang G, Li S, et al. Endovascular stent-graft treatment for stanford type A aortic dissection. European Journal of Vascular and Endovascular Surgery. 2011;**42**:787-794. DOI: 10.1016/j.ejvs.2011.08.015 0000700612

[78] Kato M, Kuratani T, Kaneko M, Ohtake H, Minatoya K, Sawa Y. The results of stent-grafting of the aortic arch aneurysms and dissections. Journal of Vascular Surgery. 2002;**36**(6):1136-1141

[79] Kreibich M, Rylski B, Kondov S. The transapical implantation of an endovascular valve-carrying conduit into the ascending aorta of a pig. Asvide. 2018;**5**:285

[80] Ghoreishi M, Chahal D, Shah A, et al. First-in-human endovascular aortic root repair (Endo-Bentall) for acute type A dissection. Circulation: Cardiovascular Interventions. 2023;**16**(10):e013348

Chapter 4

Genetic Aortic Disease: Unraveling the Genetic Landscape of Marfan and Related Syndromes

Takayuki Okada, Chika Sato, Sayoko Haruyama, Saki Shimada, Phạm Thị Xuyên, Hiroyasu Tsukaguchi and Tadaaki Koyama

Abstract

Marfan syndrome is a common monogenic disorder of connective tissue, which primarily affects the cardiovascular, skeletal, and ocular systems, with an incidence of 1 in 10,000. Recent advances in studies on genetic aortic disorders, Marfan, and related disorders have clarified the genetic factors underlying these conditions. Such knowledge will help to develop diagnostic strategies, preventive approaches, and precision medicine. Clinical and genetic studies with Marfan syndrome and related disorders have deciphered the complexities of genetic determinants and their clinical relevance by interpreting the diverse findings including variants of uncertain significance (VUS). Cutting-edge diagnostic techniques and next-generation sequencing facilitate the identification of pathogenic and/or predisposing factors, which significantly increase the potential for early intervention and personalized treatment. By summarizing current research, this review provides valuable insights into the pathophysiology and management of genetic aortic disorder, paving the way for future research and clinical advancements in cardiovascular medicine.

Keywords: genetic landscape, Marfan syndrome, diagnostic strategies, preventive strategies, precision medicine, variants of uncertain significance

1. Introduction

The recent innovation of genetic technology has allowed us to clarify the role of genetic factors in the pathogenesis of aortic dissection and life-threatening cardiovascular conditions. Marfan syndrome is related to genetic disorders primarily affecting the connective tissues. The prototypic, most common form is Marfan syndrome, 70% of which is caused by the dominant mutations in the Fibririn 1 (*FBN1*) gene, encoding the elastic fibers particularly enriched in the aortic walls and ciliary bodies. The cardinal clinical features of Marfan syndrome are cystic dilation in the aortic outlet, lens dislocation, and skeletal deformities of the spine and extremities (Ghent Criteria) (**Figure 1** and **Table 1**). Recent studies have unveiled a broader genetic landscape underlying aortic

IntechOpen

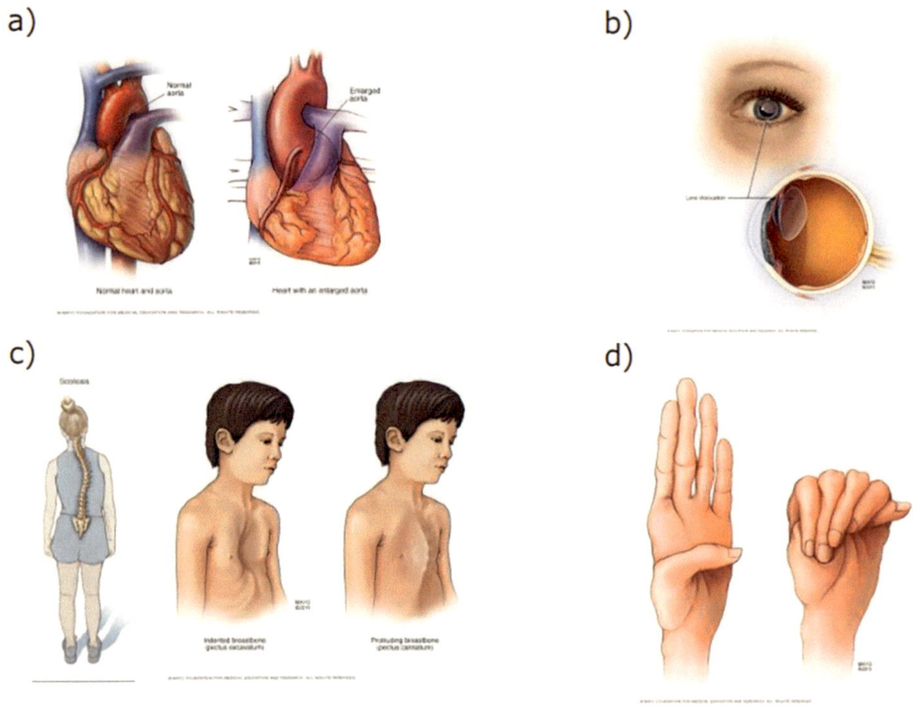

Figure 1.
Clinical features of Marfan syndrome. (a) Aortic root aneurysm, (b) ectopia lentis, (c) Scoliosis, chest wall deformities, (d) thumb sign, wrist sign. Images are referred to: MAYO CLINIC. https://www.mayoclinic.org/diseases-conditions/marfan-syndrome/symptoms-causes/syc-20350782, with permission.

disorders and their diverse clinical phenotypes beyond those traditionally described for Marfan syndrome. This review aims to better understand the multifaceted nature of aortic dissection, exploring the complex interplay between genetic predisposition, diagnostic modalities, preventive strategies, and precision medicine. Based on the up-to-date evidence, this chapter will provide a comprehensive overview of the current understanding of aortic dissection and its implications for clinical practice.

2. Unraveling the genetic landscape

2.1 Genetic factors of Marfan and related syndromes

About 70% of the Marfan syndrome was caused by the mutations in Fibririn-1(*FBN1*) gene. Recent studies have elucidated the role of diverse genetic factors in predisposing individuals to aortic dissection, other than the classic causative genes of Marfan syndrome, Fibrilin-1 (*FBN1*)(**Table 2**). These factors encompass mutations in genes involved in vascular smooth muscle function, extracellular matrix remodeling, and inflammatory pathways (**Figure 2**).

- *ACTA2* Mutations: Alpha-actin-2 (ACTA2) mutations have emerged as culprits for familial thoracic aortic aneurysms and dissections (FTAAD: MIM 607086). These mutations disrupt the contractile function of vascular smooth muscle cells, leading to arterial wall fragility and predisposition to dissection [5].

In the absence of family history
1. Ao $(Z \geqq 2)$ + EL → MFS
2. Ao $(Z \geqq 2)$ + Bonafide *FBN1* mutation → MFS
3. Ao $(Z \geqq 2)$ + Systemic features $(7 \geqq pts)$ → MFS*
4. EL + *FBN1* with known Ao → MFS
• EL with or without Systemic features AND with an *FBN1* not known with Ao or no *FBN1* → ELS
• Ao (Z<2) AND Systemic features (5 ≧ pts with at least one skeletal feature) without EL → MASS
• MVP AND Ao (Z<2) AND Systemic features (<5 pts) without EL → MVPS
In the presence of family history
5. EL+ FH of MFS (as defined above(1)-(4)) → MFS*
6. Systemic features $(7 \geqq pts)$ + FH → MFS*
7. Ao (Z ≧ 2 above 20 years old, ≧ 3 below 20 years) FH of MFS (as defined above(1)-(4)) → MFS*

*Ao: Aortic diameter at the sinuses of Valsalva above indicated Z-score or aortic root dissection, EL: Ectopia lentis, MFS: Marfan syndrome, ELS: Ehlers-Danlos syndrome, MASS: myopia, mitral valve prolapse, borderline (Z < 2) aortic root dilatation, striae, skeletal Endings phenotype, MVPS: mitral valve prolapse syndrome, FH: Family history. *Where aortic root dilatation (Z ≥2) or dissection is present but ectopia lentis is absent and the FBN1 genetic results status is either unknown or negative, an MFS diagnosis is confirmed by the presence of sufficient systemic findings (≥7 points, according to the proposed scoring system) [1]. However, MS-related conditions features such as Shprintzen-Goldberg syndrome(SGS), Loeys-Dietz syndrome (LDS) or vascular EDS must be excluded by performing appropriate alternative genetic testing (TGFBR1/2, COL3A1, and other relevant genetic testing) as well as biochemical collagen study.*
The Ghent criteria are worldwide used in helping physicians to diagnose MFS appropriately. New NGS techniques allow the detection of FBN1 variants in up to 97% of Marfan patients who fulfil the Ghent criteria. The current Ghent criteria have excellent specificity to predict individuals with FBN1 variants. Ref. [1].

Table 1.
Revised Ghent criteria for diagnosis of Marfan syndrome and related conditions.

Systemic features	**Score**
Wrist AND thumb sign (wrist or thumb sign)	3(1)
Pectus carinatum deformity (pectus excavatum or chest asymmetry)	2(1)
Hindfoot deformity (plain pes planus)	2(1)
Pneumothorax	2
Dural ectasia	2
Protrusio acetabuli	2
Reduced upper segment/lower segment ratio + increased arm/height + no severe scoliosis	1
Scoliosis or thoracolumbar kyphosis	1
Reduced elbow extension	1
Facial features (3/5) : dolichocephaly, enophthalmos, downslanting palpebral fissures, malar hypoplasia, retrognathia	1
Skin striae	1
Myopia > 3 diopters	1
Mitral valve prolapse (all types)	1
Maximum total: 20 points; score ≧ 7 indicates systemic involvement	

A systemic score calculator and a complete description of each component evaluation can be found at the Marfan Foundation website.

Table 2.
Scoring for systemic features of Marfan syndrome.

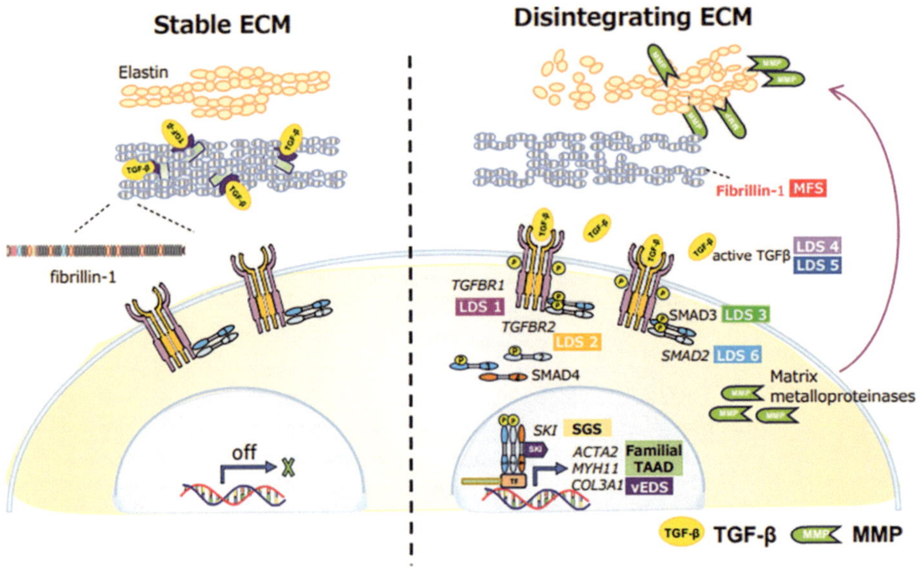

Figure 2.
The TGFβ signaling pathway in genetic connective tissue disorders. Altered TGFβ signaling plays a major role in the pathology of Marfan syndrome (MFS) and related diseases. Connective tissue diseases are associated with specific TGFβ signaling effectors (black boxes). The effects of TGFβ signaling pathways in elastic fiber remodeling are compared under normal and the disease status of genetic connective tissue disorders, including Marfan syndrome (MFS) and Loeys-Dietz syndromes (LDS). Under normal conditions, the large latent complex LTBP, which is covalently cross-linked to fibrillin, sequesters the small latent TGF-β complexes into the fibrils. Tissue injuries induce the release of active TGF-β from latent complex and/or conformational change activating the TGF-β receptor binding site. Binding of active TGF-β with the TGF-β receptor type II leads to the phosphorylation and recruitment of TGF-β receptor type I into a heteromeric receptor complexes. The serine/threonine kinase activity of the activated complex phosphotylates Smad2 and Smad3 that both bind to Smad4 and translocate into the nucleus to enhance gene transcription of Pro-inflammatory factor, for example, MMP MFS: Marfan syndrome, LDS: Loeys Dietz syndrome, TADD: thoracic aortic aneurysm/dissection, vEDS: Ehlers-Danlos syndrome, vascular type, SGS: Shprintzen-Goldberg syndrome. Refs. [2–4].

- *MYH11* Mutations: Mutations in the *MYH11* gene, encoding the smooth muscle myosin heavy chain, are associated with familial thoracic aortic aneurysms and dissections (FTAAD: MIM 607086). These mutations impair smooth muscle contractility, compromising the structural integrity of the aortic wall [6].

- *TGFBR1/TGFBR2* Mutations: Defects in the transforming growth factor-beta (TGF-β) receptor genes, *TGFBR1* and *TGFBR2*, have been identified in individuals with Loeys-Dietz syndrome (609,192, 610,168) characterized by thoracic aortic aneurysms and dissections., as well as skeletal defects. Dysregulated TGF-β signaling contributes to abnormal extracellular matrix remodeling and vascular smooth muscle cell proliferation [7].

In our Clinical Genetics Center of the KMU hospital, the genetic testing panel for these 15 genes causative of genetic aortic disorders is provided in collaboration with the Kazusa DNA laboratory (KMU homepage; https://hp.kmu.ac.jp/treatment/departments/clinical_genetics/marfan/). The results will be returned to the patients and referral doctors within 2 months and will be explained to the patient and family in aid of genetic counseling.

2.2 Importance of genetic risk assessment

Genetic risk assessment allows the identification of individuals at risk for aortic dissection and guiding clinical management. Comprehensive genetic evaluation includes thorough family history assessment, genetic testing, and interpretation of genetic variants.

- Family history assessment: A taking of detailed family history helps clarify the transmission patterns suggestive of hereditary connective tissue disorders or familial clustering of aortic diseases. Individuals with affected relatives may benefit from targeted genetic testing and surveillance [8].

- Genetic testing modalities: Advances in genetic testing technologies, including next-generation sequencing (NGS) and whole-exome sequencing (WES), enable the comprehensive analysis of genes associated with aortic dissection. These modalities facilitate the identification of pathogenic variants and variants of uncertain significance (VUS) [9], according to the American College of Medical Genetics and Genomics (ACMG) criteria (**Table 3**).

Gene	Phenotype	Hereditary	OMIM #
FBN1	Marfan syndrome	AD	134797
TGFBR1	Loeys-Dietz syndrome 1 (LDS1)	AD	190181
TGFBR2	Loeys-Dietz syndrome 2 (LDS2)	AD	190182
SMAD3	Loeys-Dietz syndrome 3 (LDS3)	AD	603109
TGFB2	Loeys-Dietz syndrome 4 (LDS4)	AD	190220
TGFB3	Loeys-Dietz syndrome 5 (LDS5)	AD	190230
SMAD2	Loeys-Dietz syndrome 6 (LDS6)	AD	601366
FBN2	Congenital Contracturai Arachnodactyly (Beals syndrome)	AD	612570
COL3A1	Ehlers-Danlos syndrome, vascular type (vEDS)	AD	120180
COL1A1	Ehlers-Danlos syndrome, arthrochalasia type (aEDS)	AD	120150
ACTA2	Familial thoracic aortic aneurysm/dissection (Familial TAAD)	AD	102620
MYH11	Familial thoracic aortic aneurysm/dissection (Familial TAAD)	AD	160745
MYLK	Familial thoracic aortic aneurysm/dissection (Familial TAAD)	AD	600922
PRKG1	Familial thoracic aortic aneurysm/dissection (Familial TAAD)	AD	176894
PMEPA1	Familial thoracic aortic aneurysm/dissection (Familial TAAD)	AD	606564
EFEMP2	EFEMP2-Related Cutis Laxa	AR	604633
FLNA	X-Linked Otopalatodigital Spectrum Disorders	XL	300017
SLC2A10	Arterial Tortuosity Syndrome	AR	606145

A list of 18 genes of Marfan and related syndrome, for which are sequenced in the Marfan sequence panel (Kazusa DNA Research Institute), are shown.
FBN1: Fibrilin-1, TGFBR1: Transforming Growth Factors beta receptor 1, TGFBR2: Transforming Growth Factors beta receptor 2, SMAD3: SMAD family member 3, TGFB2: Transforming Growth Factors beta 2, TGFB2: Transforming Growth Factors beta 3, SMAD2: SMAD family member 2, FBN2: Fibrilin-2, COL3A1: collagen type III alpha 1 chain, COL1A1 : collagen type I alpha 1 chain, ACTA2: Actin alpha 2 smooth muscle, MYH11: Myosin heavy chain 11, smooth muscle, MYLK: Myosin light chain kinase, PRKG1:. protein kinase cGMP-dependent 1, PMEPA1: prostate transmembrane protein, androgen induced 1, EFEMP2-. EGF containing fibulin extracellular matrix protein 2, FLNA: filamin A, SLC2A10: solute carrier family 2 member 10.

Table 3.
Genes involved in genetic aortic diseases.

- Interpretation of genetic variants: The interpretation of genetic variants, particularly VUS, poses challenges in clinical decision-making. Multidisciplinary collaboration involving geneticists, cardiologists, and genetic counselors is essential to contextualize genetic findings and allow an accurate risk assessment [10].

2.3 Variants of uncertain significance (VUS)

Variants of uncertain significance (VUS) represent genetic alterations whose pathogenicity is not definitively proven (**Figure 3** and **Table 4**). The pathogenic relevance of VUS must be carefully evaluated, considering various parameters, including population allele frequency, evolutionary conservation, functional studies, and phenotype-genotype cosegregation.

- Challenges in interpretation: VUS may pose a significant challenge for clinicians when making therapeutic decisions due to the uncertainty surrounding their clinical significance. These variants often show ambiguous or conflicting evidence regarding their pathogenicity, necessitating the collection of more phenotype-genotype data and additional functional assay [13].

- Clinical implications: The identification of VUS prompts the patients to undergo regular surveillance and genetic counseling. Patients harboring VUS may require regular clinical follow-up and examination to monitor disease progression and complications and reassess the significance of the variants regularly by searching the updated database [14].

- Research efforts: Ongoing research efforts aim to elucidate the clinical significance of VUS through functional studies (transfection of variants in mammalian cells, generating the animal model by use of genome editing technology, CRISPR-Cas9), large-scale sequencing initiatives, and data-sharing platforms. Collaborative endeavors are essential to generate robust evidence and refine the pathogenicity of VUS [15].

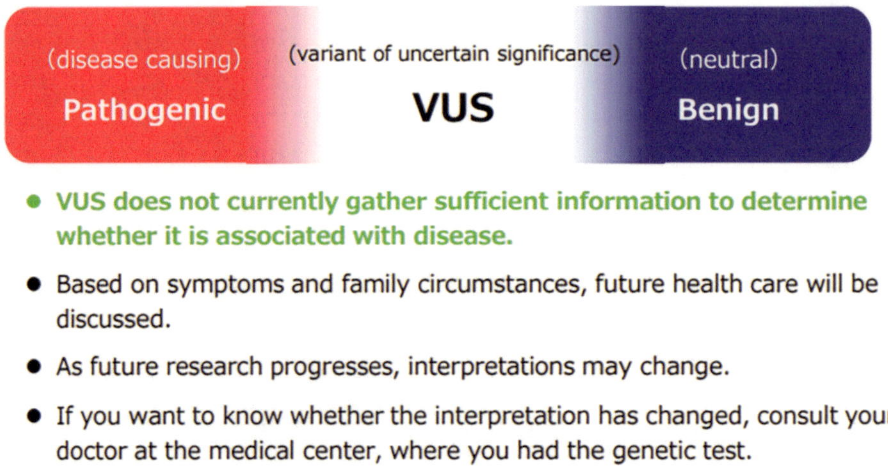

Figure 3.
Interpretation of variant of uncertain significance (VUS). Variants of uncertain significance (VUSs) exist along a spectrum between the benign and suspected pathogenicity. Judgement of UVS may alter to the either category, depending upon the accumulating data about genotype-phenotype, and functional expression. Ref. [11].

Sequence variant interpretation	Resources for interpretation
Pathogenic	• Population data
Likely pathogenic	• Computational and predictive data
Variant of uncertain significance (VUS)	• Functional data
Likely benign	• Segregation data
Benign	• De novo data
	• Allelic data
	• other database (Reputable source)
	• other data (Found in case with an alternate cause. Patient's phenotype or family history highly specific for gene.)

The genetic variants are classified into five classes of interpretation based upon the resources from interpretations. Interpretations need an integrative, multidisciplinary collaboration with experts in clinical phenotypes, family and population genetics, in silico and experimental studies. Systematic assessment for the relevance of VUS is discussed on a regular basis in expert panel of international consortium in Clin-Gen (FBN1 Variant Curation Expert Panel FBN1 Variant Curation Expert Panel—ClinGen—Clinical Genome Resource Ref. [12]).

Table 4.
Interpretation of sequence variants.

3. Novel gene identification and analytical techniques

3.1 State-of-the-art mutation identification

Advanced genetic sequencing technologies, WES or Whole-genome sequencing (WGS), have revolutionized the identification of genetic variants causing aortic dissection. These techniques offer unparalleled sensitivity and specificity in detecting rare and novel pathogenic variants.

- Next-generation sequencing (NGS): NGS platforms enable the rapid and cost-effective sequencing of large genomic regions, facilitating the identification of rare variants implicated in aortic dissection. Whole-genome sequencing (WGS) and whole-exome sequencing (WES) are particularly valuable for uncovering novel disease-causing genes [16]. The limitations of the technology we have so far are only able to sequence a short fragment (150-200 base-pair). Recently, a single molecule, long-read sequence will read 5 to 10 Mega bases all at once become available (NovaSeqXPlus, Pac-Bio, GridION, PromethION, Nanopore) (**Figure 4**).

- Functional genomics approaches: Functional omics approaches, including transcriptomics, epigenomics, and proteomics, provide insights into the molecular mechanisms underlying aortic dissection. These techniques could elucidate gene expression patterns, regulatory networks, and protein interactions, which are implicated in the pathogenesis of aortic disorders [18].

3.2 Clinical applications of genetic analysis

The integration of genetic analysis into clinical practice has translational implications from bed-sed to bedside to improve the diagnosis, prognosis, and management of aortic dissection. Genetic testing informs risk stratification, guides therapeutic decision-making, and facilitates personalized medicine approaches.

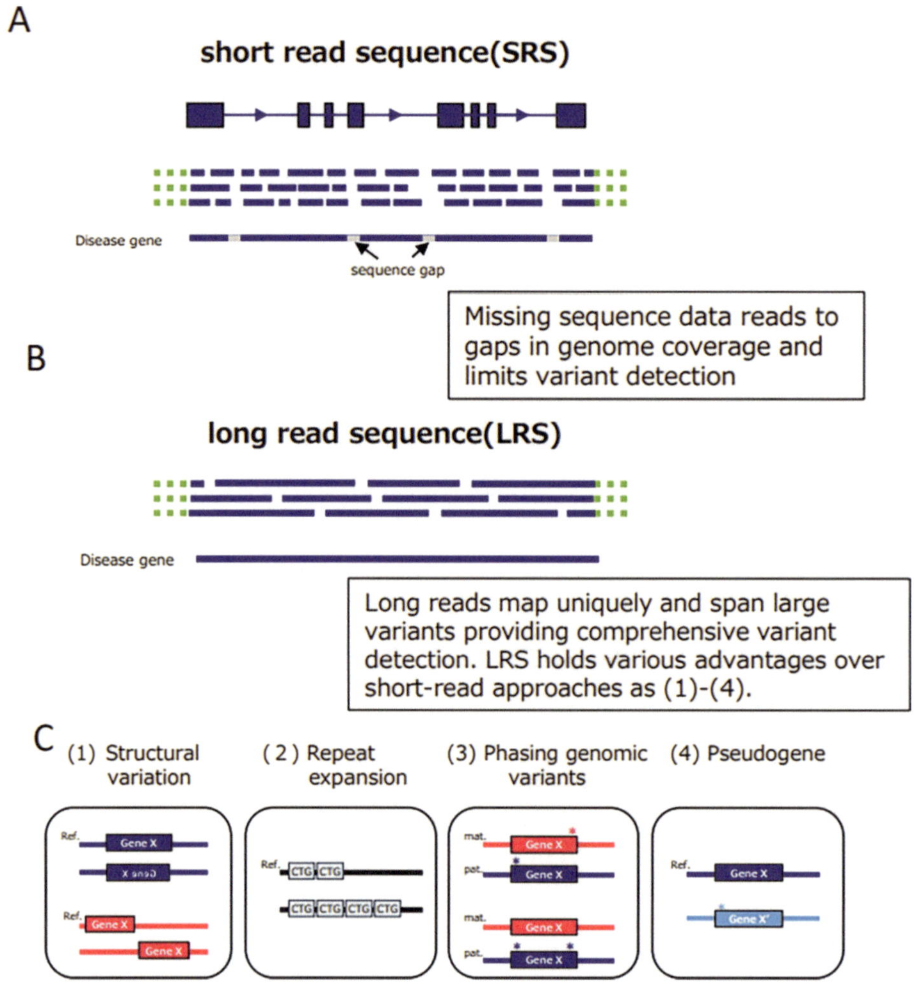

Figure 4.
Comparison of NGS technology of short read sequence vs. long read sequence. A, short read, B, Ling read, C, advantage of the long reads. The predominant difference between LRS and the conventional SR-NGS approaches is a significant increase in read length. In contrast to short reads (150-300 bp), LRS allows much longer sequence on average over 10kb in one single read, thereby requiring less read depth to cover the target gene. Ref. [17].

- Risk stratification: Genetic testing enables the identification of individuals at increased risk for aortic dissection based on their genetic profile. High-risk individuals may benefit from enhanced surveillance, early intervention, and targeted preventive measures [19].

- Therapeutic decision-making: Identification of specific genetic variants will help therapeutic decision-making, particularly in the selection of pharmacological agents and surgical interventions. For example, aortic disease patients who have the pathogenic *FBN1* variants are recommended to replace the dissected aortic lesions by the vascular graft rather than by stent implantation to avoid recurrent rupture of the genetically fragile aortic wall. Moreover, asymptomatic carriers of *FBN1* variants would be better to take regular check-ups (CT or US) to prevent or earlier intervene in aortic diseases. Precision medicine approaches will allow tailored treatments based on personal molecular defects and will thus improve patient outcomes [20].

- Family screening and counseling: Genetic analysis will allow a risk assessment for their family members beyond the proband, leading to better family health care by offering cascade screening and genetic counseling. Family members who are found to carry pathogenic variants can benefit from early detection, proactive management, and informed reproductive planning [21].

4. Diagnosis and early intervention

4.1 Role of imaging techniques

Advanced imaging modalities play a crucial role in the early diagnosis and risk stratification of aortic dissection. Computed tomography angiography (CTA), magnetic resonance imaging (MRI), and transesophageal echocardiography (TEE) offer high sensitivity and specificity in detecting aortic lesions.

- Computed tomography angiography (CTA): CTA is a cornerstone of imaging for aortic dissection, providing detailed visualization of the aortic locations, expansion, and nature of pathology. Multidetector-row CT scanners offer rapid acquisition times and high spatial resolution, enabling accurate diagnosis and characterization of dissection morphology [22].

- Magnetic resonance imaging (MRI): MRI is valuable for assessing the locations, extent, and complications of aortic dissection, particularly in patients with contraindications to iodinated contrast agents or radiation exposure. MRI provides multiplanar imaging, tissue characterization, and functional assessment, aiding in treatment planning and follow-up [23].

- Transesophageal echocardiography (TEE): TEE offers real-time imaging of the aorta with high spatial resolution and sensitivity, making it indispensable for intraoperative and perioperative monitoring of aortic dissection. TEE-guided interventions facilitate the accurate placement of endovascular stent grafts and assessment of aortic valve function [24].

4.2 Clinical evaluation

Clinical evaluation is of fundamental importance for the initial assessment of patients with suspected aortic disorders, guiding diagnostic workup, risk stratification, and therapeutic decision-making. Key clinical features suggestive of aortic dissection include severe chest or back pain, pulse deficits, neurologic deficits, and a widened mediastinum on chest radiography.

- Diagnostic algorithms: Clinical practice guidelines, such as the 2022 ACC/AHA Guideline for the Diagnosis and Management of Aortic Disease, provide evidence-based algorithms for the diagnosis and management of aortic dissection, emphasizing the importance of integrating the clinical findings, imaging studies, and biomarkers. These algorithms facilitate timely decision-making and optimize patient outcomes [25, 26].

- Risk stratification models: Risk stratification models, such as the Stanford and DeBakey classifications, categorize aortic dissections based on spatial expansion and anatomical involvement of branch vessels. These models help treatment decisions and prognostication, guiding the selection of surgical or conservative management strategies [27].

- Multidisciplinary approach: A multidisciplinary approach involving cardiologists, cardiothoracic surgeons, vascular surgeons, and radiologists is essential for the comprehensive evaluation and management of aortic dissection. Collaborative care ensures timely diagnosis, risk assessment, and coordinated treatment planning [28].

5. Advancements in treatment

5.1 Surgical techniques

Surgical intervention remains the cornerstone of treatment for acute and chronic aortic dissection, aiming to prevent complications, relieve symptoms, and restore aortic wall integrity. Evolving surgical techniques and devices continue to improve outcomes and expand treatment options.

- Open surgical repair: Traditional open surgical repair involves excision of the dissected aortic segment and replacement with a prosthetic graft, often combined with aortic valve repair or replacement. Despite the recent advances in endovascular therapy, open repair remains a gold standard for complex dissections and connective tissue disorders [29].

- Endovascular stent grafting: Endovascular stent grafting offers a less invasive alternative to open surgery for select patients with aortic dissection, particularly those with distal or limited disease. Thoracic endovascular aortic repair (TEVAR) provides rapid hemostasis, reduced perioperative morbidity, and shorter hospital stays compared to open repair [30].

- Hybrid approaches: Hybrid approaches combine open surgical techniques with endovascular stent grafting to address complex aortic pathology. These procedures allow customized treatment strategies, improving the postoperative outcomes in patients with challenging anatomy or comorbidities [31].

5.2 Evidence-based algorithms

Clinical practice guidelines provide evidence-based algorithms for the diagnosis and management of aortic dissection, summarizing the up-to-date research evidence and expert consensus recommendations. These guidelines could offer structured approaches to risk assessment, diagnostic evaluation, and treatment selection, promoting standardized care and improved patient outcomes.

- American College of Cardiology/American Heart Association Guidelines: The ACC/AHA guidelines 2022 provide comprehensive recommendations for the diagnosis and management of thoracic aortic diseases, incorporating input from multiple specialty societies and expert panels. These guidelines emphasize risk stratification, imaging protocols, and treatment algorithms tailored to personalized patient's demands [32].

- European Society of Cardiology (ESC) Guidelines: The european society of cardiology guidelines offer evidence-based recommendations for the diagnosis and management of aortic diseases including aortic dissection, thoracic aortic aneurysms, and aortic valve disease. These guidelines advocate for a multidisciplinary approach to patient care, highlighting the importance of risk factor modification, genetic counseling, and long-term surveillance. By promoting adherence to standardized protocols and best practices, these guidelines aim to optimize patient outcomes and reduce the burden of aortic disease-related morbidity and mortality [33].

6. Perspective and emerging trends

6.1 Harnessing genomic data

The integration of genomic data into clinical practice holds immense promise to deepen our understanding of aortic dissection and improving patient care. Large-scale genomic studies, such as genome-wide association studies (GWAS) and collaborative consortia, are elucidating the genetic architecture of aortic disease and identifying novel disease-causing genes and pathways.

- Precision medicine approaches: Precision medicine approaches leverage genomic data to tailor treatments to the underlying molecular defects, optimizing therapeutic efficacy and minimizing adverse effects. Targeted therapies, gene editing technologies, and regenerative medicine strategies offer innovative avenues for personalized medicine in aortic dissection [34].

- Predictive modeling: Computational modeling and machine learning algorithms analyze genomic, clinical, and imaging data to predict disease onset, progression, and response to therapy. These predictive models would enable risk stratification, treatment selection, and prognostication, guiding precision medicine interventions and improving patient outcomes [35].

6.2 Advancements in preventive medicine

Preventive medicine strategies play a crucial role in mitigating the risk of aortic dissection and improving the public health outcomes. Lifestyle modifications, pharmacological interventions, and genetic screening programs offer opportunities for primary and secondary prevention of aortic diseases.

- Risk factor modification: Targeted interventions aimed at modifiable risk factors, such as hypertension, smoking, and dyslipidemia, can attenuate the progression of aortic disease and reduce the incidence of a life-threatening aortic dissection. Comprehensive risk factor management, including lifestyle modifications and pharmacotherapy, is essential for primary prevention [36].

- Genetic screening programs: Population-based genetic screening programs identify individuals at increased risk for hereditary connective tissue disorders and familial aortic diseases, facilitating early detection and intervention. Cascade screening of at-risk family members enables proactive management and preventive strategies, reducing the burden of aortic dissection on affected families [24].

6.3 Patient-centered care

Patient-oriented care emphasizes shared decision-making, personalized treatment plans, and holistic support for patients and their families. Encouraging patients with knowledge, resources, and psychosocial support enhances treatment adherence, improves health outcomes, and fosters resilience in the face of chronic illness.

- Patient education and empowerment: Comprehensive patient education programs provide individuals with the information, skills, and resources needed to actively participate in their care. Health literacy, self-management strategies, and shared decision-making tools will guide patients correctly to make informed choices and advocate for their health needs [37].

- Psychosocial support services: Psychosocial support services, including counseling, peer-support groups, and community resources, address the emotional, social, and practical needs of patients with aortic diseases and their families. These services promote resilience, coping skills, and quality of life, fostering holistic well-being across the disease continuum [38].

7. Precision medicine approaches

7.1 Personalized therapeutic strategies

Precision medicine approaches aim to tailor therapeutic strategies to the respective patient's genetic profile, clinical characteristics, and disease phenotype. Personalized interventions optimize treatment efficacy and minimize adverse effects.

- *Genotype-guided therapy*: Genotype-guided therapy involves selecting pharmacological agents and surgical interventions based on the patient's genetic mutations and molecular pathways implicated in aortic dissection. This approach enhances therapeutic precision and efficacy.

- *Biomarker-guided management*: Biomarker-guided management utilizes specific biomarkers to monitor disease progression, assess therapeutic response, and guide treatment adjustments. Biomarkers of vascular inflammation, extracellular matrix turnover, and hemodynamic stress offer insights into the disease state and therapeutic efficacy.

7.2 Future directions and innovations

The field of precision medicine in aortic disorders continues to evolve, driven by ongoing research and technological innovations. Future directions will include the integration of multi-omics data, the development of novel therapeutic targets, and the implementation of advanced diagnostic tools.

- *Multi-omics integration:* Integrating multi-omics data, including genomics, transcriptomics, proteomics, and metabolomics, offers a comprehensive understanding of the molecular underpinnings of aortic dissection. Multi-omics approaches facilitate the identification of novel biomarkers, therapeutic targets, and disease pathways.

- *Gene editing and therapy:* Genome editing technologies, such as CRISPR-Cas9, hold promise for correcting pathogenic mutations and restoring normal cellular function. Gene therapy approaches aim to deliver therapeutic genes or modulate gene expression to mitigate the effects of deleterious mutations.

- *Artificial intelligence and machine learning:* Artificial intelligence (AI) and machine learning (ML) algorithms have the potential to revolutionize the diagnosis, risk stratification, and management of aortic dissection. These technologies enable the analysis of complex data sets, identification of predictive patterns, and development of personalized treatment algorithms.

8. Conclusion

The unrevealing of the genetic landscape in common aortic diseases expands our view of Marfan syndrome, encompassing a diverse array of genetic mutations and molecular pathways. Advances in diagnostic strategies, including genetic testing and preventive strategies, have improved our approach to managing this condition. Precision medicine will open a promising avenue for improving patient outcomes, although challenges still remain, particularly in cases involving variants of uncertain significance (VUS). Addressing these challenges is crucial for optimizing patient care and extending life expectancy. Ongoing research and multidisciplinary collaboration are essential for further elucidation of the complexities of aortic dissection and translating scientific discoveries into clinical practice.

Acknowledgements

The authors would like to acknowledge the support of Tomoka Sato, Saeko Haruyama, Saki Shimada, Center for Clinical Genetics, and Kansai Medical University Hospital for their contributions to this work. We are grateful for the support from the Japan Society for the Promotion of Science (JSPS) Grant-in-Aid for Scientific Research (Grant No. 19 K09254 and 24 K12002).

Conflict of interest

The authors declare no conflict of interest.

Author details

Takayuki Okada[1*], Chika Sato[2], Sayoko Haruyama[3], Saki Shimada[2], Phạm Thị Xuyên[4], Hiroyasu Tsukaguchi[2] and Tadaaki Koyama[1]

1 Department of Cardiovascular Surgery, Kansai Medical University, Hirakata, Japan

2 Clinical Genetics Center, Kansai Medical University, Hirakata, Japan

3 Department of Medical Ethics and Medical Genetics, Kyoto University of School of Public Health, Kyoto, Japan

4 Health Management Department, University of Health Sciences, Vietnam National University, Ho Chi Minh, Vietnam

*Address all correspondence to: okada0525@gmail.com

References

[1] Loeys BL, Dietz HC, Braverman AC, Callewaert BL, De Backer J, Devereux RB, et al. The revised Ghent nosology for the Marfan syndrome. Journal of Medical Genetics. July 2010;**47**(7):476-485. DOI: 10.1136/jmg.2009.072785

[2] Chen PY, Qin L, Simons M. TGFβ signaling pathways in human health and disease. Frontiers in Molecular Biosciences. 1 Jun 2023;**10**:1113061. DOI: 10.3389/fmolb.2023.1113061

[3] Verstraeten A, Alaerts M, Van Laer L, Loeys B. Marfan Syndrome and Related Disorders: 25 Years of Gene Discovery. Hum Mutation. Jun 2016;**37**(6):524-531. DOI: 10.1002/humu.22977

[4] Ramachandra CJ, Mehta A, Guo KW, Wong P, Tan JL, Shim W. Molecular pathogenesis of Marfan syndrome. International Journal of Cardiology. 2015;**187**:585-591. DOI: 10.1016/j.ijcard.2015.03.423

[5] Milewicz DM, Regalado E. Heritable thoracic aortic disease overview. In: Adam MP, Ardinger HH, Pagon RA, et al., editors. GeneReviews®. [Internet]. Seattle (WA): University of Washington, Seattle; 1993. Available from: https://www.ncbi.nlm.nih.gov/books/NBK1120/

[6] Guo DC, Regalado E, Casteel DE, Santos-Cortez RL, Gong L, Kim JJ, et al. Recurrent gain-of-function mutation in PRKG1 causes thoracic aortic aneurysms and acute aortic dissections. American Journal of Human Genetics. 2013;**92**(1):194-203. DOI: 10.1016/j.ajhg.2012.12.015. Epub 2013 Feb 7

[7] Dietz HC, Cutting CR, Pyeritz RE, Maslen CL, Sakai LY, Corson GM, et al. Marfan syndrome caused by a recurrent de novo missense mutation in the fibrillin gene. Nature. 1991;**352**(6332):337-339. DOI: 10.1038/352337a0

[8] Loeys BL, Chen J, Neptune ER, Judge DP, Podowski M, Holm T, et al. A syndrome of altered cardiovascular, craniofacial, neurocognitive and skeletal development caused by mutations in TGFBR1 or TGFBR2. Nature Genetics. 2005;**37**(3):275-281. DOI: 10.1038/ng1511. Epub 2005 Feb 20

[9] De Backer J, Loeys B, Leroy B, Coucke P, Dietz H, De Paepe A. Utility of molecular analyses in the exploration of extreme intrafamilial variability in the Marfan syndrome. Clinical Genetics. 2007;**72**(1):188-198. DOI: 10.1111/j.1399-0004.2007.00859.x

[10] Renard M, Callewaert B, Baetens M, Campens L, MacDermot K, Fryns JP, et al. Novel MYH11 and ACTA2 mutations reveal a role for enhanced TGFβ signaling in FTAAD. International Journal of Cardiology. 2013;**168**(2):1323-1331. DOI: 10.1016/j.ijcard.2012.12.082. Epub 2013 Jan 21

[11] Kim SW, Kim B, Kim Y, Lee KA. Re-evaluation of a Fibrillin-1 Gene Variant of Uncertain Significance Using the ClinGen Guidelines. Annals of Laboratory Medicine. 1 May 2024;**44**(3):271-278. DOI: 10.3343/alm.2023.0152. Epub 2023 Oct 16. PMID: 37840311; PMCID: PMC10813823

[12] Standards and guidelines for the interpretation of sequence variants: A joint consensus recommendation of the American College of Medical Genetics and Genomics and the Association for Molecular Pathology. Genetics in Medicine. 2015;**17**(5):405-424. DOI: 10.1038/gim.2015.30

[13] Mátyás G, Alonso S, Patrignani A, Marti M, Arnold E, Magyar I, et al. Large genomic fibrillin-1 (FBN1) gene deletions provide evidence for true haploinsufficiency in Marfan syndrome. Human Genetics. 2007;**121**(3-4):223-232. DOI: 10.1007/s00439-006-0307-5 Epub 2007 Jan 17

[14] Wooderchak-Donahue WL, VanSant-Webb C, Tvrdik T, Plant P, Lewis T, Stocks J, et al. Clinical utility of a next generation sequencing panel assay for Marfan and Marfan-like syndromes featuring aortopathy. American Journal of Medical Genetics. Part A. 2015;**167A**(8):1747-1757. DOI: 10.1002/ajmg.a.37068. Epub 2015 Apr 9

[15] Lindsay ME, Schepers D, Bolar NA, Doyle JJ, Gallo E, Fert-Bober J, et al. Loss-of-function mutations in TGFB2 cause a syndromic presentation of thoracic aortic aneurysm. Nature Genetics. 2012;**44**(8):922-927. DOI: 10.1038/ng.2349

[16] Regalado ES, Guo DC, Estrera AL, Buja LM, Milewicz DM. Acute aortic dissections with pregnancy in women with ACTA2 mutations. American Journal of Medical Genetics. Part A. 2014;**164A**(4):1065-1070. DOI: 10.1002/ajmg.a.36371. Epub 2014 Feb 20

[17] Mantere T, Kersten S, Hoischen A. Long-Read Sequencing Emerging in Medical Genetics. Frontiers in Genetics. 7 May 2019;**10**:426. DOI: 10.3389/fgene.2019.00426

[18] Pannu H, Fadulu VT, Chang J, Lafont A, Hasham SN, Sparks E, et al. Mutations in transforming growth factor-beta receptor type II cause familial thoracic aortic aneurysms and dissections. Circulation. 2005;**112**(4):513-520. DOI: 10.1161/circulationaha.105.537340. Epub 2005 Jun 27

[19] Wuyts W, Dietz HC, Van Laer L, Loeys B, De Backer J. Marfan syndrome: From gene to therapy. Current Opinion in Pediatrics. 2005;**17**(6):659-667. DOI: 10.1097/01.mop.0000184353.27128.f5

[20] Renard M, Callewaert B, Malfait F, Campens L, Sharif S, del Campo M, et al. Thoracic aortic-aneurysm and dissection in association with significant mitral valve disease caused by mutations in TGFB2. International Journal of Cardiology. 2013;**168**(2):1455-1456. DOI: 10.1016/j.ijcard.2013.03.019. Epub 2013 Mar 25

[21] Regalado ES, Guo DC, Villamizar C, Avidan N, Gilchrist D, McGillivray B, et al. Exome sequencing identifies SMAD3 mutations as a cause of familial thoracic aortic aneurysm and dissection with intracranial and other arterial aneurysms. Circulation Research. 2011;**109**(6):680-686. DOI: 10.1161/circresaha.111.248161. Epub 2011 Apr 7

[22] Coady MA, Rizzo JA, Goldstein LJ, Elefteriades JA. Natural history, pathogenesis, and etiology of thoracic aortic aneurysms and dissections. Cardiology Clinics. 1999;**17**(4):615-635. DOI: 10.1016/s0733-8651(05)70145-4

[23] Nienaber CA, Clough RE, Sakalihasan N, Suzuki T, Gibbs R, Mussa F, et al. Aortic dissection. Nature Reviews Disease Primers. 2016;**2**:16053. DOI: 10.1038/nrdp.2016.53

[24] Hagan PG, Nienaber CA, Isselbacher EM, Bruckman D, Karavite DJ, Russman PL, et al. The international registry of acute aortic dissection (IRAD): New insights into an old disease. Journal of the American Medical Association. 2000;**283**(7):897-903. DOI: 10.1001/jama.283.7.897

[25] Eagle KA, Isselbacher EM, DeSanctis RW. Diagnosis and

management of aortic dissection. The New England Journal of Medicine. 1993;**328**(8):553-559. DOI: 10.1056/NEJM199302253280807

[26] Isselbacher EM, Preventza O, Hamilton Black J 3rd, Augoustides JG, Beck AW, Bolen MA, et al. Peer Review Committee Members. 2022 ACC/AHA guideline for the diagnosis and management of aortic disease: A report of the American Heart Association/American College of Cardiology joint committee on clinical practice guidelines. Circulation. 2022;**146**(24):e334-e482. DOI: 10.1161/CIR.0000000000001106. Epub 2022 November 2. PMID: 36322642; PMCID: PMC9876736

[27] Olsson C, Thelin S, Ståhle E, Ekbom A, Granath F. Thoracic aortic aneurysm and dissection: Increasing prevalence and improved outcomes reported in a nationwide population-based study of more than 14,000 cases from 1987 to 2002. Circulation 2006;**114**(24):2611-8. DOI: 10.1161/circulationaha.106.630400. Epub 2006 Oct 2

[28] Pape LA, Awais M, Woznicki EM, Suzuki T, Trimarchi S, Evangelista A, et al. Presentation, diagnosis, and outcomes of acute aortic dissection: 17-year trends from the international registry of acute aortic dissection. Journal of the American College of Cardiology. 2015;**66**(4):350-358. DOI: 10.1016/j.jacc.2015.05.029

[29] Tsai TT, Trimarchi S, Nienaber CA. Acute aortic dissection: Perspectives from the international registry of acute aortic dissection (IRAD). European Journal of Vascular and Endovascular Surgery. 2009;**37**(2):149-159. DOI: 10.1016/j.ejvs.2008.11.021. Epub 2008 Dec 31

[30] Sueyoshi E, Sakamoto I, Hayashi K, Yamaguchi T, Imada T. Growth rate of aortic diameter in patients with type B aortic dissection during the chronic phase. Circulation. 14 Sep 2004;**110**(11 Suppl. 1):II256-II261. DOI: 10.1161/01.CIR.0000138386.48852.b6. PMID: 15364872

[31] Di Eusanio M, Trimarchi S, Patel HJ, Hutchison S, Suzuki T, Peterson MD, et al. Clinical presentation, management, and short-term outcome of patients with type A acute dissection complicated by mesenteric malperfusion: Observations from the international registry of acute aortic dissection. The Journal of Thoracic and Cardiovascular Surgery. 2013;**146**(2):323-328. DOI: 10.1016/j.jtcvs.2013.04.011. Epub 2013 May 28

[32] Dake MD, Kato N, Mitchell RS, Semba CP, Razavi MK, Shimono T, et al. Endovascular stent-graft placement for the treatment of acute aortic dissection. The New England Journal of Medicine. 1999;**341**(20):1546-1552. DOI: 10.1056/NEJM199911183412102

[33] Chen Y, Gao W, Yang M, Meng Z. Clinical characteristics and outcomes of Stanford type A acute aortic dissection complicated by cerebral infarction: A retrospective study. Journal of Cardiothoracic Surgery. 2020;**15**(1):64. DOI: 10.1186/s13019-020-01099-9

[34] Milewicz DM, Guo DC, Tran-Fadulu V, Lafont AL, Papke CL, Inamoto S, et al. Genetic basis of thoracic aortic aneurysms and dissections: Focus on smooth muscle cell contractile dysfunction. Annual Review of Genomics and Human Genetics. 2008;**9**:283-302. DOI: 10.1146/annurev.genom.8.080706.092303

[35] Zhang L, Zhou Y, Wu W, Hou L, Chen X, Ma Y, et al. The clinical and genetic features in a cohort of Chinese patients with aortic dissection. Heart, Lung & Circulation. 2016;**25**(7):683-690.

DOI: 10.1016/j.hlc.2015.12.012. Epub 2016 Jan 12

[36] Mészáros I, Mórocz J, Szlávi J, Schmidt J, Tornóci L, Nagy L, et al. Epidemiology and clinicopathology of aortic dissection. Chest. 2000;**117**(5):1271-1278. DOI: 10.1378/chest.117.5.1271

[37] Tang L, Zheng J, Sun L, Song Y, Liu L, Qiao T, et al. Potential of novel biomarkers in diagnosis, risk stratification, and prognosis of acute aortic dissection. Disease Markers. 2020;**2020**:2097971. DOI: 10.1155/2020/2097971

[38] Zhu J, Li G, Xiong H, Xu Z. Changes in biomechanical properties of the ascending aorta and main pulmonary artery in acute aortic dissection: A clinical study. Experimental and Therapeutic Medicine. 2019;**17**(3):2173-2177. DOI: 10.3892/etm.2019.7204. Epub 2019 Jan 16

Chapter 5

Role of Transesophageal Echocardiography in Surgical Treatment of Aortic Dissection

Kazumasa Orihashi

Abstract

Acute type A aortic dissection is a life-threatening condition frequently complicated by rupture and/or malperfusion, which can occur at any time. While computed tomography (CT) is the gold standard for preoperative diagnostic imaging to develop the optimal surgical strategy, transesophageal echocardiography (TEE) is invaluable in the operating room. TEE compensates for the limitations of CT by providing real-time information, enabling timely and accurate management of unexpected events such as rupture, perfusion-related dissection, or new malperfusion in the coronary, cerebral, and visceral arteries. These critical events, often occurring out of sight of the surgical field, can go unrecognized by surgeons, anesthesiologists, or perfusionists. TEE acts as a navigational radar in an airport control tower, guiding experienced pilots through complex situations. However, the effectiveness of TEE depends on the operator's ability to use it at the optimal timing and target the correct anatomical structures. This chapter aims to elucidate the methodology, timing, and specific assessments required for TEE to optimize intraoperative management of aortic dissection, ensuring the best possible outcomes for patients.

Keywords: acute aortic dissection, transesophageal echocardiography, perfusion, extracorporeal circulation, complications

1. Introduction

Acute type A aortic dissection (ATAAD) is often complicated by rupture and/or malperfusion, significantly worsening the prognosis of patients. According to the "Annual Report" published annually by the Japanese Association for Thoracic Surgery, the operative mortality of ATAAD was as high as 18.4% in 2000. However, by 2020, this figure had decreased to 5.7% [1]. This improvement is attributed to advancements in computed tomography (CT)—the gold standard for diagnostic imaging—refinements in surgical strategies, and the development of endovascular interventions [2]. The advent of 320-row CT has revolutionized diagnostic imaging by enabling the acquisition of whole-body images within seconds. It allows for the visualization of any plane, the creation of three-dimensional images, and the extraction of particular structures such as the aorta. These capabilities facilitate surgical planning based on objective, technologist-independent information, thereby improving surgical outcomes. However, there are situations where CT may not provide sufficient

IntechOpen

information for strategy formulation, particularly in cases of unstable hemodynamics due to shock or cardiac arrest, or when only limited images from preceding institutions are available. Furthermore, the definitive limitation of CT is that it becomes impractical once surgical treatment has commenced.

Transesophageal echocardiography (TEE) can compensate for this limitation. TEE provides not only morphological and kinetic information but also real-time hemodynamic data without radiation exposure or the need for contrast agents. The surgical strategies can be refined based on TEE-derived information [3]. However, the quality of TEE assessment can vary significantly among examiners. To address this variation, this chapter summarizes the standardized role of TEE in the management of ATAAD.

2. Flow of TEE assessment in the perioperative period

Figure 1 illustrates the flow of TEE assessment in the perioperative period. Initially, the surgeon formulates surgical and extracorporeal circulation (ECC) strategies based on CT-derived information. Incorporating additional data obtained from TEE—such as entry position, presence of bleeding, aortic regurgitation (AR), and malperfusion—the surgeon then finalizes the surgical plan. TEE-derived information is invaluable not only for strategy formulation but also for intraoperative assessment in the event of unexpected complications such as rupture or new malperfusion. Although such incidents are rare, data acquisition becomes extremely challenging once they occur. Therefore, it is advisable to complete a comprehensive TEE assessment beforehand. Given the unpredictability of such events, the author typically completes this assessment as quickly as possible, usually within 10 minutes.

Various events can occur in the perioperative period. One common event is sudden hypotension before ECC is established, often caused by vasodilation due to anesthesia

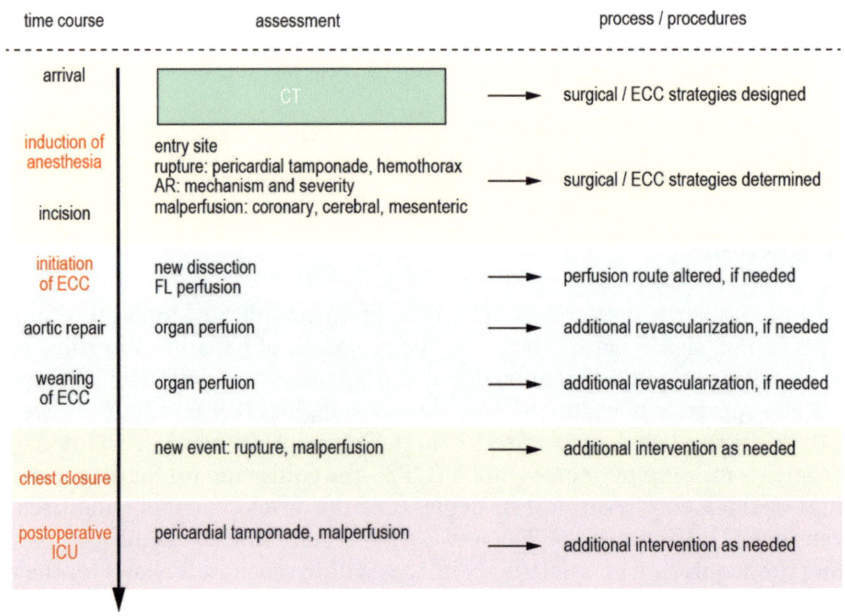

Figure 1.
Time Course of Assessments and Consequential Processes or Procedures. CT: computed tomography, ECC: extracorporeal circulation, ICU: intensive care unit.

induction, but it can also result from myocardial ischemia, rupture, or dissection extension to the subclavian artery, all of which should be evaluated by TEE. Another critical event is the development of a new dissection or false lumen perfusion at the initiation of ECC. New complications can also arise after weaning from ECC, as illustrated by two cases later in this chapter. In the postoperative intensive care unit, pericardial tamponade or new malperfusion events may occur. In each scenario, a definitive "0 or 1" judgment is required. Even with extensive experience, decisions based on probability are not reliable; thus, TEE is employed to make definitive "0 or 1" decisions.

3. Intraoperative hypotension and ECC management

In cases of unexpected hypotension or an unusual decrease in the ECC system's reservoir level, probable bleeding should be investigated. Before sternotomy, the free spaces, including the pericardial and pleural cavities, should be examined (**Figure 2a**). These areas can be assessed within seconds by rotating the TEE probe 90–120 degrees to the left and right.

Figure 2b depicts TEE images of a case where the patient's blood pressure suddenly dropped to 30 mmHg before the skin incision. The TEE image revealed marked pericardial tamponade, prompting an urgent sternotomy. Although the heart was fibrillating on

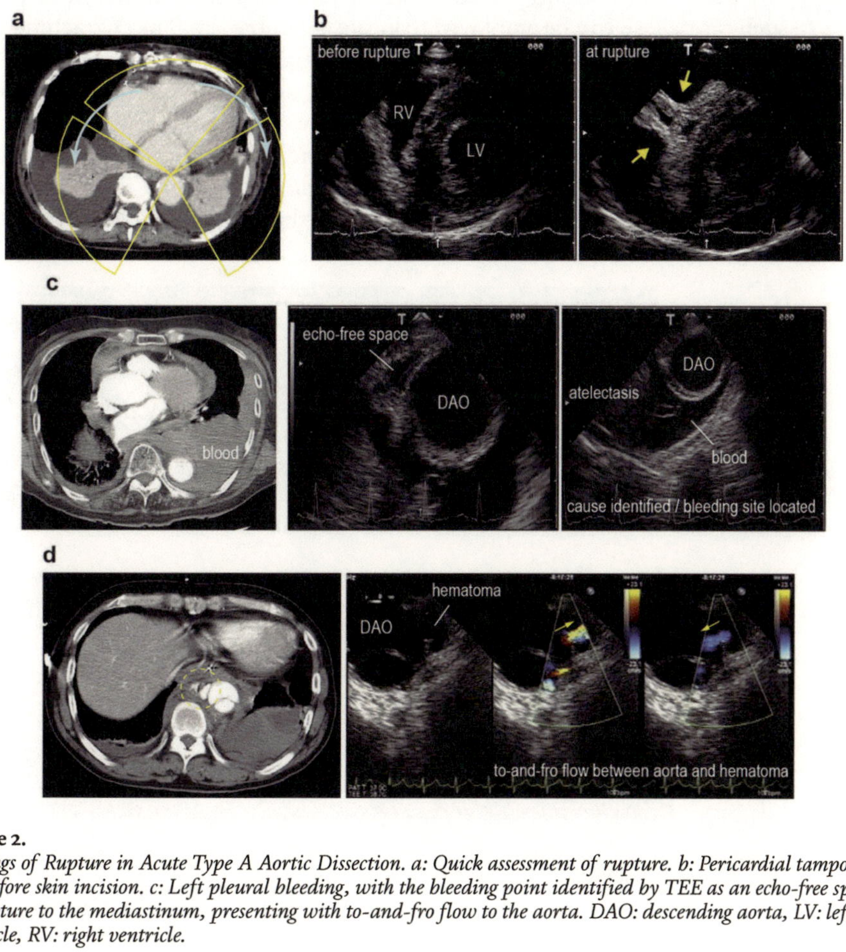

Figure 2.
Findings of Rupture in Acute Type A Aortic Dissection. a: Quick assessment of rupture. b: Pericardial tamponade just before skin incision. c: Left pleural bleeding, with the bleeding point identified by TEE as an echo-free space. d: Rupture to the mediastinum, presenting with to-and-fro flow to the aorta. DAO: descending aorta, LV: left ventricle, RV: right ventricle.

pericardiotomy, ECC was initiated while the heart was massaged. The surgical treatment proceeded as planned, and the patient was discharged without complications.

Figure 2c presents the CT and TEE findings of an 86-year-old female patient transferred in shock, associated with a left hemothorax [4]. CT was performed after draining 500 mL of blood, but neither the cause nor the bleeding site was identified. Due to recurrent shock, the patient underwent emergency open surgery. TEE revealed a type B aortic dissection and an echo-free space in the mediastinum adjacent to the aorta, indicating the bleeding site. Only 10 cm of the corresponding aorta was replaced. Although stent grafting might be an option, the bleeding site might not be located via aortography, necessitating broad stent graft placement, potentially leading to paraplegia. TEE aids in minimizing the length of coverage. In another case, a 58-year-old male patient (**Figure 2d**) presented with shock following mediastinal bleeding. TEE showed a to-and-fro flow between the mediastinum and the aorta, with the entry site 3 cm distal to it. Due to the rupture site's proximity to the diaphragm and unknown Adamkiewicz artery level, only the minimal aorta segment including the rupture site was replaced to prevent paraplegia. Both patients had uneventful postoperative courses.

4. Identifying the entry site in aortic dissection with TEE

It is not uncommon for the entry site of an aortic dissection to be unidentified on CT images. In such cases, TEE can be employed to locate the entry site. The characteristic TEE finding for an entry site is an "interrupted intimal flap with blood flow through it." However, visualizing the distal portion of the ascending aorta or the infrarenal portion of the abdominal aorta can be challenging. When the entry site is not visible, it is advisable to assess the direction of blood flow in the false lumen of the aortic arch. The location of the entry site can be inferred based on the direction of this flow. If the blood flow in the false lumen is antegrade, the entry site is likely in the ascending aorta (**Figure 3a**).

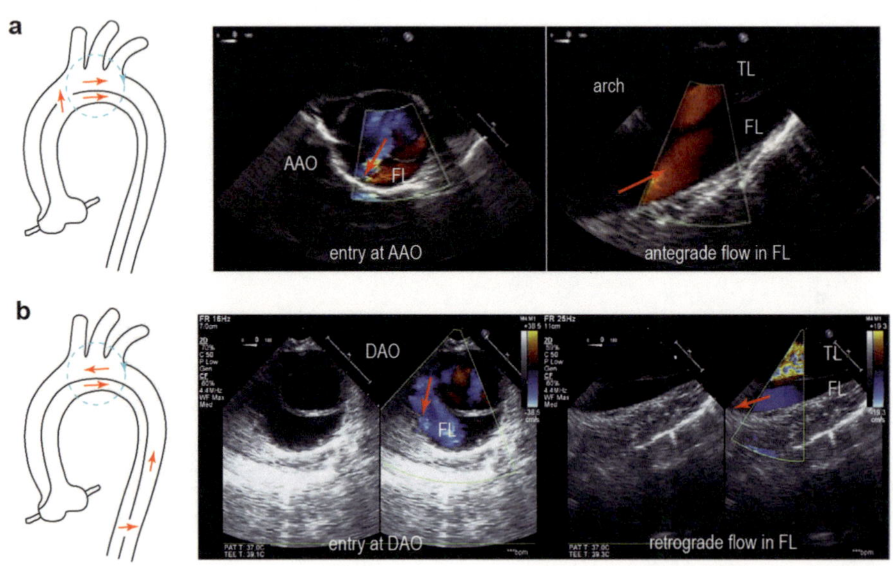

Figure 3.
Locating Entry Site by TEE Findings. a: An entry in the ascending aorta (AAO) generating antegrade flow in the false lumen (FL) of the aortic arch. b: An entry in the descending aorta (DAO) causing retrograde flow in the FL of the aortic arch. TL: true lumen.

Conversely, if the flow is retrograde, the entry site is likely in the distal portion of the aorta (**Figure 3b**). This approach can help pinpoint the entry site more accurately and assist in the formulation of appropriate surgical strategies.

5. Aortic regurgitation

Acute aortic regurgitation caused by ATAAD significantly burdens the heart, often leading to pulmonary edema even in young patients before they can be taken to the operating room. There are three primary mechanisms of AR in this context (**Figure 4a**) [5].

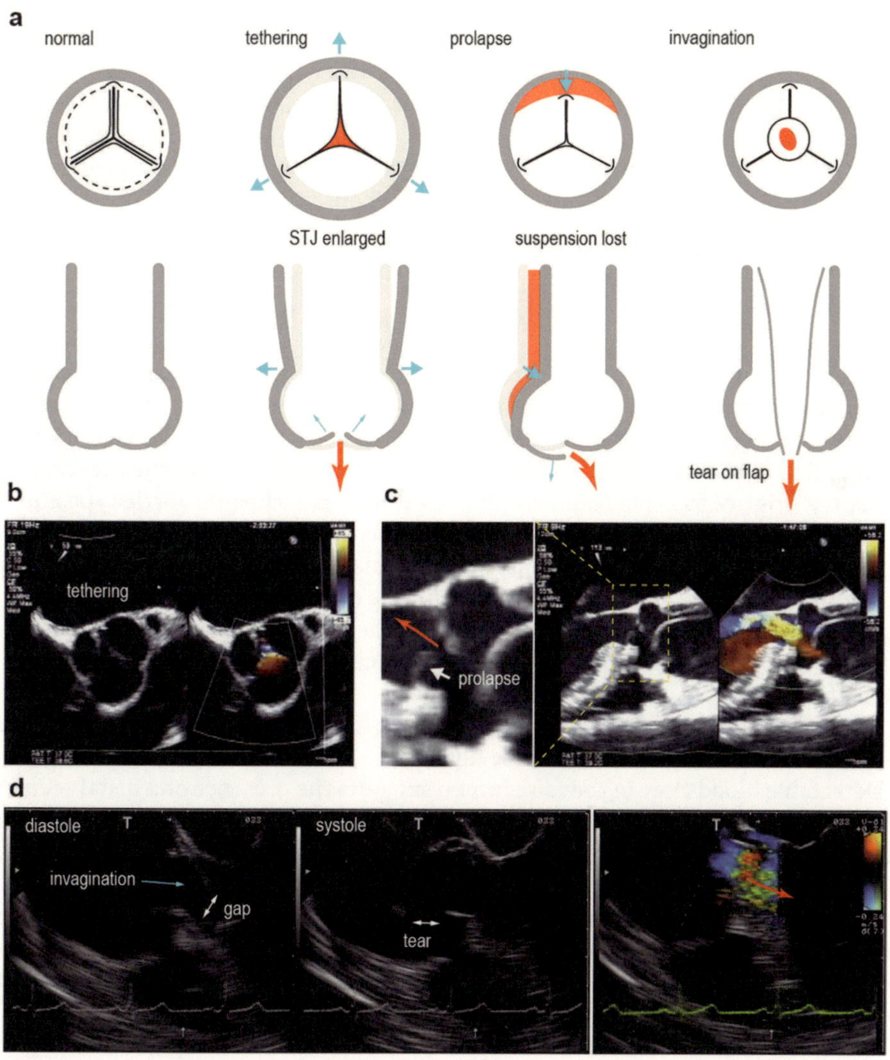

Figure 4.
Mechanisms of Aortic Regurgitation. a: Three types of mechanisms. b: Enlargement of the ascending aorta and sinotubular junction (STJ) causing tethering of commissures, forming a triangular regurgitant orifice. c: Dissection of the Valsalva sinus wall loosening the suspension of commissures, leading to cusp prolapse. d: Highly mobile flap with tear invaginating into the aortic valve causing incompetent valve closure.

1. Tethering of commissures: This occurs due to the enlargement of the ascending aorta and the sinotubular junction, preventing the cusps from coapting at the center. This results in a triangular regurgitant orifice and a central regurgitant jet (**Figure 4b**).

2. Prolapse of cusps: Prolapse occurs when the suspension of the commissures is lost due to the dissection of the aortic wall, leading to an eccentric regurgitant jet (**Figure 4c**).

3. Intimo-intimal intussusception: Rarely, a highly mobile intimal flap in the ascending aorta results in intimo-intimal intussusception or invagination into the aortic valve [6–10]. If there is a tear on the invaginated flap, regurgitation ensues (**Figure 4d**). This type of AR can also be associated with myocardial ischemia [6].

Even moderate-to-severe AR may be addressed with repair rather than valve replacement. Repair strategies include resolving tethering by normalizing the size of the sinotubular junction during stump reconstruction or correcting the prolapse of the cusps by suspending the commissure to the reconstructed aortic wall.

6. Malperfusion

In ATAAD, any branch artery can be compromised by malperfusion. However, TEE primarily assesses the coronary arteries, arch branch arteries, and visceral arteries. The mechanism of malperfusion involves the "compressed true lumen by an expanded false lumen," influenced by the entry blood flow and the presence of reentry (**Figure 5a**). There are two types of branch occlusion: aortic type and branch type (**Figure 5b**). In the aortic type, the intimal flap is pressed against the opposite wall, obstructing the branch orifice. This mechanism also affects the flap in the proximal aorta, reducing blood flow in the true lumen. In the branch type, the dissection extends into the branch artery, where the expanded false lumen compresses the true lumen. While the mechanisms are similar, the site of obstruction differs.

TEE findings indicative of malperfusion include (1) a true lumen smaller than the false lumen and (2) no flow in the false lumen.

Detectable blood flow in the false lumen suggests the presence of a distal reentry, indicating that the target organ is perfused from either lumen and is not malperfused. In the superior mesenteric artery (SMA), significant malperfusion occurs when the true lumen is smaller than half of the entire lumen, likely because branch arteries from the SMA become obstructed, similar to the aorta. New malperfusion can arise at the initiation of ECC due to altered pressure gradients between the lumina. TEE's role is to detect these changes. While CT visualizes the entire pathway from the aorta to the target organ, TEE has a limited visualization area. Therefore, intraoperative assessment of perfusion status integrates TEE with other modalities to evaluate perfu sion at four zones: (1) Aortic zone; (2) Branch zone; (3) Peripheral zone; and (4) Tissue zone (**Figure 5c**).

As illustrated in this figure, the majority of the assessment is performed using TEE.

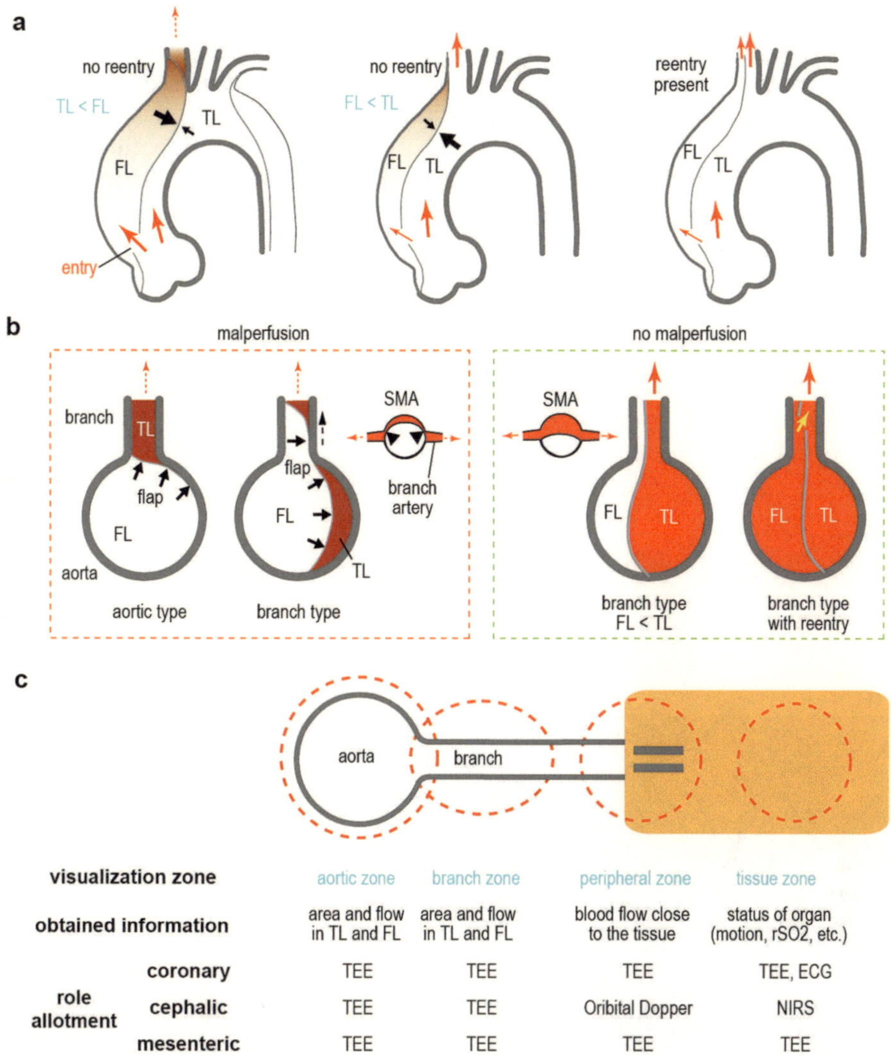

Figure 5.
Mechanisms, Types, and Assessment of Malperfusion. a: Absence of reentry and predominant flow into the false lumen (FL) causing malperfusion. b: Two types of malperfusion: aortic type and branch type, differentiated by TEE findings. c: Four zones to assess perfusion and specific modalities for each organ. ECG: electrocardiogram, NIRS: near-infrared spectroscopy, rSO2: regional oxygen saturation, SMA: superior mesenteric artery, TEE: transesophageal echocardiography.

6.1 Malperfusion of coronary arteries

Malperfusion of the coronary arteries is initially assessed by examining ventricular contraction (tissue zone) and subsequently by detailed examination of each coronary artery. Unlike typical myocardial infarction, where obstruction occurs within the coronary arteries, in ATAAD, obstruction typically occurs at the orifice and proximal portions of the coronary arteries (aortic and branch zones), making TEE assessment feasible. **Figure 6a** schematically illustrates the types of coronary artery malperfusion. The horizontal row depicts the morphological changes in the coronary artery and intima, while the vertical column shows the degree of dissection extension and the presence or absence of ischemia. When an entry tear is located in the ascending aorta, dissection rarely extends into the coronary artery, typically remaining at the orifice due to similar pressures in the true and false lumina. Conversely, if the entry is distal to the aortic arch, the false lumen pressure increases, exceeding the true lumen pressure, potentially leading to coronary artery dissection or orifice occlusion.

Figure 6b presents examples of left coronary artery dissection. In most cases, the left coronary artery remains intact (left), but occasionally it is occluded at

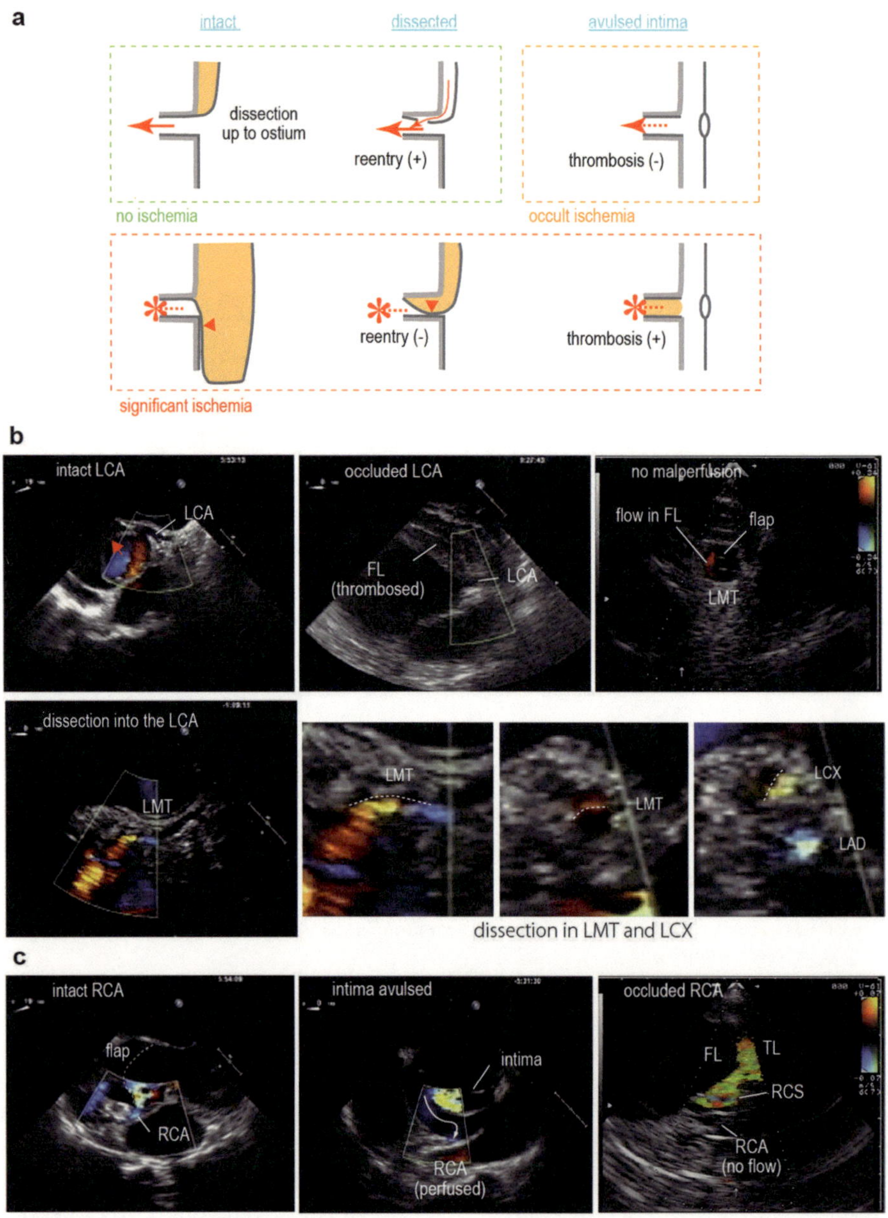

Figure 6.
Coronary Malperfusion. a: Types of dissection and occurrence of malperfusion. b: Findings in the left coronary artery (LCA). c: Findings in the right coronary artery (RCA). FL: false lumen, LAD: left anterior descending artery, LCX: left circumflex artery, LMT: left main truncus, RCS: right coronary sinus, TL: true lumen.

the orifice (center), necessitating prompt perfusion restoration. If a flow signal is detectable in the false lumen, distal perfusion is maintained (right). However, branch-type dissections, shown in the lower row, may lead to subsequent malperfusion onset.

Figure 6c illustrates right coronary artery dissection. Typically, the dissection extends beyond the sinotubular junction but stops at the orifice. Due to the right coronary artery's small diameter and its location on the outer curvature of the ascending aorta, dissection rarely extends into the artery, although the intima may be avulsed at the orifice. In such cases, the coronary artery is perfused via the false lumen, complicating cardioplegic solution infusion post-aortotomy. Hence, revascularization of the right coronary artery before aortotomy is advisable. This crucial information should be communicated to the surgeon. The rightmost figure shows an aortic-type occlusion of the right coronary artery. Impaired perfusion in this scenario must be conveyed to the surgical team.

There are reports suggesting that 3D-TEE is useful for coronary artery assessment [11, 12]. However, the author prefers using 2D and xPlane modes, employing 3D imaging only for understanding the spatial relationship of the coronary arteries.

6.2 Malperfusion of arch branch arteries

The treatment strategies for cases with occluded arch vessels remain controversial. Direct cannulation and perfusion to the occluded right common carotid artery have been attempted with fairly good results, as evidenced by meta-analyses [13–16]. However, occlusion of the right common carotid artery does not necessarily result in cerebral ischemia. Cerebral perfusion is supplied by the bilateral internal carotid and vertebral arteries, which converge to form the basilar artery, and subsequently the circle of Willis. This compensatory system can offset the occlusion of a single vessel. Nonetheless, this system may not provide sufficient blood supply under the conditions of pulseless perfusion with relatively low perfusion pressure during ECC.

To address this challenge, the author has developed a three-stage monitoring protocol for cerebral perfusion (**Figure 7a**) [17]. Near-infrared spectroscopy (NIRS) is used for continuous monitoring of regional oxygen saturation in the bilateral frontal lobes (rSO_2), indicating perfusion from the carotid artery system (tissue zone). If rSO_2 levels drop below 55–60% [18] or if inadequate perfusion of the carotid artery system is suspected, orbital Doppler is employed (peripheral zone). The orbital Doppler technique involves placing a linear probe on the eyelid and visualizing the eye horizontally in a slightly inward direction. With the fundus at the 6-o'clock position, the blood flow signal in the optic nerve (central retinal artery) can be detected. The velocity range below 10 cm/sec is suitable for this purpose. Pulsed-wave Doppler provides information on pulsatility and velocity [19]. Detectable flow signal in the central retinal artery, despite occlusion of the ipsilateral carotid artery, indicates effective collateral circulation via the circle of Willis [20]. The ophthalmic artery, originating from the internal carotid artery, reflects perfusion in the carotid artery system. This artery can usually be detected even at perfusion pressures as low as 30 mmHg. A sustained absence of detectable flow in the ophthalmic artery is associated with cerebral infarction, while a lack of flow in the central retinal artery is linked to higher brain dysfunction such as delirium [21]. Orbital Doppler scanning should be completed within 10 seconds under hypothermia to avoid potential heat injury to the cornea.

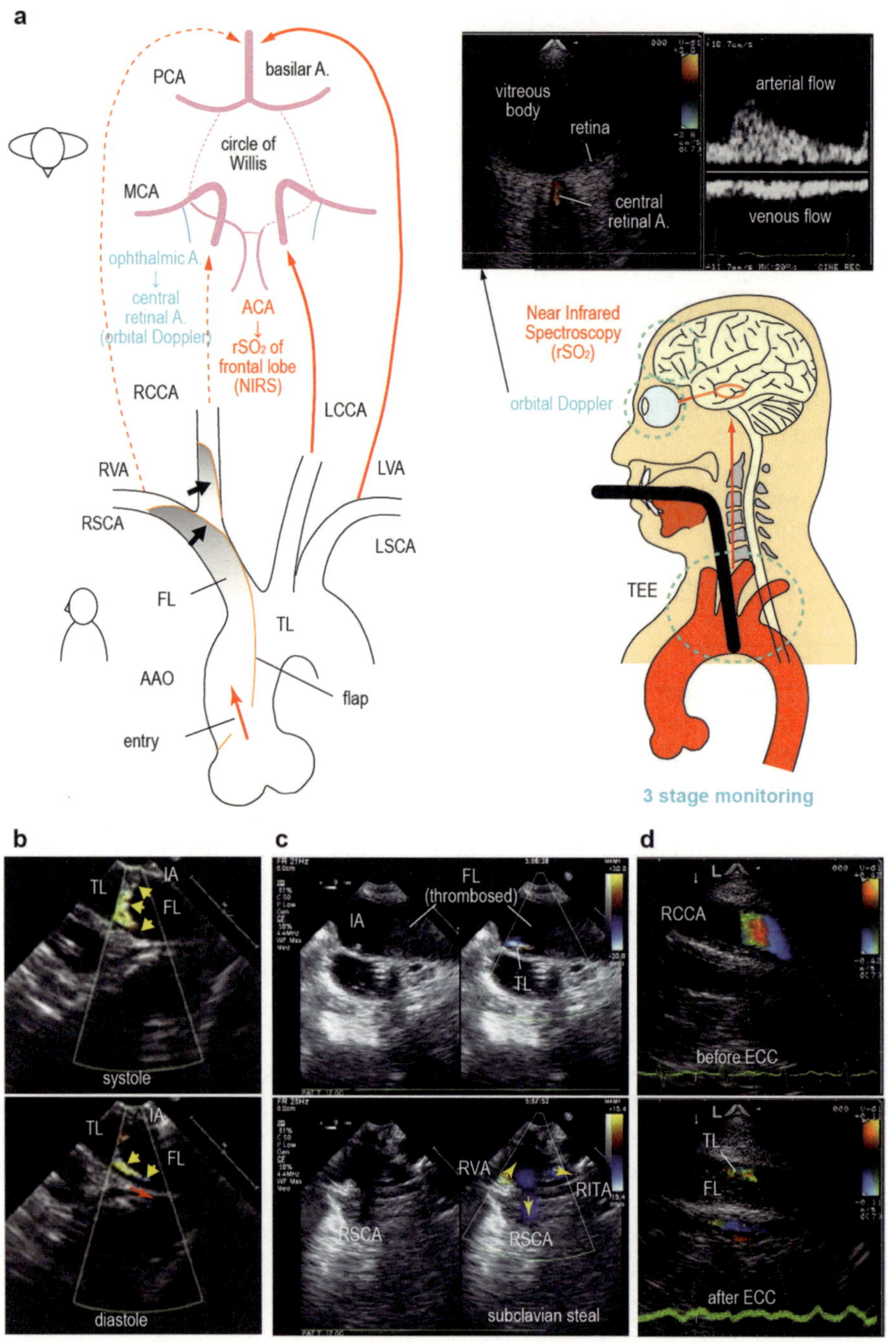

Figure 7.
Cerebral Malperfusion. a: Cerebral perfusion system, normal and malperfused, and three-stage monitoring. b: Balloon-like flap in the innominate artery (IA) with to-and-fro movement. c: Narrowed true lumen (TL) in the IA leading to subclavian steal. d: New dissection in the right common carotid artery (RCCA) after extracorporeal circulation (ECC). AO: ascending aorta, ACA: anterior cerebral artery, FL false lumen, LCCA: left common carotid artery, LSCA: left subclavian artery, LVA: left vertebral artery, MCA: middle cerebral artery, NIRS: near-infrared spectroscopy, PCA: posterior cerebral artery, RCCA: right common carotid artery, RITA: right internal thoracic artery, RSCA: right subclavian artery, rSO2: regional oxygen saturation, RVA: right vertebral artery.

If cerebral malperfusion is suspected based on orbital Doppler findings, perfusion in the upstream branch arteries is examined using TEE (branch zone). One example is the malposition of a cannula for selective cerebral perfusion [22]. Although visualizing arch branch arteries with TEE can be challenging due to interference from the trachea, techniques such as using a fluid-filled balloon placed in the trachea have been reported [23]. However, most of these arteries can be visualized by lateral bending of the TEE probe and scanning from the side of the trachea [24]. Despite the need for specific manipulation techniques and anatomical knowledge, TEE provides valuable information on cerebral perfusion, particularly in treating ATAAD. In cases with an entry tear in the ascending aorta, the dissection often extends to the innominate artery, occasionally causing significant stenosis. Artificial perfusion from the right axillary artery typically recanalizes the innominate artery, although not always [25]. Real-time information on perfusion status is critical for this assessment. **Figure 7b** shows a balloon-like flap in the innominate artery with pulsatile to-and-fro movement. During systole, blood narrowly passes around it to perfuse the distal region, a finding not detectable by CT. **Figure 7c** illustrates the branch-type occlusion of the innominate artery, where antegrade flow in the right subclavian and right internal thoracic artery is present, but flow in the right vertebral artery is retrograde, indicating "subclavian steal" syndrome. Following aortic repair, all flows became antegrade. **Figure 7d** shows changes in the right common carotid artery; while it was patent before ECC, the true lumen collapsed post-ECC, likely due to dissection extension from the anastomosis site. Although this information covers limited areas, integrating these small data points provides a comprehensive understanding of the perfusion status.

6.3 Malperfusion of visceral arteries

Mesenteric ischemia remains a challenging problem, often characterized by difficult diagnosis and the need for timely treatment [26, 27]. Real-time information obtained at the bedside is crucial for addressing this issue, which prompted the author to develop TEE visualization techniques for assessing visceral arteries (**Figure 8a** aorta and branch zone) [28].

To visualize these arteries, the TEE probe is advanced with the short-axis view of the descending aorta in sight. As the probe progresses, the vertebra, initially at the 4-o'clock position, moves to the 6-o'clock position around the level of the esophageal hiatus (TH10). The celiac artery appears at about 2 inches below (TH12), followed by the superior mesenteric artery (SMA) 1 inch further down (L1), and finally the renal arteries at L2 (**Figure 8a**). Scanning at a 90-degree plane provides a sagittal section of these arteries. The celiac artery branches perpendicularly from the anterior wall of the aorta and quickly divides into three arteries, while the SMA courses dorsally along the aorta. Although maintaining the image of the aorta on the screen requires upper and lateral bending of the probe, this technique yields valuable information on visceral perfusion [29–31].

Figure 8b depicts an aortic-type occlusion of the SMA with a patent celiac artery, while **Figure 8c** shows both arteries occluded, suggesting potential hepatic ischemia. **Figure 8d** illustrates a branch-type malperfusion with a flow signal only in the narrow true lumen. In all these cases, the intestine was necrotic. Given that the intestine is a muscular organ, malperfusion can be suspected by observing its morphology and kinetics (tissue zone). **Figure 8e** (left) shows ischemic intestines with a dilated

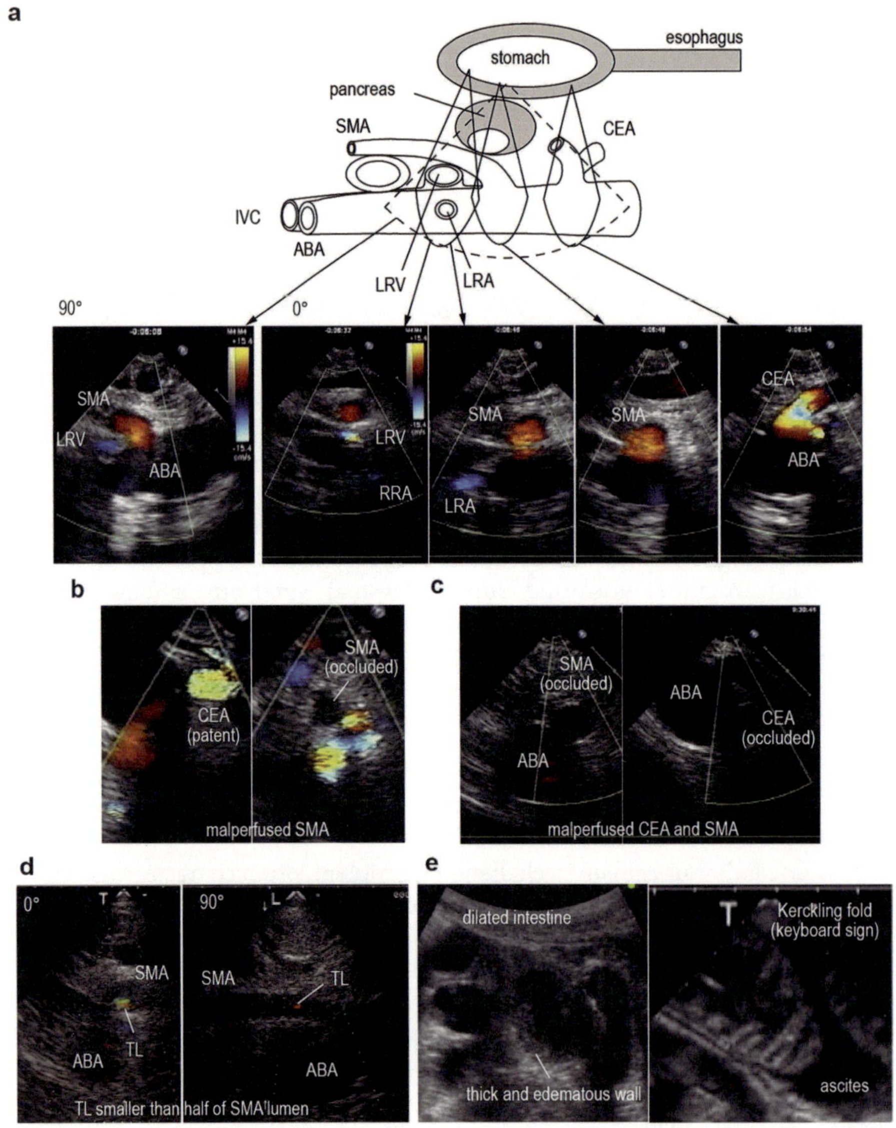

Figure 8.
Visceral Malperfusion. a: TEE visualization of visceral arteries, scanned from the stomach posteriorly in the horizontal or sagittal plane. b: Aortic type malperfusion of superior mesenteric artery (SMA), with patent celiac artery (CEA). c: Occlusion of both arteries. d: Branch type malperfusion of SMA with compressed true lumen (TL). e: Intestinal ischemia presenting with dilatation, edematous wall and folds, and ascites. ABA: abdominal aorta, FL: faluse lumen, IVC: inferior vena cava, LRA: left renal artery, LRV: left renal vein, RRA: right renal artery.

lumen, thick edematous walls, and reduced peristalsis. Immediate evaluation of the SMA is critical because the window for salvaging the intestine is only about 4 hours. The right image shows a typical finding of a necrotic intestine with markedly dilated loops and visible Kerckring's folds in the presence of abundant ascites, indicating the need for immediate laparotomy and resection.

These findings can also be obtained using surface ultrasonography. It is essential to utilize every available modality to gather comprehensive information and accurately assess the situation.

7. Initiation of ECC

ECC-induced dissection is rare, with an incidence of less than 0.3%, but its mortality is notably high, ranging from 20–48% [32, 33]. While ultrasound technologies can aid in rescuing patients [34], timely assessment is crucial. The author has encountered two such cases, both of whom were successfully rescued likely because the dissections were immediately detected with TEE and promptly treated. In the first case, aortic arch dissection occurred following perfusion from the right axillary artery. TEE revealed a linear image passing through the arch (**Figure 9a**) [35]. Despite the immediate cessation of the pump, the dissection had already extended to the descending aorta, reducing the true lumen to a slit-like structure. There was no unusual increase in perfusion pressure. In the second case, dissection appeared in the descending aorta approximately 10 seconds after initiating femoral arterial perfusion. TEE visualized the gradual prominence of a very thin intima at the 8–12 o'clock position, with slightly echogenic fine dots in the false lumen, which eventually occupied the entire aortic lumen (**Figure 9b**) [36]. In both cases, perfusion was redirected through an alternative route, perfusion in the individual branch arteries was checked, and the aorta was repaired. Both patients were discharged without significant sequelae.

If these occurrences had not been recognized, aortic-type malperfusion could have led to multiple organ failure, potentially being diagnosed as "stroke or hepatic failure of unknown reason." The need for TEE assessment is apparent by the fact that no one else had recognized these events. TEE is only useful if employed at the right time and for the appropriate assessment. Importantly, dissection is difficult to recognize on TEE images after it has passed, but capturing the decisive moment is critical. Monitoring the downstream area of perfusion with TEE is essential.

Another significant event at this stage is false lumen perfusion, where perfused blood predominantly enters the false lumen through a reentry, causing aortic-type malperfusion due to increased pressure in the false lumen. Although there is an ongoing debate about the best perfusion strategy to prevent false lumen perfusion [37–40], the author believes there is no single "best" strategy as situations vary in individual cases. The optimal approach is to "perfuse first and modify it as needed according to the result" [41]. To ascertain the "result" of initial perfusion, it is necessary to monitor the downstream area with TEE (**Figure 9c**).

This issue tends to occur in cases of retrograde type A dissection with the entry point in the abdominal aorta. **Figure 9d** illustrates changes in the descending aorta in one such case. The patient's blood pressure suddenly dropped, and TEE clarified the reason. Before femoral arterial perfusion, blood flow was present only in the true lumen with spontaneous echo contrast (SEC) in the false lumen. Upon initiating perfusion, the true lumen collapsed, and the SEC in the false lumen moved upward and disappeared. Systemic perfusion was established via the left subclavian artery, and the scheduled repair was completed. **Figure 9e** shows TEE findings in the ascending aorta, which was filled with SEC following systemic perfusion, without any changes in other monitors. This indicated an enlarged false lumen. As coronary perfusion was maintained through the gap around the thin flap and there was no decrease in rSO_2, cooling continued and aortic replacement was performed. Both cases had uneventful postoperative courses without complications.

Recently, cannulation to the dissected arch has been reported [42–45]. The author used this technique in one ECC-induced dissection case, and TEE was instrumental in detecting erroneous entry of the guidewire into the false lumen or unintendedly deep placement.

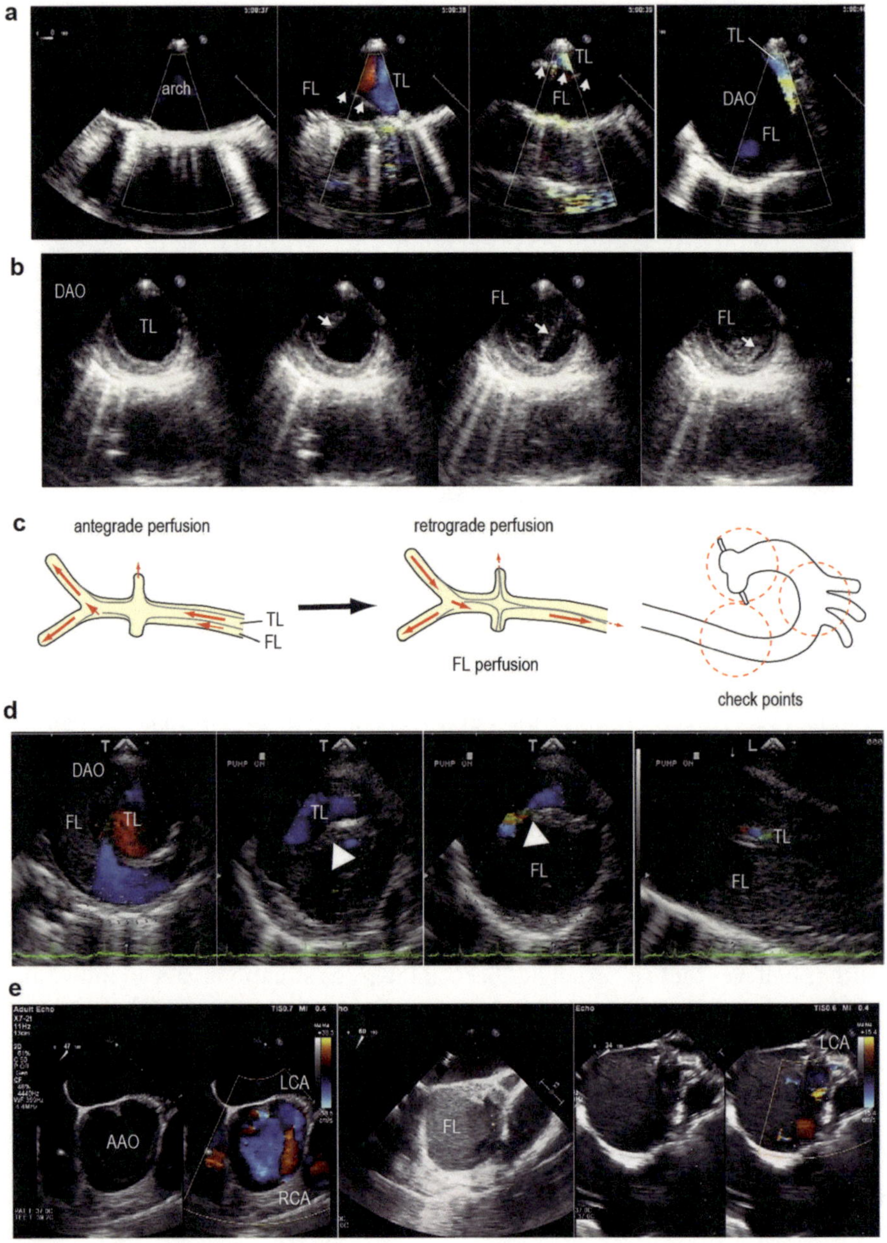

Figure 9.
Events at the Initiation of Artificial Perfusion. a: Perfusion-induced dissection in the arch, with the intimal flap passing. b: New dissection in the descending aorta (DAO) with a very thin flap. c: Mechanism of false lumen (FL) perfusion. d: FL perfusion detected in DAO. e: FL perfusion detected in ascending aorta (AAO), with perfusion to the left coronary artery (LCA) detectable. RCA: right coronary artery, TL: true lumen.

8. After weaning from ECC

Two cases of unexpected events after ECC are presented. In one case (**Figure 10a**), the patient experienced a sudden drop in blood pressure just before chest closure, despite an otherwise uneventful course [46]. TEE revealed dyskinesia in the anterior

DOI: http://dx.doi.org/10.5772/intechopen.1005684

wall of the left ventricle and no detectable blood flow in the left coronary artery. Immediate re-initiation of ECC and revascularization of the left coronary artery with a saphenous vein graft were performed. TEE showed a thickened Valsalva sinus wall, indicating a newly developed dissection extending from the proximal anastomosis site, leading to an occlusion of the left coronary ostium. The Valsalva sinus wall near the anastomosis was reinforced with a pair of pledgets to prevent further extension of the dissection (**Figure 10b**). Perfusion in the left coronary artery recovered, and the patient had an uneventful postoperative course (**Figure 10c**). In another case, dissection initially extended into the left coronary artery, but the true lumen was predominant (**Figure 10d**). However, during weaning from ECC, the false lumen gradually enlarged to nearly 50% of the lumen and then occupied more than half before chest closure. Despite these changes, the left ventricle maintained normal contraction. Due to the progressive changes in the coronary artery, coronary artery stenosis was assessed via coronary angiography, which revealed more than 95% stenosis of the left main trunk. Coronary revascularization was performed, and the patient had an uneventful postoperative course. If the left coronary artery had not been monitored

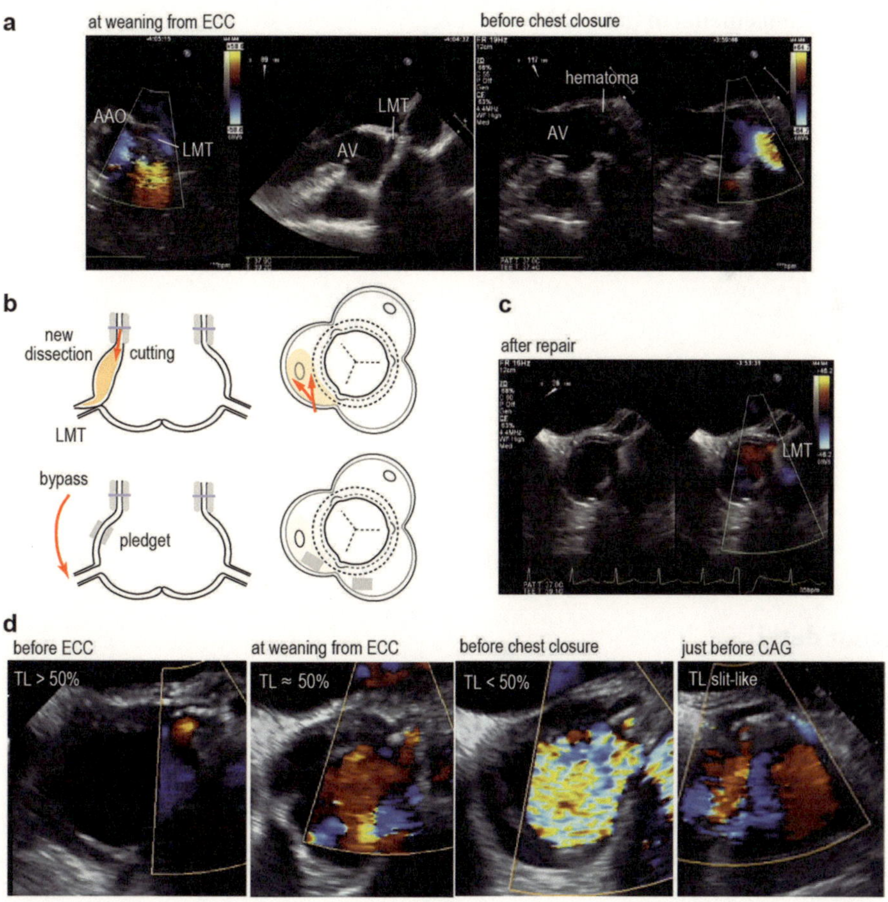

Figure 10.
Unexpected Events After Weaning from Extracorporeal Circulation (ECC). a: Occlusion of left main truncus (LMT) before chest closure. b: Possible mechanism of occlusion and subsequent treatment. c: Restored flow in LMT. d: Progressive compression of LMT lumen. AAO: ascending aorta, AV: aortic valve, CAG: coronary angiography.

with TEE, the patient might have experienced sudden shock or cardiac arrest in the ICU, with findings similar to those in the first case.

9. Conclusions

In this chapter, various applications of TEE for managing ATAAD are discussed, including visualization techniques, assessment timing, and target structures. Although TEE requires significant time and effort, the information it provides is crucial for rescuing patients and avoiding complications. This parallels surgical training where practice and experience lead to better outcomes. Despite recent improvements in surgical outcomes, reported mortality rates only reflect patients who undergo surgery. The real prognosis, including those who do not receive surgical treatment, is likely worse, with many survivors suffering from sequelae. Future directions should focus on the following: (1) prevention of ATAAD and (2) precision strategies in surgical treatment. The latest guidelines have, for the first time, addressed the issue of prevention [2]. The personal strategies described in this chapter are a work in progress and will continue to be refined. The author hopes this chapter serves as a catalyst for further advancements in the field.

Author details

Kazumasa Orihashi
Kochi Medical School, Nankoku, Japan

*Address all correspondence to: orihashik@kochi-u.ac.jp

References

[1] Committee for Scientific Affairs, The Japanese Association for Thoracic Surgery, Matsumiya G, Sato Y, Takeuchi H, et al. Thoracic and cardiovascular surgeries in Japan during 2020: Annual report by the Japanese Association for Thoracic Surgery. General Thoracic and Cardiovascular Surgery. 2024;**72**:61-94

[2] Ogino H, Iida O, Akutsu K, Chiba Y, Hayashi H, Ishibashi H, et al. JCS/JSCVS/JATS/JSVS 2020 guideline on diagnosis and treatment of aortic aneurysm and aortic dissection. Circulation Journal. 2023;**87**:1410-1621

[3] Thorsgard ME, Morrissette GJ, Sun B, et al. Impact of intraoperative transesophageal echocardiography on acute type-A aortic dissection. Journal of Cardiothoracic and Vascular Anesthesia. 2014;**28**:1203-1207

[4] Orihashi K, Sueda T, Okada K, Imai K. Identification of intramural hematoma and the site of aortic rupture by transesophageal echocardiography. The Journal of Thoracic and Cardiovascular Surgery. 2008;**136**:1089-1091

[5] Patel PA, Bavaria JE, Ghadimi K, et al. Aortic regurgitation in acute type-A aortic dissection: A clinical classification for the perioperative echocardiographer in the era of the functional aortic annulus. Journal of Cardiothoracic and Vascular Anesthesia. 2018;**32**:586-597

[6] Pan H, Sun W. Stanford type A acute aortic dissection with proximal intimo-intimal intussusception: A case report and literature review. Journal of Cardiothoracic Surgery. 2021;**16**:201

[7] Nakamura R, Honda K, Yuzaki M, Nishimura Y. Severe aortic regurgitation with intimal intussusception secondary to Debakey type I aortic dissection. Echocardiography. 2020;**37**:652-653

[8] Armour T, Armour S, Reddy P, Brinster D. Type A dissection involving intimo-intimal intussusception through the aortic valve. A & A Case Reports. 2015;**5**:21-24

[9] Thunberg CA, Ramakrishna H. Echocardiographic detection of intimo-intimal intussusception in a patient with acute Stanford type A aortic dissection. Annals of Cardiac Anaesthesia. 2015;**18**:227-230

[10] Hara H, Tanabe K, Tanimoto S, et al. Aortic regurgitation due to back-and-forth intimal flap movement detected by both multidetector computed tomography and transesophageal echocardiography. Journal of Cardiology Cases. 2013;**7**:e161-e163

[11] Sasaki S, Watanabe H, Shibayama K, et al. Three-dimensional transesophageal echocardiographic evaluation of coronary involvement in patients with acute type A aortic dissection. Journal of the American Society of Echocardiography. 2013;**26**:837-845

[12] Wang CJ, Rodriguez Diaz CA, Trinh MA. Use of real-time three-dimensional transesophageal echocardiography in type A aortic dissections: Advantages of 3D TEE illustrated in three cases. Annals of Cardiac Anaesthesia. 2015;**18**:83-86

[13] Gimibuchi T, Seto T, Naito K, et al. Strategies to improve outcomes for acute type A aortic dissection with cerebral malperfusion. European Journal of Cardio-Thoracic Surgery. 2021;**59**:666-673

[14] Minatoya K. Aggressive strategy to save the brain in a case of acute aortic dissection. Journal of Cardiac Surgery. 2021;**36**:3981-3982

[15] Sugiyama K, Watanuki H, Futamura Y, et al. Impact of direct carotid artery perfusion in acute type A aortic dissection involving the common carotid artery. General Thoracic and Cardiovascular Surgery. 2021;**69**:1467-1475

[16] He K, Qin X, Li M, et al. Two surgical strategies (early carotid reperfusion vs. central aortic repair-first) of acute type A aortic dissection complicated with cerebral malperfusion syndrome: A meta-analysis and systematic review. BMC Cardiovascular Disorders. 2024;**24**:239

[17] Orihashi K. Cerebral malperfusion in acute aortic dissection. Surgery Today. 2016;**46**:1353-1361

[18] Orihashi K, Sueda T, Okada K, Imai K. Near-infrared spectroscopy for monitoring cerebral ischemia during selective cerebral perfusion. European Journal of Cardio-Thoracic Surgery. 2004;**26**:907-911

[19] Orihashi K, Matsuura Y, Sueda T, et al. Flow velocity of central retinal artery and retrobulbar vessels during cardiovascular operations. The Journal of Thoracic and Cardiovascular Surgery. 1997;**114**:1081-1087

[20] Kondo N, Hirose N, Kihara K, Orihashi K. Cerebral perfusion in debranching thoracic endovascular aortic repair monitored by orbital ultrasonography. The Journal of Thoracic and Cardiovascular Surgery. 2019;**158**:e81-e83

[21] Orihashi K, Matsuura Y, Sueda T, et al. Clinical implication of orbital ultrasound monitoring during selective cerebral perfusion. The Annals of Thoracic Surgery. 2001;**71**:673-677

[22] Orihashi K, Sueda T, Okada K, Imai K. Malposition of selective cerebral perfusion catheter is not a rare event. European Journal of Cardio-Thoracic Surgery. 2005;**27**:644-648

[23] Jansen Klomp WW, Peelen LM, Brandon Bravo Bruinsma GJ, et al. Modified transesophageal echocardiography of the dissected thoracic aorta; a novel diagnostic approach. Cardiovascular Ultrasound. 2016;**14**:28

[24] Orihashi K, Matsuura Y, Sueda T, et al. Aortic arch branches are no longer blind zone for transesophageal echocardiography: A new eye for aortic surgeons. The Journal of Thoracic and Cardiovascular Surgery. 2000;**120**:466-472

[25] Orihashi K, Sueda T, Okada K, Takahashi S. Compressed true lumen in the innominate artery: A pitfall of right axillary arterial perfusion in acute aortic dissection. The Journal of Thoracic and Cardiovascular Surgery. 2009;**137**:242-243

[26] Sfeir PM, Issa K, Ayoub CM. Mesenteric malperfusion syndromes in type A aortic dissection: Current management strategies. Journal of Cardiothoracic and Vascular Anesthesia. 2021;**35**:3711-3719

[27] Moral S, Avegliano G, Cuéllar H, et al. Usefulness of transesophageal echocardiography in the evaluation of celiac trunk and superior mesenteric artery involvement in acute aortic dissection. Journal of the American Society of Echocardiography. 2021;**34**:327-335

[28] Orihashi K, Matsuura Y, Sueda T, et al. Abdominal aorta and visceral arteries visualized with transesophageal echocardiography during operations on the aorta. The Journal of Thoracic and Cardiovascular Surgery. 1998;**115**:945-947

[29] Orihashi K, Sueda T, Okada K, Imai K. Perioperative diagnosis of mesenteric ischemia in acute aortic dissection by transesophageal echocardiography. European Journal of Cardio-Thoracic Surgery. 2005;**28**:871-876

[30] Orihashi K. Malperfusion in acute type A aortic dissection: Unsolved problem. The Annals of Thoracic Surgery. 2013;**95**:1570-1576

[31] Orihashi K. Mesenteric ischemia in acute aortic dissection. General Thoracic and Cardiovascular Surgery. 2018;**66**:557-564

[32] Leontyev S, Borger MA, Legare JF, et al. Iatrogenic type A aortic dissection during cardiac procedures: Early and late outcome in 48 patients. European Journal of Cardio-Thoracic Surgery. 2012;**41**:641-646

[33] Fleck T, Ehrlich M, Czerny M, Wolner E, Grabenwoger M, Grimm M. Intraoperative iatrogenic type A aortic dissection and perioperative outcome. Interdisciplinary CardioVascular and Thoracic Surgery. 2006;**5**:11-14

[34] Singh A, Mehta Y. Intraoperative aortic dissection. Annals of Cardiac Anaesthesia. 2015;**18**:537-542

[35] Yamamoto M, Nishimori H, Tashiro M, Orihashi K. Triple ultrasonography for iatrogenic acute aortic dissection caused by axillary arterial perfusion. Interactive Cardiovascular and Thoracic Surgery. 2017;**25**:995-997

[36] Orihashi K, Kihara K, Yamamoto M, Nishimori H. Iatrogenic subintimal aortic dissection that disappeared without a trace. European Journal of Cardio-Thoracic Surgery. 2017;**52**:825-826

[37] Chang Y, Lin H, Qian D, et al. Comparison of single axillary vs. dual arterial cannulation for acute type A aortic dissection: A propensity score matching analysis. Frontiers in Cardiovascular Medicine. 2022;**9**:809493

[38] Guo J, Wang Y, Zhu J, et al. Right axillary and femoral artery perfusion with mild hypothermia for aortic arch replacement. Journal of Cardiothoracic Surgery. 2014;**9**:94

[39] Hussain A, Uzzaman M, Mohamed S, Khan F, Butt S, Khan H. Femoral versus axillary cannulation in acute type A aortic dissections: A meta-analysis. Journal of Cardiac Surgery. 2021;**36**:3761-3769

[40] Tong G, Zhuang DL, Sun ZC, Chen SR, Fan RX, Sun TC. Femoral artery cannulation as a safe alternative for aortic dissection arch repair in the era of axillary artery cannulation. Journal of Thoracic Disease. 2021;**13**:671-680

[41] Orihashi K, Sueda T, Okada K, Imai K. Detection and monitoring of complications associated with femoral or axillary arterial cannulation for surgical repair of aortic dissection. Journal of Cardiothoracic and Vascular Anesthesia. 2006;**20**:20-25

[42] Ma H, Xiao Z, Shi J, Liu L, Qin C, Guo Y. Aortic arch cannulation with the guidance of transesophageal echocardiography for Stanford type A aortic dissection. Journal of Cardiothoracic Surgery. 2018;**13**:106

[43] Gegouskov V, Manchev G, Danov V, Stoitsev G, Iliev S. Direct cannulation of

ascending aorta versus standard femoral artery cannulation in acute aortic dissection type A. The Heart Surgery Forum. 2018;**21**:E139-E144

[44] Brinster DR, Parrish DW, Meyers KS, Reddy P, Kasirajan V. Central aortic cannulation for Stanford type A aortic dissection with the use of three-dimensional and two-dimensional transesophageal echocardiography. Journal of Cardiac Surgery. 2014;**29**:729-732

[45] Attaran S, Safar M, Saleh HZ, Field M, Kuduvalli M, Oo A. Cannulating a dissecting aorta using ultrasound-epiaortic and transesophageal guidance. The Heart Surgery Forum. 2011;**14**:E373-E375

[46] Orihashi K, Takasaki T, Ozawa M, Sueda T. Intraoperative occlusion of left coronary ostium after aortic repair detected by transesophageal echocardiography. The Journal of Thoracic and Cardiovascular Surgery. 2011;**142**:e205-e206

Chapter 6

Combined Ultrasound in Screening for Aortic Dissection: The Fate of the Residual False Lumen after Surgery

André Timóteo Sapalo

Abstract

Because of its frequency and unusual appearance, aortic dissection (AD) is a rare and potentially fatal disorder marked by the dynamic progression of pressure loads. Aortic dissection (AD) is a rare and potentially fatal disorder marked by the dynamic progression of pressure loads. The diagnosis of AD can be challenging. This chapter explores contemporary challenges in screening for aortic dissection using ultrasound parameters. It discusses advancements in the TEM classification of dissection, enhancing its robustness to provide more comprehensive information for surgeons, cardiologists, and hemodynamicists regarding therapeutic strategies and predicting the success of treatment approaches. Additionally, the chapter highlights the utility of measuring peak systolic velocity, end-diastolic flow, pulsatility index (PI), resistivity index (RI), and cardio-ankle vascular index (CAVI) as reliable tools for assessing vascular compliance and local and systemic hemodynamic changes both before and after surgery. Emphasis is also placed on the importance of routine monitoring of the patent false lumen with ultrasound to prevent the advancement of residual volume into the intimal layers of the arteries post-surgery, thereby reducing the risk of aneurysm formation, segmental growth of the distal aorta, and the need for subsequent aortic reoperations.

Keywords: aortic dissection, aortic dissection surgery, classification of dissection, hypothermic total circulatory arrest, cardiopulmonary bypass, transesophageal echocardiography, transthoracic echocardiography, ultrasound

1. Introduction

Aorta dissection (AD), which is characterized by the rupture of the aorta wall's intimal layer, is a common condition but is still regarded as rare due to its prevalence of 1–3%. Every 100,000 individuals experience an aortic dissection about three times a year [1]. With 5-year survival rates in acute cases of type A and type B dissections ranging from 55 to 85% and surgical mortality rates as low as 12%, AD currently represents a substantial clinical challenge [2–4]. The mortality rate is initially approximately 1% per hour without treatment, increasing to 50% by the third day [5]. Even after successful surgery, complications related to AD contribute to 31–66% of deaths in type B cases, which typically have a lower risk compared to type A aortic dissection [6–9].

Consequently, clinical decision-making regarding the use of an endovascular approach requires an understanding of the anatomical adaptations and hemodynamic consequences in response to the pathophysiological changes observed in AD. To achieve this, the disease is categorized based on the location of the intimal layer rupture and the extent of aortic involvement within the segments. Currently, several clinically accepted classification systems exist, with the DeBakey classification being commonly employed, delineating the condition into four types [10, 11].

2. There hemodynamic alterations and pathophysiology of aortic dissection

Our thorough understanding of the pathogenesis of this disease currently has several gaps. Conditions that put more stress on the endothelium wall are assumed to be linked to its beginning. Uncontrolled hypertension, pheochromocytoma, substance abuse (drugs, cocaine, etc.), aortic coarctation, and various connective tissue disorders, including Turner syndrome, familial thoracic aortic aneurysm and dissection syndrome, Loeys-Dietz syndrome, Marfan syndrome, and Ehlers-Danlos syndrome Type IV, are among these conditions [12].

2.1 Pressure stress in the aorta

Most cases of AD are associated with pressure stress, particularly in older patients [13]. It is crucial to keep in mind that systemic vascular resistance, intravascular volume, and cardiac output (CO) all affect systolic blood pressure in order to comprehend this. In the meantime, venous compliance, intravascular volume, and right atrial pressure control systemic venous pressure. These hemodynamic parameters are significantly affected by sodium balance [14]. Expansion of the interstitial compartment can directly reduce venous compliance, thereby impacting overall cardiovascular function [15].

In some cases, despite normal renal ultrastructure, patients exhibit persistent sodium and water retention, possibly due to mechanisms termed 'reverse failure' or 'direct failure'. Reverse failure is typically observed in patients with preserved ejection fraction and left ventricular (LV) remodeling, where there is inadequate baroreceptor sensing of elevated circulating volume [16, 17]. Conversely, hypovolemia can lead to cardiac chamber overload, resulting in venous congestion and increased capillary pressure. This promotes interstitial fluid accumulation along with plasma volume depletion, stimulating renal sodium and water retention, thereby exacerbating systolic blood pressure to the extent of inducing intimal dissection in the most vulnerable regions affected by elevated pressure [18, 19].

Conversely, hypertension is associated with LV remodeling and reduced LV end-diastolic volume. Consequently, many patients with chronic, poorly controlled hypertension have preserved ejection fraction and reduced stroke volume. In these instances, inadequate tissue perfusion, including renal blood flow, impairs normal sodium excretion. Both theories of pressure emphasize the significant impact of elevated pressure on the aortic artery walls, reducing cardiac output and activating neurohormonal responses [20].

Elevated intracardiac pressures, characteristic of chronic hypertension, usually result in the production of natriuretic peptides, notably brain and atrial, which cause diuretic and natriuretic responses [21]. Mechanosensitive nerve terminals in the heart chambers and cardiopulmonary system, as well as malfunctioning baroreceptors in the carotid sinus and aortic arch, can disrupt signaling at afferent sensing locations in the cardiopulmonary system and affect natriuresis [22].

Both baroreceptors and cardiopulmonary arterial reflexes are compromised in chronic hypertension, which results in improper tonic regulation of sympathetic outflow and subsequent sympathetic nervous system (SNS) activation [23]. This promotes renal retention of salt and water despite volume expansion by causing the secretion of antidiuretic hormone (ADH) and the release of renin [24].

It is now well-established that when pressure stress on the aortic walls exceeds their resistance, it is a strong indicator of eventual aortic dilation and dissection. To further elucidate this, it is important to note that AD occurs when the layers of the aortic wall separate due to the infiltration of high-pressure arterial blood. Therefore, high shear stress in the aorta, combined with a defect in the aortic media, contributes to this process.

Thus, shear stress is caused by the rapid increase in luminal pressure per unit time (dP/dt) resulting from cardiac systole [25]. As the aorta extends from the heart, an increasing proportion of the kinetic energy from left ventricular systole is stored in the aortic wall as potential energy, which facilitates the forward propagation of cardiac output during diastole. This conversion of kinetic to potential energy also attenuates shear stress [26]. The ascending aorta is most vulnerable to dissection, also known as type A dissection, since it experiences the most dramatic changes in pressure. Aortic media degeneration is a typical aspect of aging, but it occurs more quickly in people who have Turner syndrome, inflammatory arteritis, bicuspid aortic valves, or hereditary connective tissue abnormalities [27].

Blood can propagate either proximally or distally through the aortic media when the aortic intima is damaged, forming a false lumen that can potentially connect with the aorta's real lumen [28]. Blood may flow through the true lumen, the false lumen, or both [29]. The propagation of the dissection significantly contributes to the morbidity associated with AD by disrupting blood flow through branch vessels or by directly affecting the pericardium or aortic valve. Over time, the dissection may traverse the entire aortic wall, leading to aortic rupture and exsanguination [30].

2.2 Endothelial stress and reduced vascular compliance

The most well-established pathophysiological etiology for aortic dissection is vascular dysfunction. Because the aorta is subjected to considerable pressure stresses, there has been a hypothesis that comorbid disorders such as high blood pressure, diabetes, obesity, and aging could produce various macro- and microvascular alterations in the arteries [31]. As previously noted, these comorbidities could be a component of a systemic proinflammatory state that shows up as increased plasma levels of soluble ST2, pentraxin-3, and tumor necrosis factor-alpha (TNFα) and interleukin-6 (IL-6) [32] (**Figure 1**).

Thus, as circulating biomarkers become available in the bloodstream, mechanical stimuli are engaged through the baroreflex (shear stress), and hormonal stimuli are activated through the chemoreflex (vasoactive chemicals). This activation

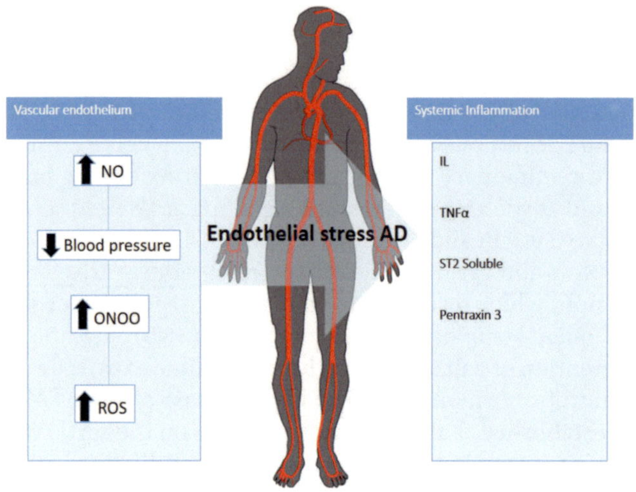

Figure 1.
A brief overview of the mechanisms underlying increased inflammatory responses during cardiopulmonary bypass is presented. The closed-loop circulation is interfered with when the circulatory system is linked to cardiopulmonary bypass. This disruption causes nitric oxide (NO) levels to rise and blood pressure to drop. It also initiates mechanical stimuli through the baroreflex (shear stress) and hormonal stimuli through the chemoreflex (vasoactive hormones). Elevated NO levels can react with oxygen to produce the potent oxidant peroxynitrite (ONOO). Nitric oxide synthase is harmed by this mechanism, which reduces NO's bioavailability.

results in the release of vasodilatory substances such as prostacyclin, nitric oxide (NO), endothelium-derived hyperpolarizing factor, and C-type natriuretic peptide. Vasoconstrictor medications that are produced concurrently include angiotensin II (Ang II), thromboxane A2, endothelin, and reactive oxygen species (ROS). Furthermore, NO, NF-κB, E-selectin, and vascular cell adhesion molecule (VCAM) are examples of inflammatory modulators that control vascular homeostasis. Additionally, the expression of VCAM and E-selectin promotes monocyte migration to the subendothelial area by releasing transforming growth factor-beta (TGFβ).

On the other hand, TGFβ causes fibroblasts to mature into myofibroblasts and promotes the build-up of collagen in the interstitial space. The primary cause of oxidative stress is peroxynitrite (ONOO-), which is created when superoxide (O_2^+) and nitric oxide (NO) mix. Remember that ONOO is a strong free radical that can harm nitric oxide synthase enzymes and the vascular endothelium, which lowers the amount of accessible NO. Therefore, it is believed that increased levels of $ONOO^-$ are primarily responsible for the fragility of the aortic intima.

Protein kinase G (PKG) activity is lowered by soluble guanylate cyclase (sGC) activity, which is lowered by decreased NO levels and ONOO production in cardiomyocytes. This series of events results in hypophosphorylation of titin, which raises the resting tension in cardiomyocytes. The subsequent activation of pro-hypertrophic impulses causes cardiomyocyte hypertrophy.

Because of this, the aorta endothelium is more vulnerable to the cytotoxic effects of relatively high amounts of reactive oxygen species (ROS). One of the primary causes of aortic aneurysm and dissection is well recognized to be the inflammatory response associated with increased production of reactive oxygen species (ROS), such as superoxide and hydrogen peroxide. Leukocytes produce these dangerous substances, which lead to vascular tissue deterioration and inflammation. Moreover, superoxide is produced by the three main cell types of the aortic wall: fibroblasts, endothelial cells, and smooth muscle cells (SMCs). Furthermore, current studies have demonstrated that ROS activates matrix metalloproteinases (MMPs), which in turn causes vascular SMCs to die [33, 34].

2.3 The cascade of coagulation

A sequence of successive chemical processes that result in the creation of a blood clot is referred to as the "coagulation cascade." A number of coagulation factors, numbered from component I to XIII, essentially mediate this process. Each of these factors is essential in initiating the next component in the sequence. Prolonged bleeding may result from the lack or insufficiency of any of these components, which can have a substantial influence on the ability and rate of coagulation [35, 36].

Prior to blood vessel damage, interactions between the vessel walls and circulating platelets, mediated by adhesive proteins, are activated. This interaction initiates the formation of an initial platelet plug. The subendothelial region, which is rich in thrombogenic molecules like collagen, tissue factor, von Willebrand factor, and laminin, is crucial for initiating the coagulation cascade following arterial damage. It is interesting to note that platelets adhere strongly to collagen and von Willebrand factor that are present in the subendothelial region as opposed to the intact vascular endothelium [37, 38].

There are three primary phases in the homeostatic regulation of the coagulation cascade [39]:

1. *Platelet adhesion:* Von Willebrand factor (VWF) is exposed after vascular injury and serves as a link between platelet surface receptors (GPIb) and endothelial collagen. This interaction promotes platelet adhesion.

2. *Platelet secretion*: The three types of granules present in platelets are α-granules, dense granules, and lysosomes. The widely dispersed α-granules include a variety of proteins, such as fibrinogen, coagulation factors, VWF, and growth factors. Calcium and other substances needed for platelet activation and subsequent coagulation are released when the granules attach.

3. The stability and hardness of the platelet aggregation depend on thrombine A2 (TXA2), which is released by active platelets and enhances platelet activation. Platelet aggregation is further enhanced by ADP, which binds to GpIIb/IIIa receptors to facilitate fibrinogen deposition. This process results in the generation of thrombin, which changes fibrinogen into fibrin, strengthening the original platelet plug and designating the secondary hemostasis stage.

Nitric oxide (NO), a component that is fundamentally released by endothelial cells, macrophages, and platelets, plays a regulatory role in hemostasis. With a short half-life of 3 to 5 seconds, NO inhibits platelet activation and promotes vasodilation. Similarly, prostacyclin, synthesized by endothelial cells, exerts inhibitory effects on platelet function, contributing to vascular homeostasis and preventing excessive clot formation [40, 41].

In the context of aortic dissection, there is a disruption of the coagulation cascade. Antithrombotic medications are therefore frequently used in these patients to prevent or manage common cardiovascular disorders, including coronary artery disease, peripheral vascular atherosclerosis, and atrial fibrillation. Two main classes of oral antithrombotic drugs are available: antiplatelet agents and anticoagulants. Aspirin and P2Y12 inhibitors, either alone or in combination with dual antiplatelet therapy (DAPT), are commonly prescribed antiplatelet agents. Among oral anticoagulants, vitamin K antagonists (VKAs) and direct oral anticoagulants (DOACs) are frequently utilized [42].

Consequently, bleeding is a common and serious complication in patients with aortic dissection, often necessitating extensive administration of blood products and clotting factor concentrates. Notably, bleeding is associated with a high incidence of perioperative coagulation disorders. In patients with coagulopathic aortic dissection, hospital mortality rates of up to 20% have been reported [43].

3. Combined ultrasound and TEM classification in screening for aortic dissection

Therefore, AD requires a comprehensive evaluation that extends beyond the anatomical and geometric assessments of the aortic artery, as categorized by the Stanford and DeBakey classifications [44]. Emerging evidence suggests that the site of rupture can also lead to complex myocardial perfusion challenges and affect other target organs. Consequently, the recently introduced TEM classification seeks to expand the evaluation of dissection by not only considering the area of rupture but also assessing cardiovascular involvement in the context of perfusion difficulties (**Figure 2**).

AD is a potentially life-threatening condition, underscoring the critical need for prompt diagnosis to enhance patient outcomes and survival rates. Diagnostic imaging techniques, such as computed tomography angiography (CTA), magnetic resonance angiography (MRA), and ultrasound, are essential for achieving diagnostic accuracy and facilitating follow-up.

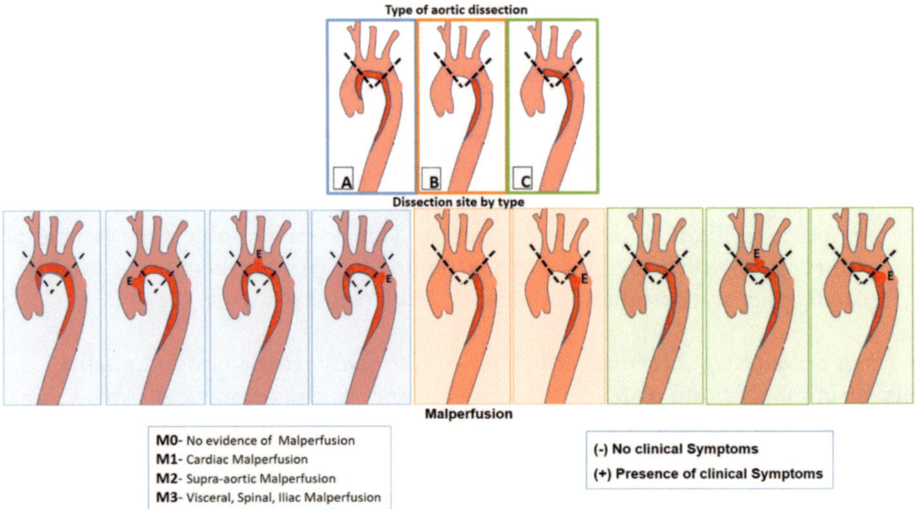

Figure 2.
TEM classification in terms of the rupture of the intimal layer of the aorta, they are classified as follows: E0—No entry tear identified; E1—Entry tear in the ascending aorta between the aortic valve and proximal to the brachiocephalic trunk; E2—Entry tear in the aortic arch between the brachiocephalic trunk and the left subclavian artery; E3—Entry tear in the descending aorta distal to the left subclavian artery.

The surgical management of AD is heavily dependent on several factors, including the extent of the dissection, the location of the primary inflow rupture, and the presence of compromised organ perfusion. There is a significant need for a precise classification system that integrates various imaging modalities with interpretation and treatment strategies. The introduction of the TEM classification has notably advanced these efforts, particularly by enhancing the utility of ultrasound in this context.

The primary therapeutic objective in AD is to exclude the primary lesion from circulation, which can be achieved through surgical resection or alternative methods such as transcatheter procedures. This decision critically influences the presence or absence of malperfusion.

The TEM classification system was developed to provide a more accurate and comprehensive assessment of the disease complexity and patient classification in AD. This system not only enhances the understanding of disease mechanisms but also aids in making informed decisions regarding the extent of surgical intervention and prognosis prediction. As illustrated in **Figure 1**, the classification of malperfusion is as follows:

- *M0*: No radiological or clinical evidence of malperfusion.

- *M1*: Cardiac malperfusion, characterized by dissection involving at least one main coronary artery, with or without evidence of ischemia (M1+ or M1-), such as electrocardiographic changes or elevated serum cardiac enzymes.

- *M2*: Supra-aortic malperfusion, involving dissection of at least one supra-aortic vessel or collapse of the true lumen of the aortic arch, with or without clinical symptoms of cerebral malperfusion (e.g., stroke) or upper limb malperfusion (e.g., pulse deficit, pain, pallor, paresthesia).

- *M3*: Visceral or lower limb malperfusion, characterized by dissection involving at least one visceral, renal, or iliac artery, or collapse of the true lumen of the aorta, leading to functional closure of at least one descending visceral, renal, or iliac artery. This may occur with or without clinical symptoms of cerebral (e.g., stroke) or upper limb malperfusion (e.g., pulse deficit, pain, pallor, paresthesia), or symptoms related to descending iliac artery involvement, such as intestinal ischemia (e.g., abdominal pain, ileus, bloody diarrhea), renal dysfunction (e.g., anuria, signs of renal failure), or poor perfusion of the lower limbs (e.g., pulse deficit, pain, pallor, paresthesia).

In our most recent study, titled *Correlation Between Echocardiographic Variables and TEM Classification in Aortic Dissection*, we demonstrated that the Global Longitudinal Strain (GLS) echocardiographic myocardial deformation technique is a reliable parameter for assessing myocardial malperfusion, providing greater accuracy compared to electrocardiographic changes, which may not always be apparent. Our findings revealed a strong correlation between GLS and poor perfusion in the E1 and M1-, E1 and M1- Bi, and E2 and M2+ categories (**Figure 3**).

Similarly, we demonstrated a strong correlation between biomarkers of vascular serum dysfunction, such as smooth muscle myosin heavy chain (smMHC) and soluble endothelial cell adhesion molecule (sELAF), and the vascular Doppler ultrasound spectral profile, particularly through the pulsatility index. This index is a key parameter for assessing malperfusion in target organs distal to the heart (**Figure 4**).

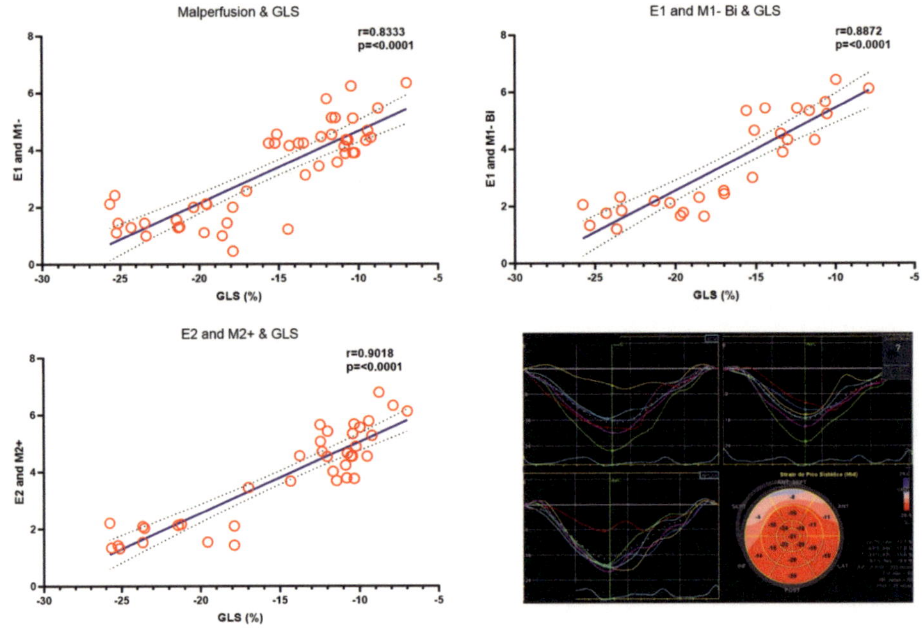

Figure 3.
E1 and M1-: Intimal layer rupture in the ascending aorta with cardiac malperfusion; E1 and M1- Bi: Intimal layer rupture in the ascending aorta with cardiac malperfusion and a bicuspid aortic valve; E2 and M2+: Aortic arch rupture with evidence of supra-aortic malperfusion.

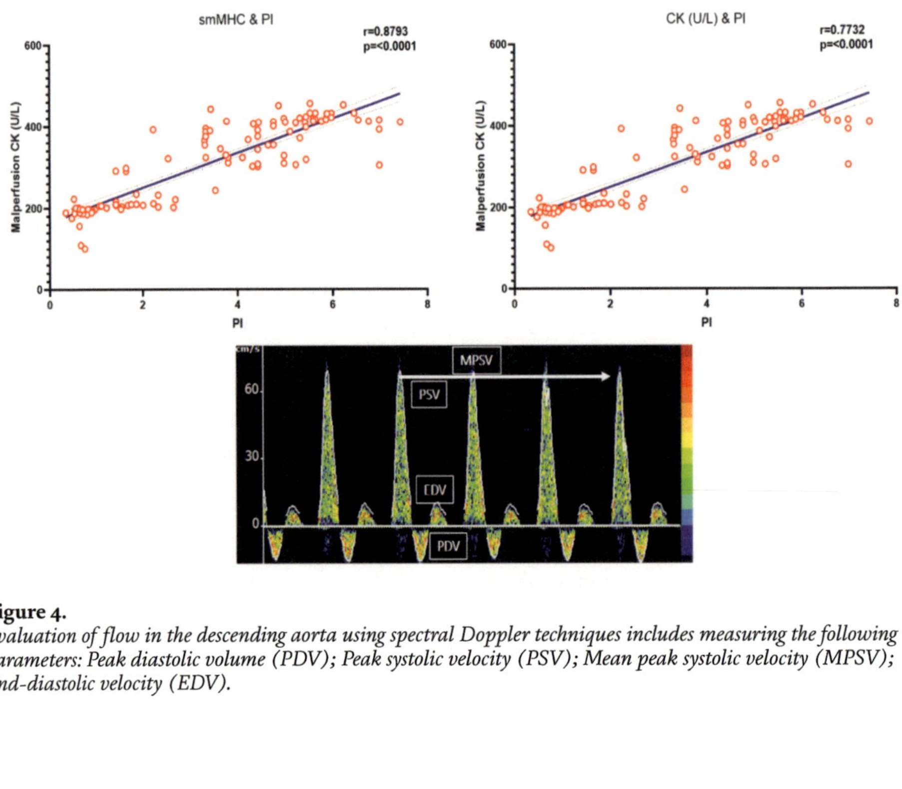

Figure 4.
Evaluation of flow in the descending aorta using spectral Doppler techniques includes measuring the following parameters: Peak diastolic volume (PDV); Peak systolic velocity (PSV); Mean peak systolic velocity (MPSV); End-diastolic velocity (EDV).

Thus, this new finding underscores the value of the TEM classification as an invaluable tool for the comprehensive assessment of aortic dissection. It extends beyond simple anatomical evaluation and surgical feasibility studies to encompass predictions of surgical outcomes and potential postoperative complications. Its capacity to integrate various diagnostic modalities highlights its crucial role in guiding clinical decision-making and enhancing patient management strategies.

3.1 Dop echocardiographic technique for assessing myocardial malperfusion in aortic dissection

The following outlines a technique for assessing myocardial deformation using speckle tracking. Given that aortic dissection is a rare and emergency condition, and because ultrasound is inherently technique-dependent and susceptible to various errors, it is crucial that all echocardiographic images are collected prospectively. This approach ensures optimal image quality and consistency by having the same certified ultrasound examiner conduct all assessments. In our study, images used to evaluate deformation caused by myocardial malperfusion before and after surgical repair were acquired using a GE Vivid E95 ultrasound system. The images were recorded with electrocardiogram (ECG) tracings over at least three consecutive cardiac cycles. All images were obtained at a frame rate of 55–90 frames per second and subsequently reviewed offline using EchoPac software (version 112, GE Vingmed Ultrasound AS), in accordance with the recommended guidelines [45].

Myocardial deformation in the presence of perfusion deficits was assessed using two-dimensional deformation analysis based on the three apical views of the left ventricle (LV). Whenever feasible, the second of the three cardiac cycles acquired was selected for analysis. Strain measurements were derived from the "full thickness" (or meso) of the myocardium, and final systolic values were recorded, excluding post-systolic strain measurements. The reference time point was manually established at the onset of the QRS complex. End-systole was defined as the moment of aortic valve closure, identified through the Doppler velocity signal in the LV outflow tract while measuring LV global longitudinal strain (GLS). The LV was segmented into 18 segments according to the methodology described by Voigt et al. [46].

3.2 Doppler vascular ultrasound

Recent advancements in vascular ultrasound technology now enable the assessment of hemodynamic profiles using Doppler techniques. This capability facilitates the documentation of blood flow quality, allowing for the identification of variables indicative of potential hemodynamic impairment and arterial contractility [47–49]. This tool permits the comprehensive mapping of blood flow profiles, including peak systolic velocity, end-diastolic flow, PI, and RI, thereby providing valuable insights into both the quantity and quality of blood flow over specific time intervals [50, 51].

In our recent study, significant differences were observed in arterial compliance following AD surgery when assessed distally in the region of the dissected artery. Initially, Doppler spectrum images of these arteries displayed a triphasic morphology with high pulsatility, characterized by narrow systolic peaks, flow reversal at the onset of diastole, and the absence of flow at the end of diastole (**Figure 5**). After

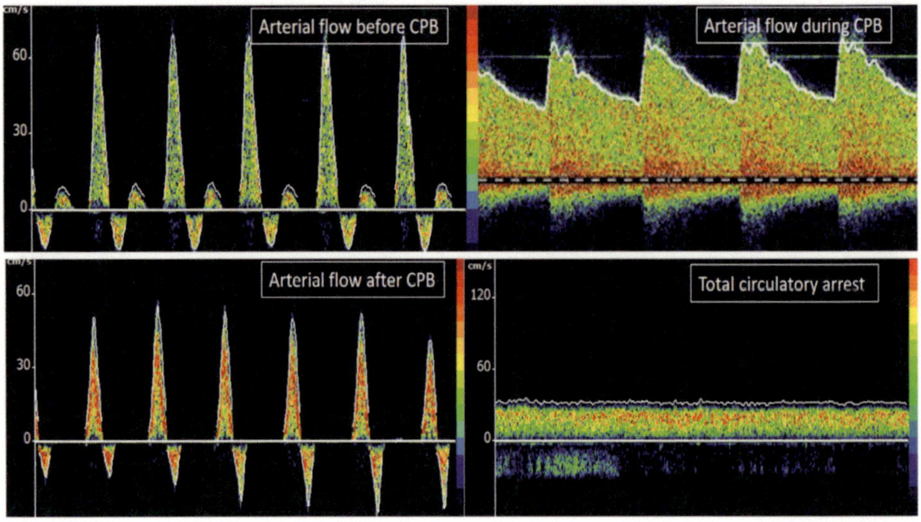

Figure 5.
Blood flow pattern. Before during and after aortic dissection surgery.

cardiopulmonary bypass (CPB), the flow pattern transitioned to a biphasic configuration, marked by reduced pulsatility, broad systolic peaks, and the absence of end-diastolic flow (**Figure 5**).

It is crucial to note the impact of these flow patterns. Although patients initially exhibited an arterial flow pattern, during CPB, the pump flow is continuous. During the dissection procedure, with the induction of deep hypothermia, arterial compliance, and hemodynamic functions must be preserved to facilitate the surgeon's activities in non-bleeding vessels (**Figure 5**).

For the sake of scientific reproducibility, vascular function ultrasound was performed using the same equipment employed to assess myocardial deformation, as previously described. Continuous wave Doppler spectral profile mapping was acquired from the suprasternal window, enabling assessment of the flow profile in the ascending aorta. To achieve this, the patient was positioned supine, and the transducer was placed superior to the manubrium of the sternum. The probe's index marker should be oriented toward the left shoulder, with the face of the transducer positioned nearly parallel to the neck. This approach provides an anatomical view of the ascending aorta, the aortic arch, and the proximal segments of the descending aorta. The subcostal window is optimal for analyzing the thoracic aorta.

In all cases, it is essential to correct the angle of incidence of the ultrasound beams. Adjusting the angle to align the ultrasound beams with the flow direction is crucial for accurately capturing and processing the signals. This facilitates the quantification of blood flow parameters, such as peak systolic velocity (PSV), resistivity index (RI), and pulsatility index (PI), along with temporal characterization.

4. Deep hypothermic circulatory arrest in aortic dissection surgery

Cooling the body, referred to as hypothermia, is a valuable technique in heart surgery. There are four levels of hypothermia: mild, moderate, deep, and profound. While deep hypothermia typically involves cooling the body to temperatures below

28°C, in cardiac surgery, it is often achieved at temperatures below 20°C 50. Deep hypothermia is employed not only to facilitate the surgical procedure but primarily to protect the brain and vital organs from ischemic damage resulting from interrupted blood flow. By slowing metabolic processes, deep hypothermia reduces the demand for oxygen and energy, thereby making it safer to temporarily halt blood circulation during cardiac surgery. Despite its long history, deep hypothermia remains a critical component of certain heart surgeries [52].

Understanding the physiological and mechanistic complexities of hypothermia is challenging due to the involvement of intricate systemic and cellular processes. The benefits of hypothermia during CPB are based on the hypothesis that the duration of safe circulatory arrest is inversely related to body temperature. In this context, "safe" refers to a period of circulatory arrest during which no detrimental effects are observed on the structure and function of internal organs, particularly the brain, which is highly vulnerable to ischemia [53].

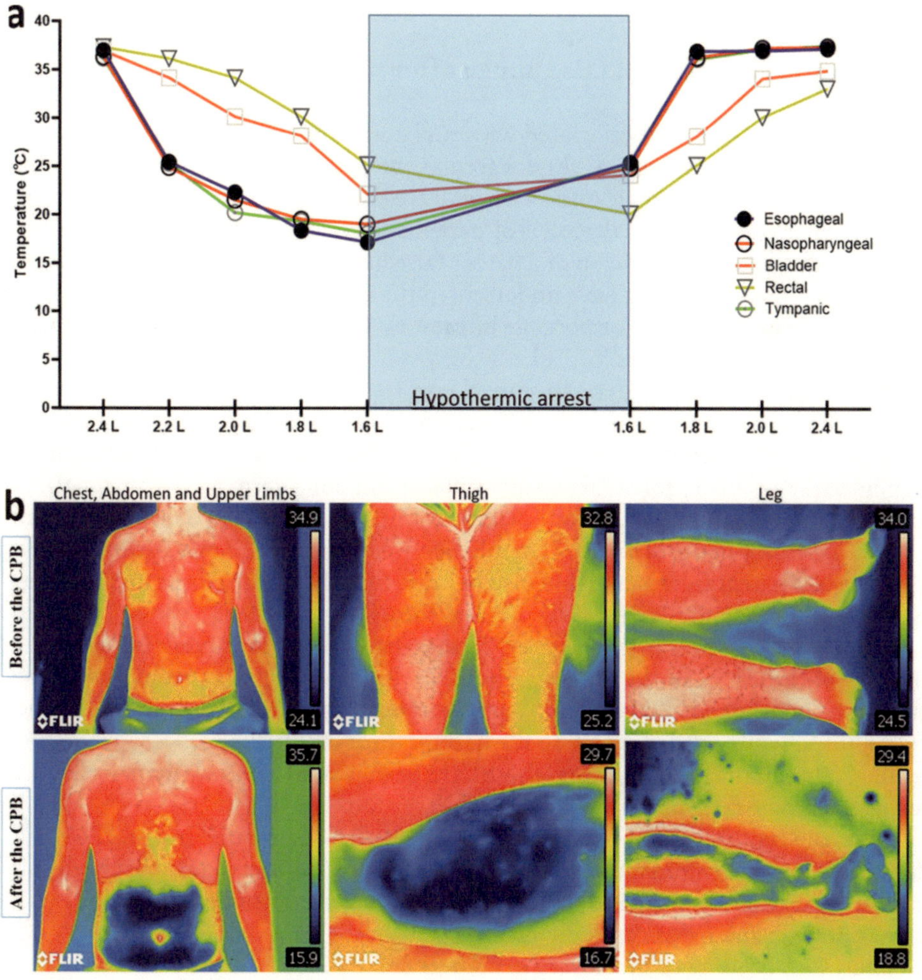

Figure 6.
(a) Graphical summary depicting the temperature drop using different thermometers and the flow adjustment of the centrifugal pump in liters (L). (b) Thermographic image showing body temperature before and after CPB.

In our most recent study, we demonstrated a thermal disparity when comparing different temperature measurement sites during the rewarming phase in patients undergoing AD surgery. Specifically, esophageal, nasopharyngeal, and tympanic thermometers exhibited significantly faster cooling and rewarming rates compared to rectal and bladder thermometers (**Figure 6a**). This discrepancy can initially be attributed to the lower temperatures recorded by the latter, which may be influenced by factors such as fecal matter in the rectal region, creating an inhomogeneous thermal environment, and the humid conditions in the bladder due to urine excretion.

However, our results extend beyond the traditional analysis of temperature using conventional parameters. Segmental mapping with a thermographic machine, as depicted in **Figure 6b**, corroborates the temperatures observed in the bladder and rectal regions, indicating that cooling and rewarming processes in these areas are indeed slower. This slower response may be influenced by factors such as the density of surrounding organs and tissues, vascular compliance, and the distance between these deeper sites and the primary heat sources, such as the heart or the continuous flow pump used in CPB.

5. The fate of the residual false lumen after surgery

The high mortality rate associated with surgical therapy has prompted research into alternative approaches [54]. Endovascular therapy has emerged as a viable option for patients with type B aortic dissection who are too unstable for traditional surgery [55]. Recent studies indicate that 12% of patients experience mortality after aortic AD repair due to the progression of a patent false lumen [56]. Consequently, advancements in diagnostic imaging have underscored the importance of postsurgical patient care, including monitoring for possible intramural hemorrhage, aneurysm formation, and penetrating aortic ulcers [57, 58].

It is crucial to recognize that the clinical progression of the residual false lumen can vary among different types of aortic dissection. Therefore, rigorous assessment using echocardiography is essential to mitigate the risk of false lumen progression. This highlights the necessity for stringent surveillance and long-term follow-up to evaluate surgical outcomes and monitor the potential advancement of the patent false lumen.

Routine assessments of arterial compliance are imperative, not only due to the presence of a patent false lumen but also because the AD surgery itself involves deep hypothermic circulatory arrest (DHCA) and the use of CPB [59].

In one of our case reports, we observed that many patients undergoing surgery are unaware of the extent of the false lumen, particularly when it is a chronic condition that has been deferred. Consequently, some surgical strategies merely aim to replace the ruptured vessel while relying on the natural thrombolization process of the residual false lumen. Furthermore, there have been instances where cannulation was performed in the false lumen rather than the true lumen.

Thus, the rupture region may remain undetected, as illustrated by the TEM classification, where nomenclature E0 indicates double ruptures. As a result, despite extensive surgical repair, the residual false lumen may progress and potentially develop into an aneurysm, as depicted in **Figure** 7.

Thus, CPB becomes a "necessary evil," particularly in AD surgery involving deep hypothermic circulatory arrest (DHCA). The most common alterations include metabolic and respiratory changes induced by oxidative stress, which results from the exposure of blood to non-endothelial surfaces, as well as the state of hyperexcitation

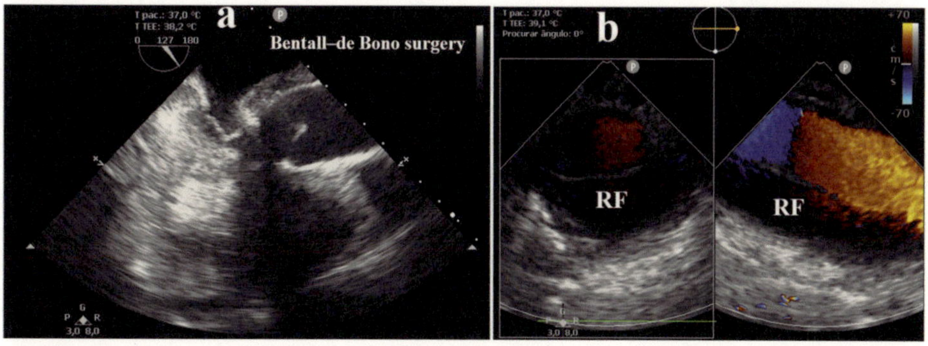

Figure 7.
(a) Bentall-De Bono aortic dissection surgery. (b) Six months later, the patient was admitted with chest pain and a suspicion of aortic aneurysms. Upon examination, it was discovered that the patent false lumen had not thrombosed and remained active.

itself [60–62]. These metabolic and perfusion deficiencies during CPB typically manifest at the vascular level. Consequently, variations in the expression and activity of nitric oxide synthase (NOS) and cyclooxygenase (COX) can influence coronary and peripheral vasomotor tone both during and after CPB [52, 63]. In addition to endothelial mechanisms, blood flow regulation is also governed by metabolic, autonomic, and myogenic mechanisms, which are primarily intrinsic characteristics of vascular smooth muscle [64].

The standard surgical approach for repairing AD typically involves replacing the aorta with a synthetic graft. This procedure often includes hypothermic circulatory arrest and selective antegrade cerebral perfusion, along with non-pulsatile flow provided by CPB pumps [65, 66]. These surgical interventions can potentially impact systemic vascular compliance and wettability. Consequently, parameters such as the PI and RI, along with the cardio-ankle vascular index (CAVI), could serve as alternative tools for monitoring patients following AD surgery.

The CAVI is a relatively recent addition to diagnostic methodologies. Originally characterized as a measure of arterial stiffness, it has evolved into a direct indicator of arterial distensibility and is now used as an independent predictor of prognostic outcomes in patients with cardiovascular disease. The CAVI enables assessment of the arterial tree from the aortic origin to the ankle [67, 68]. The index is calculated based on parameters related to arterial distensibility, which are assessed using 2D vascular ultrasound images (intraluminal volemia) and the Bramwell-Hill formula. The heart-ankle pulse wave velocity (haPWV) is determined by dividing the length (L) from the aorta to the ankle by the time (T) the pulse wave takes to travel from the aortic valve to the ankle, as illustrated in **Figure 8.**

5.1 Adverse postsurgical effects in aortic dissection

As previously highlighted, stress on the arterial walls is a defining feature of AD. Consequently, CPB is often employed during AD surgeries. The term "CPB is a necessary evil" underscores both the critical role and the inherent challenges associated with this technique. Despite its necessity, CPB is linked to significant morbidity, including complications in the pulmonary, renal, neurological, and gastrointestinal systems. Although there have been notable advancements, the primary drawbacks of CPB persist, mainly due to the adverse systemic effects triggered by inflammatory responses.

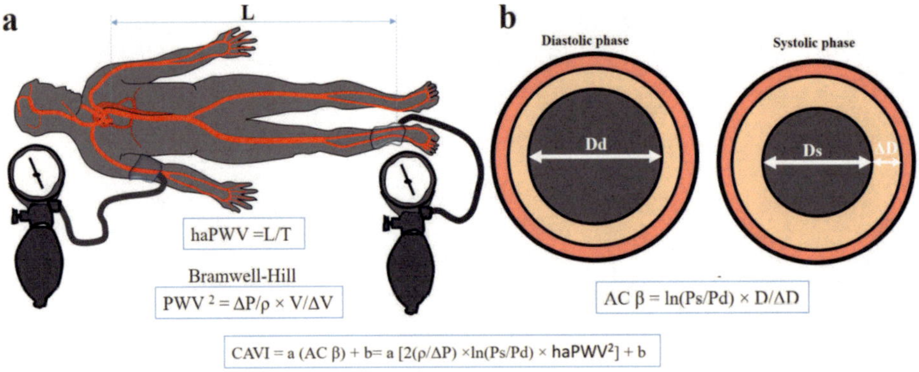

Figure 8.
(a) Illustration of pulse velocity measurement from the heart to the ankle and its respective formula (pulse wave velocity—PWV) and the corresponding Bramwell-Hill formula used to calculate pulse wave velocity (PWV). (b) Measurement of intraluminal volemia obtained by ultrasound, normally used in the aorta and carotid arteries. The combination of the two formulas makes the CAVI index a variable for screening systemic vascular resistance.

The substantial generation of reactive oxygen species (ROS) from the interaction of blood with artificial surfaces leads to a pathophysiological reaction akin to post-traumatic shock, known as post-perfusion syndrome [69, 70]. This syndrome can evolve into systemic inflammatory response syndrome, adult respiratory distress syndrome, sepsis, and ultimately result in multiple organ failure [71].

Furthermore, inflammatory responses during CPB are exacerbated by factors such as hypothermia, ischemia-reperfusion injury, endotoxemia, and the inherent surgical trauma, which activate various cellular and humoral components of the immune system [72, 73]. To address these issues, several strategies have been developed to mitigate inflammatory responses following cardiac surgery. These strategies include pharmacological interventions as well as modifications to surgical techniques and equipment. In our most recent study, we demonstrated that the use of methylene blue in patients undergoing AD surgery significantly reduces inflammatory responses, with noticeable effects observed within 24 hours (**Figure 9**).

The cascade of systemic inflammatory responses observed during CPB resembles that seen in sepsis. Patients undergoing CPB typically require prolonged ventilatory support, experience elevated postoperative bleeding, and exhibit increased capillary permeability. These conditions result in fluid shifts and the failure of multiple organs, primarily affecting the lungs, kidneys, and central nervous system.

The complex inflammatory responses during CPB arise from various factors, including the non-endothelial lining of the pump tubing, the detrimental effects of spilled pericardial blood, the cardiotomy reservoir, and blood-air interfaces. Additional contributors include significant temperature fluctuations, ischemia-reperfusion injury, complement activation, neutrophil activation with degranulation and proteolytic enzyme release, production of oxygen-derived free radicals, exposure to endotoxins, and the release of cytokines, nitric oxide, endothelin, and platelet-activating factor. Collectively, these factors contribute to a persistent and exacerbated inflammatory syndrome.

Although scientific evidence supporting the use of methylene blue (MB) is limited, it is notable that this aniline-based organic dye was originally employed for coloring and microorganism inactivation. By the late nineteenth century, it was recognized that high doses of MB could disrupt nerve fiber functions and was used as an antimalarial, for rheumatic diseases, and as a neuroleptic. As research progressed, MB

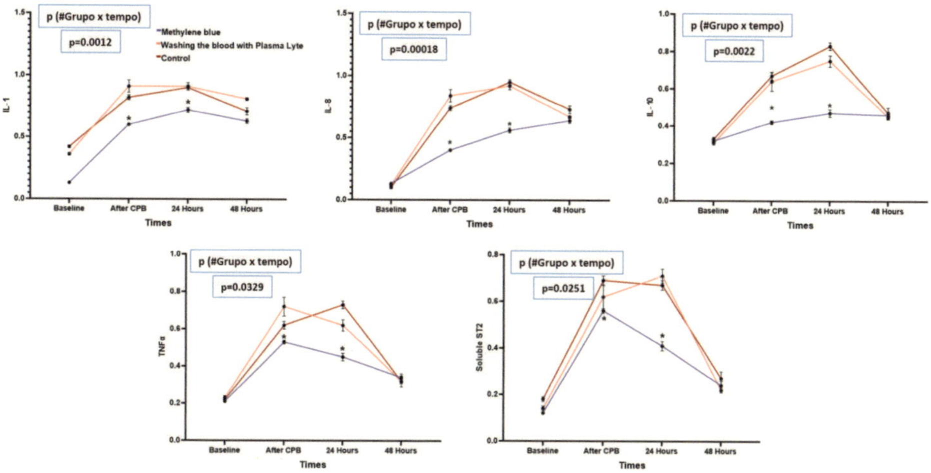

Figure 9.
Effect of methylene blue on reducing inflammatory responses to blood washing Lyte plasma was used during zero balance ultrafiltration.

was explored for its potential benefits in sepsis, shock refractory to vasoactive drugs, Alzheimer's disease, and as an antioxidant in cosmetics. Currently, its primary labeled indication is the treatment of methemoglobinemia. Our latest study has demonstrated its efficacy in mitigating sepsis following AD surgery.

6. Conclusions

In summary, AD is a life-threatening condition with severe complications. Accurate diagnosis demands a high level of clinical suspicion, as symptom variability can lead to dissection being missed in up to 39% of cases. AD is more common among the elderly, particularly those with a history of chronic hypertension. This chapter demonstrates that the TEM classification system is robust and serves as an effective tool for identifying the anatomical location of aortic rupture and associated malperfusion. This classification aids in predicting adjacent lesions related to reduced myocardial and distal perfusion, thereby guiding intervention strategies, evaluating intervention success, and anticipating potential post-intervention complications.

Doppler ultrasound of the descending aorta is presented as an excellent screening method for assessing distal malperfusion. Transesophageal echocardiography should be routinely performed in the operating room to prevent cannulation of the false lumen, which can occur when the false lumen is cannulated instead of the true lumen. Additionally, it should be included in the follow-up care of patients, particularly those with chronic conditions such as diabetes and hypertension. Finally, our findings indicate that surgery is associated with significant oxidative stress-related complications, and methylene blue appears to effectively mitigate these effects.

Acknowledgements

My heartfelt appreciation goes to Professor Minna Morreira Dias Romanos for her invaluable guidance and for granting me access to the echocardiography laboratory, where I could utilize various teaching tools without constraints. Furthermore, I am grateful for her extensive expertise in echocardiographic techniques and her insights into cardiology as a cardiologist.

Conflict of interest

The authors declare no conflict of interest.

Author details

André Timóteo Sapalo[1,2,3,4]

1 Department of Rehabilitation and Functional Performance, Health Sciences from the Ribeirão Preto Medical School of the University of São Paulo, Brazil

2 Extracorporeal Circulation and Mechanical Cardiac Assistance, Department of Surgery and Anatomy, Faculty of Medicine, Hospital das Clínicas, Brazil

3 Cardiology from the Postgraduate Program in Clinical Medicine, Echocardiography Laboratory at the Hospital das Clínicas, Faculty of Medicine, University of São Paulo, Brazil

4 The Medical Emergencies Division of the Graduate Program in Clinical Medicine at the University of São Paulo Medical School, Brazil

*Address all correspondence to: sapalo@usp.br

References

[1] Pagni S, Ganzel BL, Trivedi JR, Singh R, Mascio CE, Austin EH, et al. Early and midterm outcomes following surgery for acute type A aortic dissection. Journal of Cardiac Surgery. 2013;**28**(5):543-549. DOI: 10.1111/jocs.12170. Epub 2013 Aug 2

[2] Andersen ND, Ganapathi AM, Hanna JM, Williams JB, Gaca JG, Hughes GC. Outcomes of acute type a dissection repair before and after implementation of a multidisciplinary thoracic aortic surgery program. Journal of the American College of Cardiology. 2014;**63**(17):1796-1803. DOI: 10.1016/j.jacc.2013.10.085. Epub 2014 Jan 8

[3] Geirsson A, Ahlsson A, Franco-Cereceda A, Fuglsang S, Gunn J, Hansson EC, et al. Hospital volumes and later year of operation correlates with better outcomes in acute type A aortic dissection. European Journal of Cardio-Thoracic Surgery. 2018;**53**(1):276-281. DOI: 10.1093/ejcts/ezx231

[4] Criado FJ. Aortic dissection: A 250-year perspective. Texas Heart Institute Journal. 2011;**38**(6):694-700

[5] Grommes J, Greiner A, Bendermacher B, Erlmeier M, Frech A, Belau P, et al. Risk factors for mortality and failure of conservative treatment after aortic type B dissection. The Journal of Thoracic and Cardiovascular Surgery. 2014;**148**(5):2155-2160.e1. DOI: 10.1016/j.jtcvs.2014.03.053. Epub 2014 Apr 4

[6] Pape LA, Awais M, Woznicki EM, Suzuki T, Trimarchi S, Evangelista A, et al. Presentation, diagnosis, and outcomes of acute aortic dissection: 17-year trends from the international registry of acute aortic dissection. Journal of the American College of Cardiology. 2015;**66**(4):350-358. DOI: 10.1016/j.jacc.2015.05.029

[7] Evangelista A, Isselbacher EM, Bossone E, Gleason TG, Eusanio MD, Sechtem U, et al. Insights from the international registry of acute aortic dissection: A 20-year experience of collaborative clinical research. Circulation. 2018;**137**(17):1846-1860. DOI: 10.1161/CIRCULATIONAHA.117.031264

[8] NCD Risk Factor Collaboration (NCD-RisC). Worldwide trends in hypertension prevalence and progress in treatment and control from 1990 to 2019: A pooled analysis of 1201 population-representative studies with 104 million participants. Lancet. 2021;**398**(10304):957-980. DOI: 10.1016/S0140-6736(21)01330-1. Epub 2021 Aug 24. Erratum in: Lancet. 2022;399(10324):520. doi: 10.1016/S0140-6736(22)00061-7

[9] Sen I, Erben YM, Franco-Mesa C, DeMartino RR. Epidemiology of aortic dissection. Seminars in Vascular Surgery. 2021;**34**(1):10-17. DOI: 10.1053/j.semvascsurg.2021.02.003. Epub 2021 Feb 5

[10] De Martino A, Morganti R, Falcetta G, Scioti G, Milano AD, Pucci A, et al. Acute aortic dissection and pregnancy: Review and meta-analysis of incidence, presentation, and pathologic substrates. Journal of Cardiac Surgery. 2019;**34**(12):1591-1597. DOI: 10.1111/jocs.14305. Epub 2019 Nov 5

[11] Debakey ME, Henly WS, Cooley DA, Morris GC Jr, Crawford ES, Beall AC Jr. Surgical management of dissecting aneurysms of the aorta. The Journal of Thoracic and Cardiovascular Surgery. 1965;**49**:130-149

[12] Bachet JE, Termignon JL, Dreyfus G, Goudot B, Martinelli L, Piquois A, et al. Prevalence, cause, and results of late reoperations. The Journal of Thoracic and Cardiovascular Surgery. 1994;**108**(2):199-205; discussion 205-6

[13] Gawinecka J, Schönrath F, von Eckardstein A. Acute aortic dissection: Pathogenesis, risk factors and diagnosis. Swiss Medical Weekly. 2017;**147**:w14489. DOI: 10.4414/smw.2017.14489

[14] Stachenfeld NS. Acute effects of sodium ingestion on thirst and cardiovascular function. Current Sports Medicine Reports. 2008;**7**(4 Suppl):S7-S13. DOI: 10.1249/JSR.0b013e31817f23fc

[15] Magder S. Volume and its relationship to cardiac output and venous return. Critical Care. 2016;**20**(1):271. DOI: 10.1186/s13054-016-1438-7. Erratum in: Crit Care. 2017;21(1):16. doi: 10.1186/s13054-016-1571-3

[16] Narkiewicz K, Grassi G. Impaired baroreflex sensitivity as a potential marker of cardiovascular risk in hypertension. Journal of Hypertension. 2008;**26**(7):1303-1304. DOI: 10.1097/HJH.0b013e328305e1a5

[17] Slivnick J, Lampert BC. Hypertension and heart failure. Heart Failure Clinics. 2019;**15**(4):531-541. DOI: 10.1016/j.hfc.2019.06.007. Epub 2019 Jul 31

[18] Kreimeier U. Pathophysiology of fluid imbalance. Critical Care. 2000;**4**(Suppl_2):S3-S7. DOI: 10.1186/cc968. Epub 2000 Oct 13

[19] Dull RO, Hahn RG. Hypovolemia with peripheral edema: What is wrong? Critical Care. 2023;**27**(1):206. DOI: 10.1186/s13054-023-04496-5

[20] Safar ME, Jankowski P. Central blood pressure and hypertension: Role in cardiovascular risk assessment. Clinical Science (London, England). 2009;**116**(4):273-282. DOI: 10.1042/CS20080072

[21] Pandey KN. Emerging roles of natriuretic peptides and their receptors in pathophysiology of hypertension and cardiovascular regulation. Journal of the American Society of Hypertension. 2008;**2**(4):210-226. DOI: 10.1016/j.jash.2008.02.001

[22] Sarzani R, Spannella F, Giulietti F, Balietti P, Cocci G, Bordicchia M. Cardiac natriuretic peptides, hypertension and cardiovascular risk. High Blood Pressure and Cardiovascular Prevention. 2017;**24**(2):115-126. DOI: 10.1007/s40292-017-0196-1. Epub 2017 Apr 4

[23] Young DB, Pan YJ, Guyton AC. Control of extracellular sodium concentration by antidiuretic hormone-thirst feedback mechanism. The American Journal of Physiology. 1977;**232**(5):R145-R149. DOI: 10.1152/ajpregu.1977.232.5.R145

[24] Sica DA. Sodium and water retention in heart failure and diuretic therapy: Basic mechanisms. Cleveland Clinic Journal of Medicine. 2006;**73**(Suppl_2):S2-S7; discussion S30-3. DOI: 10.3949/ccjm.73.suppl_2.s2

[25] Siegal EM. Acute aortic dissection. Journal of Hospital Medicine. 2006;**1**(2):94-105. DOI: 10.1002/jhm.69

[26] Yap CH, Saikrishnan N, Yoganathan AP. Experimental measurement of dynamic fluid shear stress on the ventricular surface of the aortic valve leaflet. Biomechanics and Modeling in Mechanobiology. 2012;**11**(1-2):231-244. DOI: 10.1007/s10237-011-0306-2. Epub 2011 Apr 5

[27] Kiema M, Sarin JK, Kauhanen SP, Torniainen J, Matikka H, Luoto ES,

et al. Wall shear stress predicts media degeneration and biomechanical changes in thoracic aorta. Frontiers in Physiology. 2022;**13**:934941. DOI: 10.3389/fphys.2022.934941

[28] Malik ZM, Lau C, Skubas NJ. Aortic dissection: True or false? A and A Practice. 2018;**11**(5):140-143. DOI: 10.1213/XAA.0000000000000748

[29] Carrel T, Sundt TM 3rd, von Kodolitsch Y, Czerny M. Acute aortic dissection. Lancet. 2023;**401**(10378): 773-788. DOI: 10.1016/S0140-6736(22)01970-5. Epub 2023 Jan 11

[30] White A, Bozso SJ, Ouzounian M, Chu MWA, Moon MC, Canadian Thoracic Aortic Collaborative. Acute type A aortic dissection and the consequences of a patent false lumen. JTCVS Techniques. 2021;**9**:1-8. DOI: 10.1016/j.xjtc.2021.05.002

[31] Figueiredo VN, Yugar-Toledo JC, Martins LC, Martins LB, de Faria AP, de Haro MC, et al. Vascular stiffness and endothelial dysfunction: Correlations at different levels of blood pressure. Blood Pressure. 2012;**21**(1):31-38. DOI: 10.3109/08037051.2011.617045. Epub 2011 Oct 27

[32] Correia ML, Haynes WG. Arterial compliance and endothelial function. Current Diabetes Reports. 2007;**7**(4):269-275. DOI: 10.1007/s11892-007-0043-1

[33] Rajagopalan S, Meng XP, Ramasamy S, Harrison DG, Galis ZS. Reactive oxygen species produced by macrophage-derived foam cells regulate the activity of vascular matrix metalloproteinases in vitro. Implications for atherosclerotic plaque stability. The Journal of Clinical Investigation. 1996;**98**(11):2572-2579. DOI: 10.1172/JCI119076

[34] Li PF, Dietz R, von Harsdorf R. Reactive oxygen species induce apoptosis of vascular smooth muscle cell. FEBS Letters. 1997;**404**(2-3):249-252. DOI: 10.1016/s0014-5793(97)00093-8

[35] Green D. Coagulation cascade. Hemodialysis International. 2006;**10**(Suppl. 2):S2-S4. DOI: 10.1111/j.1542-4758.2006.00119.x

[36] Schenone M, Furie BC, Furie B. The blood coagulation cascade. Current Opinion in Hematology. 2004;**11**(4):272-277. DOI: 10.1097/01.moh.0000130308.37353.d4

[37] Hoffman M. Remodeling the blood coagulation cascade. Journal of Thrombosis and Thrombolysis. 2003;**16**(1-2):17-20. DOI: 10.1023/B:THRO.0000014588.95061.28

[38] Johari V, Loke C. Brief overview of the coagulation cascade. Disease-a-Month. 2012;**58**(8):421-423. DOI: 10.1016/j.disamonth.2012.04.004

[39] Palta S, Saroa R, Palta A. Overview of the coagulation system. Indian Journal of Anaesthesia. 2014;**58**(5):515-523. DOI: 10.4103/0019-5049.144643

[40] Carmeliet P, Collen D. Molecular analysis of blood vessel formation and disease. The American Journal of Physiology. 1997;**273**(5):H2091-H2104. DOI: 10.1152/ajpheart.1997.273.5.H2091

[41] Reitsma SE, Pang J, Raghunathan V, Shatzel JJ, Lorentz CU, Tucker EI, et al. Role of platelets in regulating activated coagulation factor XI activity. American Journal of Physiology. Cell Physiology. 2021;**320**(3):C365-C374. DOI: 10.1152/ajpcell.00056.2020. Epub 2021 Jan 20

[42] Vandvik PO, Lincoff AM, Gore JM, Gutterman DD, Sonnenberg FA, Alonso-Coello P, et al.

Primary and secondary prevention of cardiovascular disease: Antithrombotic therapy and prevention of thrombosis, 9th ed: American College of Chest Physicians Evidence-Based Clinical Practice Guidelines. Chest. 2012;**141**(2 Suppl):e637S-e668S. DOI: 10.1378/chest.11-2306. Erratum in: Chest. 2012 Apr;141(4):1129. Dosage error in article text

[43] Zindovic I, Sjögren J, Bjursten H, Ingemansson R, Ingimarsson J, Larsson M, et al. The coagulopathy of acute type A aortic dissection: A prospective, observational study. Journal of Cardiothoracic and Vascular Anesthesia. 2019;**33**(10):2746-2754. DOI: 10.1053/j.jvca.2019.02.013. Epub 2019 Feb 11

[44] Sherk WM, Khaja MS, Williams DM. Anatomy, pathology, and classification of aortic dissection. Techniques in Vascular and Interventional Radiology. 2021;**24**(2):100746. DOI: 10.1016/j.tvir.2021.100746. Epub 2021 Jul 26

[45] Lang RM, Badano LP, Mor-Avi V, Afilalo J, Armstrong A, Ernande L, et al. Recommendations for cardiac chamber quantification by echocardiography in adults: An update from the American Society of Echocardiography and the European Association of Cardiovascular Imaging. European Heart Journal Cardiovascular Imaging. 2015;**16**(3):233-270. DOI: 10.1093/ehjci/jev014. Erratum in: Eur Heart J Cardiovasc Imaging. 2016;17(4):412. doi: 10.1093/ehjci/jew041. Erratum in: Eur Heart J Cardiovasc Imaging. 2016 Sep;17(9):969. doi: 10.1093/ehjci/jew124

[46] Voigt JU, Cvijic M. 2- and 3-dimensional myocardial strain in cardiac health and disease. JACC: Cardiovascular Imaging. 2019;**12**(9):1849-1863. DOI: 10.1016/j.jcmg.2019.01.044

[47] Battaglia S, Danesino GM, Danesino V, Castellani S. Color Doppler ultrasonography of the abdominal aorta. Journal of Ultrasound. 2010;**13**(3):107-117. DOI: 10.1016/j.jus.2010.10.001. Epub 2010 Oct 20

[48] Farthing S, Peronneau P. Flow in the thoracic aorta. Cardiovascular Research. 1979;**13**(11):607-620. DOI: 10.1093/cvr/13.11.607

[49] Martins FF, Bassani DG, Rios DI, Resende MHF, Weisz D, Jain A, et al. Relationship of patent ductus arteriosus echocardiographic markers with descending aorta diastolic flow. Journal of Ultrasound in Medicine. 2021;**40**(8):1505-1514. DOI: 10.1002/jum.15528. Epub 2020 Oct 12

[50] Belkin MN, Kalantari S, Kanelidis AJ, Miller T, Smith BA, Besser SA, et al. Aortic pulsatility index: A novel hemodynamic variable for evaluation of decompensated heart failure. Journal of Cardiac Failure. 2021;**27**(10):1045-1052. DOI: 10.1016/j.cardfail.2021.05.010. Epub 2021 May 25

[51] Boczar KE, Boodhwani M, Beauchesne L, Dennie C, Chan KL, Wells GA, et al. Aortic stiffness, central blood pressure, and pulsatile arterial load predict future thoracic aortic aneurysm expansion. Hypertension. 2021;**77**(1):126-134. DOI: 10.1161/HYPERTENSIONAHA.120.16249. Epub 2020 Nov 30

[52] Gocoł R, Hudziak D, Bis J, Mendrala K, Morkisz Ł, Podsiadło P, et al. The role of deep hypothermia in cardiac surgery. International Journal of Environmental Research and Public Health. 2021;**18**(13):7061. DOI: 10.3390/ijerph18137061

[53] Yan TD, Bannon PG, Bavaria J, Coselli JS, Elefteriades JA, Griepp RB, et al.

Consensus on hypothermia in aortic arch surgery. Annals of Cardiothoracic Surgery. 2013;**2**(2):163-168. DOI: 10.3978/j.issn.2225-319X.2013.03.03

[54] Abbasciano RG, Koulouroudias M, Chad T, Mohamed W, Leeman I, Pellowe C, et al. Role of hypothermia in adult cardiac surgery patients: A systematic review and meta-analysis. Journal of Cardiothoracic and Vascular Anesthesia. 2022;**36**(7):1883-1890. DOI: 10.1053/j.jvca.2022.01.026. Epub 2022 Jan 31

[55] Chiu P, Miller DC. Evolution of surgical therapy for Stanford acute type A aortic dissection. Annals of Cardiothoracic Surgery. 2016;**5**(4):275-295. DOI: 10.21037/acs.2016.05.05

[56] Mesar T, Lin MJ, Kabir I, Dexter DJ, Rathore A, Panneton JM. Medical therapy in type B aortic intramural hematoma is associated with a high failure rate. Journal of Vascular Surgery. 2020;**71**(4):1088-1096. DOI: 10.1016/j.jvs.2019.07.084. Epub 2020 Feb 13

[57] Li J, Zerdzitzki M, Camboni D, Floerchinger B, Unterbuchner C, Schmid C, et al. A decade of surgical therapy in an all-comer cohort with type A aortic dissection. The Journal of Cardiovascular Surgery. 2021;**62**(4):377-384. DOI: 10.23736/S0021-9509.21.11607-6. Epub 2021 Feb 10

[58] Carroll BJ, Schermerhorn ML, Manning WJ. Imaging for acute aortic syndromes. Heart. 2020;**106**(3):182-189. DOI: 10.1136/heartjnl-2019-314897. Epub 2019 Dec 10

[59] Rogers RK, Reece TB, Bonaca MP, Hess CN. Acute aortic syndromes. Cardiology Clinics. 2021;**39**(4):495-503. DOI: 10.1016/j.ccl.2021.06.002

[60] Ziganshin BA, Elefteriades JA. Deep hypothermic circulatory arrest. Annals of Cardiothoracic Surgery. 2013;**2**(3):303-315. DOI: 10.3978/j.issn.2225-319X.2013.01.05

[61] Haji-Jafari S, Rezaei M, Azizi-Fini I, Tafti SHA, Atoof F. The effect of rewarming on hemodynamic parameters and arterial blood gases of patients after open-heart surgery: A randomized controlled trial. Journal of Vascular Nursing. 2023;**41**(1):29-35. DOI: 10.1016/j.jvn.2023.01.003. Epub 2023 Jan 28

[62] McCullough JN, Zhang N, Reich DL, Juvonen TS, Klein JJ, Spielvogel D, et al. Cerebral metabolic suppression during hypothermic circulatory arrest in humans. The Annals of Thoracic Surgery. 1999;**67**(6):1895-1899; discussion 1919-21. DOI: 10.1016/s0003-4975(99)00441-5

[63] Norwood WI, Norwood CR. Influence of hypothermia on intracellular pH during anoxia. The American Journal of Physiology. 1982;**243**(1):C62-C65. DOI: 10.1152/ajpcell.1982.243.1.C62

[64] Jonas RA, Bellinger DC, Rappaport LA, Wernovsky G, Hickey PR, Farrell DM, et al. Relation of pH strategy and developmental outcome after hypothermic circulatory arrest. The Journal of Thoracic and Cardiovascular Surgery. 1993;**106**(2):362-368

[65] Mezrow CK, Midulla PS, Sadeghi AM, Gandsas A, Wang W, Dapunt OE, et al. Evaluation of cerebral metabolism and quantitative electroencephalography after hypothermic circulatory arrest and low-flow cardiopulmonary bypass at different temperatures. The Journal of Thoracic and Cardiovascular Surgery. 1994;**107**(4):1006-1019

[66] Jassar AS, Sundt TM 3rd. How should we manage type A aortic dissection? General Thoracic and

Cardiovascular Surgery. 2019;**67**(1):137-145. DOI: 10.1007/s11748-018-0957-3. Epub 2018 Jun 20

[67] De Viti D, Dambruoso P, Izzo P, Dhojniku I, Raimondo P, Carbone C, et al. Iatrogenic acute aortic dissection in the era of minimally invasive cardiac surgery—Experience of a center and review of literature. Brazilian Journal of Cardiovascular Surgery. 2021;**36**(5):691-699. DOI: 10.21470/1678-9741-2020-0561

[68] Miyoshi T, Ito H. Arterial stiffness in health and disease: The role of cardio-ankle vascular index. Journal of Cardiology. 2021;**78**(6):493-501. DOI: 10.1016/j.jjcc.2021.07.011. Epub 2021 Aug 12

[69] Namba T, Masaki N, Takase B, Adachi T. Arterial stiffness assessed by cardio-ankle vascular index. International Journal of Molecular Sciences. 2019;**20**(15):3664. DOI: 10.3390/ijms20153664

[70] Clermont G, Vergely C, Jazayeri S, Lahet JJ, Goudeau JJ, Lecour S, et al. Systemic free radical activation is a major event involved in myocardial oxidative stress related to cardiopulmonary bypass. Anesthesiology. 2002;**96**(1):80-87. DOI: 10.1097/00000542-200201000-00019

[71] Zakkar M, Guida G, Suleiman MS, Angelini GD. Cardiopulmonary bypass and oxidative stress. Oxidative Medicine and Cellular Longevity. 2015;**2015**:189863. DOI: 10.1155/2015/189863. Epub 2015 Feb 4

[72] Rubens FD, Mesana T. The inflammatory response to cardiopulmonary bypass: A therapeutic overview. Perfusion. 2004;**19**(Suppl. 1):S5-S12. DOI: 10.1191/0267659104pf717oa

[73] Day JR, Taylor KM. The systemic inflammatory response syndrome and cardiopulmonary bypass. International Journal of Surgery. 2005;**3**(2):129-140. DOI: 10.1016/j.ijsu.2005.04.002. Epub 2005 Aug 1

Chapter 7

Surgical Management of Aortic Dissection with Aortic Arch Involvement

Giulio Pellegrini, Lorenzo Terzano and Pier Luigi Stefàno

Abstract

The extent of aortic resection for aortic dissection is still debated. Although the resection and replacement of the aortic tract involved by the intimal tear remains the gold standard treatment, the fate and the evolution of the distal false lumen are hardly predictable. In recent years, several techniques and devices have been introduced to reduce the patency of the false lumen with consequent improvement of the positive remodeling of the true lumen, allowing the surgeon to perform a surgical strategy that is the most patient-tailored possible. This chapter aims to discuss hybrid strategies and new devices with related surgical techniques, with a brief literature review, to suggest a management protocol fitting each clinical and anatomical scenario.

Keywords: aortic dissection, hybrid approach, cerebral perfusion, malperfusion syndrome, aortic arch, false lumen fate

1. Introduction

Acute aortic dissection is a life-threatening condition that can represent a challenging situation for cardiac surgeons all around the world [1, 2]. Diagnosis, surgical treatment, and management of possible complications related to aortic dissection have always been the key points of this pathology. Above all, surgical treatment and management of aortic arch dissection represent the most challenging situation [3]. In this chapter, we propose a review of the recent literature on surgical treatment of the aortic arch. We described our experience with aortic arch dissection and evaluated a possible diagnostic and surgical protocol to use for the treatment of this disease.

1.1 Epidemiology and classification

Epidemiological data upon aortic dissection is not well defined. The majority of studies published are based on small populations or autoptic data [4]. For this reason, the true incidence of aortic dissection is not yet known [5, 6]. Looking at the International Registry of Aortic Dissection (IRAD), we can assume that the mean age of patients presenting with type A acute aortic dissection is 62 +/– 14.6 years with a significant difference between men and women (two-thirds of patients were men), a proportion that did not change over 17 years [7]. If we want to focus our attention on the aortic arch, described as the anatomical region identified between Ishimaru's zones 0–2 [8, 9], few studies have been published.

Historically, aortic dissections have always been classified upon two different classification systems: The DeBakey classification and The Stanford classification. DeBakey and his colleagues identified four different types of aortic dissections. Both types I and II originate from the ascending aorta, with Type II remaining confined to the ascending tract, while Type I extends into the arch and distal aorta. Type III dissections originate after the left subclavian artery, in the descending aorta, and run toward the diaphragm for type IIIA and type IIIB extending below it in the abdominal tract [10]. The Stanford classification made by Daily and colleagues classifies aortic dissections regardless of the anatomical location of the intimal tear. The focus is represented by the involvement of the ascending tract. If the ascending aorta is affected, we are talking about type A dissection. All other dissections, where the ascending tract of the aorta is not affected, as type B. This classification system has been most widely used due to its role in clinical decision-making process. Usually, type A dissections are treated in emergency with surgical procedures on ascending aorta. On the other hand, type B dissections usually need medical treatment focused on stabilization of the pathology and surgery is confined on treatment in case of emerging complications on the dissected tract of aorta [11, 12]. In both of previous classification (Stanford and De Bakey), the presence of an intimal flap engaging both the aortic arch and the descending aorta, without intimal disruption of the ascending aorta, has not been considered (**Figures 1** and **2**) [8].

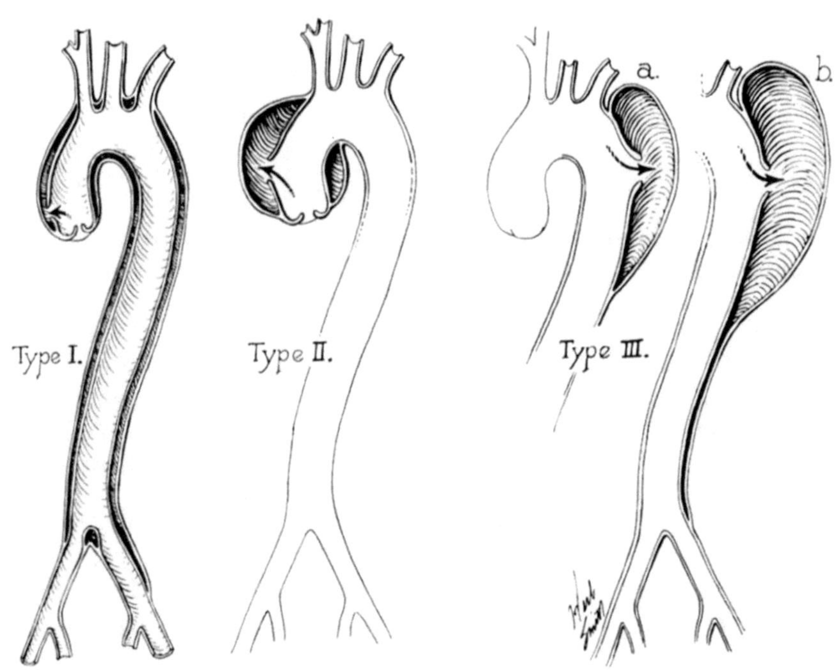

Figure 1.
De Bakey classification system.

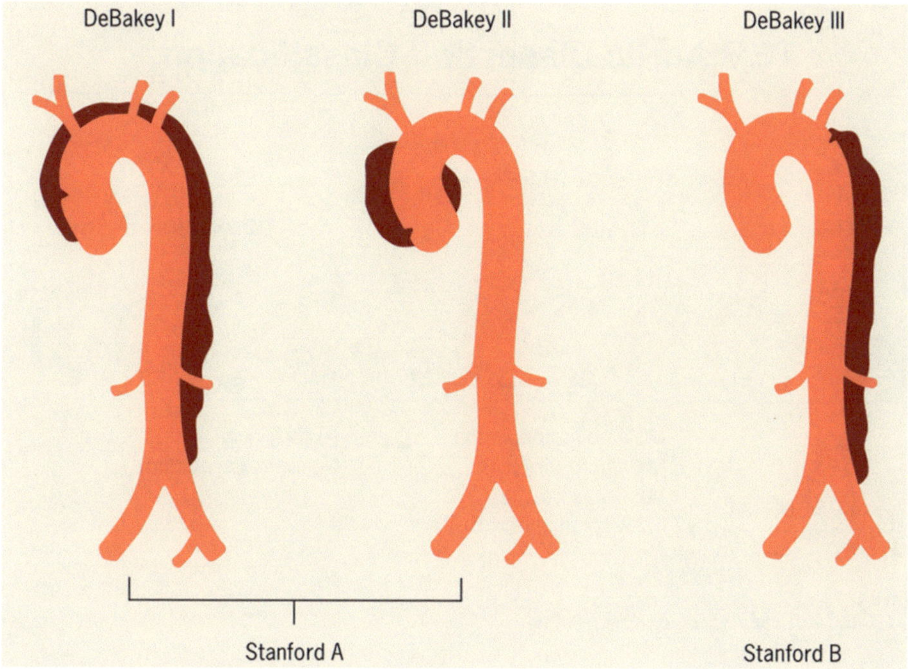

Figure 2.
Stanford classification system.

Recent literature and the most recent guidelines on the aorta tried to surpass these two systems and evaluate new ways to classify aortic dissection on a more clinical-based system [8]. Recently, the TEM (Tear, Entry, Malperfusion) classification, proposed by Sievers and colleagues, has been published. It differentiates from other classification systems by adding non-A non-B aortic dissection, first introduced by Von Segesser et al. [13] (**Figure 3**). Non-A Non-B dissections, which represent 10% of all acute aortic dissections [14], are defined as dissections with entry tear located in the descending aorta with retrograde progression into the aortic arch [13]. The location of the primary entry tear (E), which has a direct correlation with early clinical outcomes [2], and malperfusion (M) is a key point that needs to be considered in the decision-making process [15]. Different studies described that the location of entry intimal tear has a direct correlation with early surgical outcomes [14]. TEM classification has proved to be useful in clinical and surgical decision-making processes, giving additional anatomical information of the dissected tract, and focusing on organ malperfusion. These characteristics of the TEM classification system should help to decide the best surgical management of the patient and permit a correct prediction of early and late clinical outcomes. Because TEM clearly defines non-A non-B as a main category, it helps make quick clinical decisions in patients with acute dissections [15, 16]. There is currently no consensus regarding the best management of acute or subacute non-A non-B aortic dissection. In acute aortic dissection, isolated diseases of the aortic arch of any kind in adults are infrequent, as isolated surgical replacement [8]. Furthermore, if the surgical treatment of the dissected ascending aorta has been mostly standardized, the correct surgical management of the aortic arch, needed in 13–32% of ATAAD patients due to primary entry tear in Ishimaru's zones 1–2, is often center-related [17].

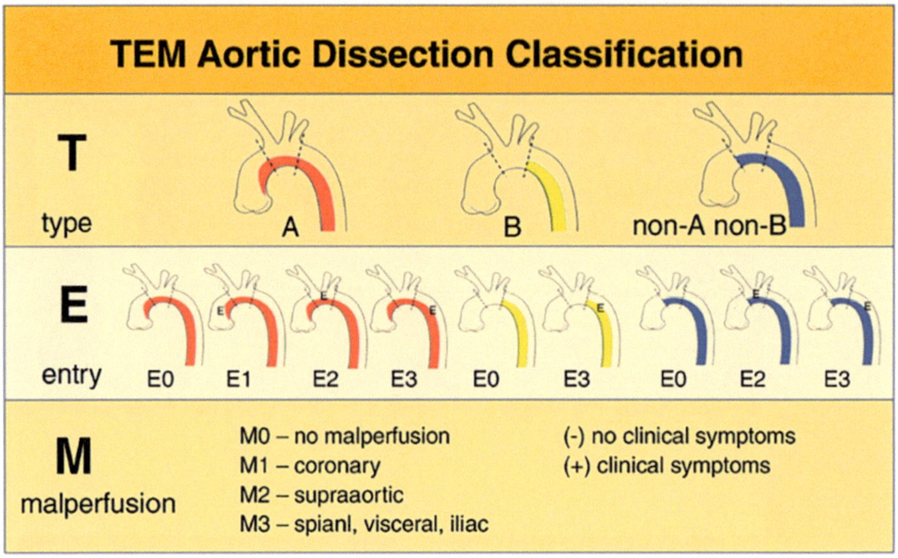

Figure 3.
TEM classification of acute aortic dissection [16].

1.2 Cerebral perfusion

Talking about aortic arch surgical treatment, a discussion about cerebral perfusion is needed. Different possibilities and techniques for cerebral protection have been proposed since the introduction of aortic arch procedures [17]. Surgical replacement of the aortic arch has become a surgical possibility, thanks to the implementation of hypothermia during circulatory arrest. The reduction of oxygen demand and metabolic activity guaranteed by lower body temperatures allows surgeon to temporarily stop circulation [14].

Referring to hypothermic circulatory arrest, the most recent EACTS guidelines on surgical treatment of the aorta redefined the correct terminology of hypothermic circulatory arrest. As it stands today, we must talk about (as reported in **Figure 4**):

- Deep hypothermia for temperature below 20°C
- Low-moderate hypothermia for temperature between 20.1 and 24°C
- High-moderate hypothermia for temperature between 24.1 and 28°C
- Mild hypothermia for temperature above 28°C [8]

Deep hypothermia permits a longer period of safe circulatory arrest, proved to be around 30 minutes, if compared to higher temperatures. In response to this longer safe period, several studies have shown that DHCA is correlated to a greater inflammatory response, greater risk of neurological damage, and higher mortality rates [18]. The first successful series of aortic arch surgical procedures using deep hypothermic circulatory arrest (DHCA) was reported in 1975 by Griepp et al. [19]. Since then, improvements and modifications have been made worldwide, ranging from Kazui [20], Bachet [21], and colleagues, who first introduced antegrade

TABLE 6 Writing Committee 2023 Consensus on Hypothermia Classification in Aortic Surgery

Category	Core Temperature (Rectal/Bladder)
Deep hypothermia	≤20°C
Low-moderate hypothermia	20.1-24°C
High-moderate hypothermia	24.1-28°C
Mild hypothermia	>28°C

Figure 4.
Definition of correct nomenclature for hypothermic circulatory arrest made by EACTS guidelines [8].

cerebral perfusion during the period of circulatory arrest, to the use of more moderate levels of hypothermia used nowadays. As it stands today, an optimal and consistent approach worldwide is still missing [20, 21]. For example, in 2017, the Society of Thoracic Surgeons reported that DHCA used to be the most common technique for circulatory arrest [22]. Nowadays, the general trend is moving, especially in Europe, toward the association of cerebral protection and warmer temperature of circulatory arrest [22]. Several studies and meta-analyses demonstrated the superiority of these surgical techniques in terms of lower early mortality and lower adverse events (**Figures 5–7**) [18, 22, 23].

1.2.1 Retrograde cerebral perfusion (RCP) and anterograde cerebral perfusion (ACP)

Retrograde cerebral perfusion, first introduced for treating air cerebral embolism, used to be the first technique that was implemented to guarantee correct cerebral protection in association with DHCA [23]. Established by cannulation of the superior vena cava (SVC), without manipulation of supra-aortic vessels, RCP guarantees cerebral perfusion through the vein system [25]. Clinical and animal trials suggested that RCP provides a small percentage of cerebral flow (10–30%) compared to baseline flow characteristics [26]. During the years, numerous concerns about RCP arose from the literature in association with the diffusion of selective anterograde perfusion.

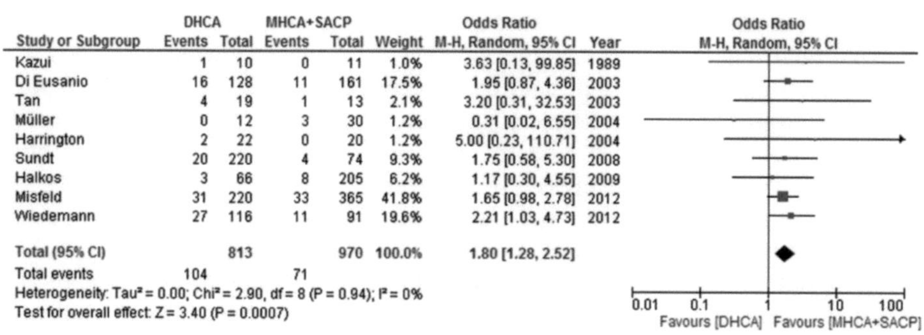

Figure 5.
Incidence comparison of postoperative stroke events during aortic arch replacement using deep hypothermic circulatory arrest alone (DHCA) or with moderate hypothermic circulatory arrest with selective antegrade cerebral protection (MHCA + SACP) made by Tian et al. [23].

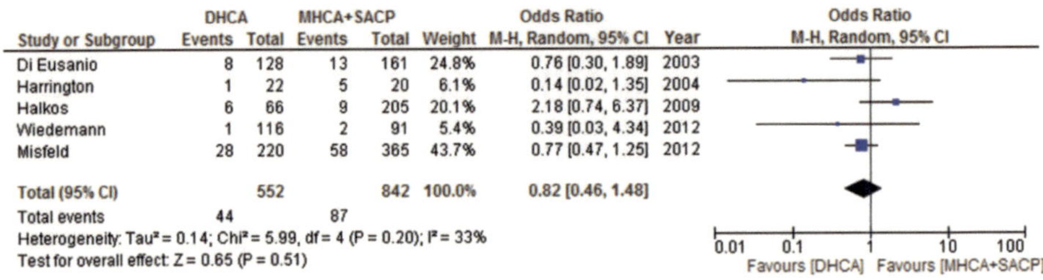

Figure 6.
Incidence comparison of postoperative temporary neurological deficit between deep hypothermic circulatory arrest alone (DHCA) and moderate hypothermic circulatory arrest with antegrade cerebral protection (MHCA+ACP) made by Tian et al. [23].

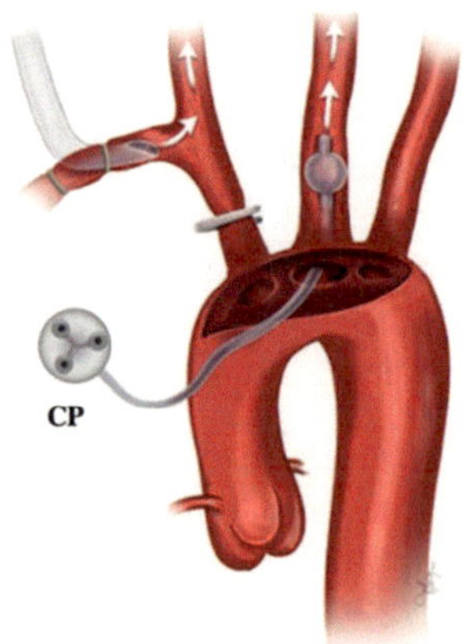

Figure 7.
Illustration of anterograde cerebral perfusion with direct cannulation of left common carotid artery as first described by Kazui et al. [24].

Several animal studies supposed that, during RCP, oxygen perfusion is not guaranteed through the cerebral parenchyma, assuming the inefficacy of this perfusion technique [27]. On the other hand, several studies with animal models challenged these concerns, defending the utility of RCP [27]. A recent meta-analysis conducted by Takagi et al. including a total of 15,365 reported no statistically significant differences in the postoperative incidence of stroke (17 studies enrolling a total of 9421 patients) and mortality (16 studies including a total of 14,452 patients). Contemporarily, a reduction in temporary neurological dysfunction (TND) was found during ACP [28].

Today, anterograde cerebral protection is the most common way of cerebral perfusion during surgical treatment on the aortic arch. Ghoreishi et al., analyzing the STS database including more than 7000 cases of Type A acute dissection, described how 71% of patients were treated using cerebral perfusion. Of these, two-thirds were ACP [28]. Several studies identified a satisfactory safe time of circulatory arrest of 80 minutes using anterograde cerebral perfusion [24].

Anterograde cerebral perfusion may be performed in different ways (unilateral cerebral perfusion and bilateral cerebral perfusion) based on the anatomical structure of the patient and possible involvement of the supra-aortic vessels by the aortic dissection. An important analysis of the eventual presence of an incomplete circle of Willis should be made based on preoperative CT to evaluate the possible necessity of direct cannulation of the left subclavian artery. Several studies found no significant differences in terms of early clinical outcomes depending on the cannulation site [29]. Ghoreishi et al. reported that, on the other hand, axillary cannulation was associated with a lower incidence of stroke, whereas femoral cannulation significantly increased the risk of stroke regardless of the cerebral perfusion strategy or the degree of hypothermia [28]. Aortic surgery centers have adopted different cerebral perfusion strategies to optimize operative results and minimize adverse neurologic outcomes [30]. Recently, the issue of using unilateral (u-ACP) or bilateral (b-ACP) ACP has been one of the most important concerns [31]. Similar results have been reported regarding mortality, stroke, TND, and renal failure rates between the two types of ACP in proximal aortic arch replacement [31]. Still debated is the effectiveness of u-ACP in total arch replacement, with b-ACP permitting longer circulatory arrest periods in safe conditions, as reported by Zierer and colleagues [32]. On the other hand, several studies found no statistical differences between unilateral and bilateral ACP upon organ perfusion [33].

2. The arch problem

Open surgery for aortic arch replacement is a challenging procedure and requires a great surgeon's experience to be performed. Moreover, aortic arch surgery is characterized by a higher operative risk with a higher rate of systemic and cerebrovascular complications, increasing early mortality. It is well known that the gold standard for the treatment of type A aortic dissection is the resection and replacement of the aortic tract with the intimal tear. Although the most frequent localization of the primary entry tear is within the ascending aorta, finding it in the distal aorta and the aortic arch is not so infrequent. When this happens, resection and replacement of the aorta must be extended to the portion where the intimal tear is located. Despite that, controversies exist about the management of the dissected aortic arch, wherever the intimal tear is located. Some authors suggest a more conservative approach, such as hemiarch replacement, to reduce procedure complexity, postoperative complications, and mortality [34]. This option improves early outcomes in terms of perioperative morbidity and mortality but does not assure similar long-term results. For this reason, other surgeons prefer a more invasive and aggressive management (e.g. total arch replacement with or without Frozen Elephant Trunk technique), regardless of the intimal tear location, to obtain a more complete result, accepting the increased procedural complexity and postoperative mortality [3].

However, some authors demonstrated similar short- and long-term outcomes of both aggressive and conservative approaches for selected patients, suggesting a more aggressive approach to treat complex arch lesions like arch aneurysms >4 cm or aortic dissection with an intimal tear at the arch unable to be excluded by hemiarch replacement [35]. It is reasonable to claim that such results are not simply reproducible because, as previously discussed, some procedures require to be performed by expert surgeons in high-volume centers to provide early and late outcomes comparable to less aggressive strategies. [36]

Whatever the strategy of choice, the aim of the surgical procedure is to save the patient's life and to achieve a regression of the dissecting process with a less invasive approach and a more complete as possible treatment of the aortic dissection, to give the patient a durable result. For this reason, although the primary strategy is to replace the aortic tract with the intimal tear, the extension of the aortic replacement is often based on institutional experience or the preferences of the surgeon.

3. Malperfusion syndrome

Acute type A aortic dissection can clinically manifest, in addition to the classic symptoms, with systemic signs due to peripheral malperfusion syndrome. We can distinguish between a static and a dynamic malperfusion. The first one could be the result of the propagation of the dissection flap into the branch vessel with resultant false lumen protrusion into the branch vessel with associated thrombosis and obstruction. Dynamic obstruction is more often the cause of malperfusion syndrome than static obstruction and is responsible for approximately 80% of cases [37].

The diagnosis of malperfusion syndrome is made, first of all, thanks to clinical manifestations of mesenteric, renal, and lower extremities ischemia (impaired solute clearance, rising creatinine, refractory hypertension, lactate elevation, peripheral pulses deficits, pain, pallor, paresthesias, poikilothermia, or paresis). Computed Tomographic Angiography, which is needed almost always to diagnose acute aortic dissection, is useful for identifying radiological signs of systemic malperfusion together with clinical signs.

This clinical entity is not only a collateral finding in the case of type A aortic dissection, but it has relevance in terms of postoperative results and patient survival. Mesenteric ischemia has been clearly identified as the second cause of death in the case of acute aortic dissection after aortic rupture [38]. For this reason, the identification of preoperative malperfusion syndrome helps the "dissection team" to decide the operative strategy and optimize the postoperative management of the patient.

4. Fate of false lumen

As discussed previously, the main target in the treatment of the aortic dissection is to replace the interested tract of the aorta to eliminate the entry tear and improve the perfusion of the true lumen, with a progressive decompression of the false lumen. But what happens distally, even if the primary entry tear has been eliminated? There is no consensus about the management of the dissected aortic tract (arch, descending aorta) without an entry tear: some surgeons prefer to limit the treatment to the tract of the aorta interested by the intimal tear; other surgeons support a more aggressive and complete treatment that involves the distal tract of the aorta as well. Nowadays, it is well known that secondary tear or reentry tear, which can supply the false lumen even after surgical correction, could be present distally to the replaced aorta (distal aortic arch, descending aorta, supra-aortic vessels), and these lesions are not so simple to identify. Furthermore, several minimal communications between the true and the false lumen have been found at the level of the distal anastomosis, as the result of micro-lacerations in the fragile tissues of a dissected aorta made by the suture line or by the needle. This phenomenon, called distal anastomosis new entry (DANE), is not so infrequent, as well as the postoperative false lumen supply by small tears in the supra-aortic vessels (**Figures 8** and **9**).

From the early postoperative period to a mid- and long-term follow-up, the presence of communication between the two lumina has been seen to be the cause of late patency of false lumen with subsequent growth of the aortic dimensions, leading to the need for reoperation with a higher operative risk and perioperative mortality [39].

An interesting study from Tamura et al. investigated the influence of patent false lumen (PFL) caused by DANE on long-term outcomes. PFL caused by DANE showed

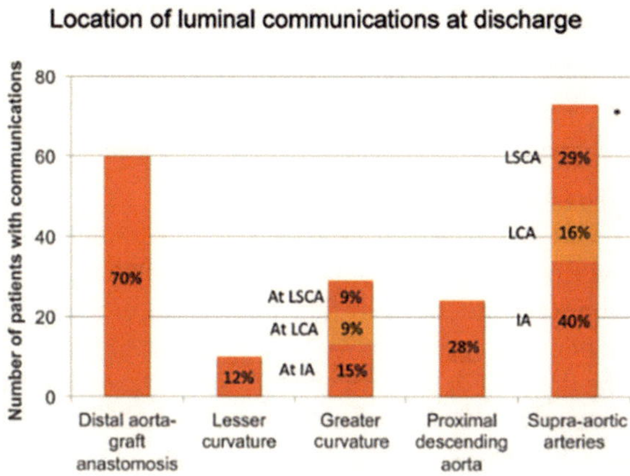

Figure 8.
Rate of communication between true and false lumen. LSCA: left subclavian artery; LCA: left carotid artery; IA: innominate artery [39].

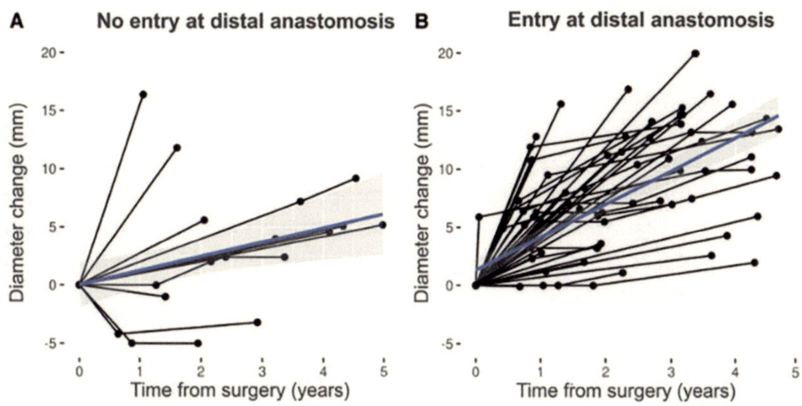

Figure 9.
Interaction between DANE and aortic growth rate (A, B) [39].

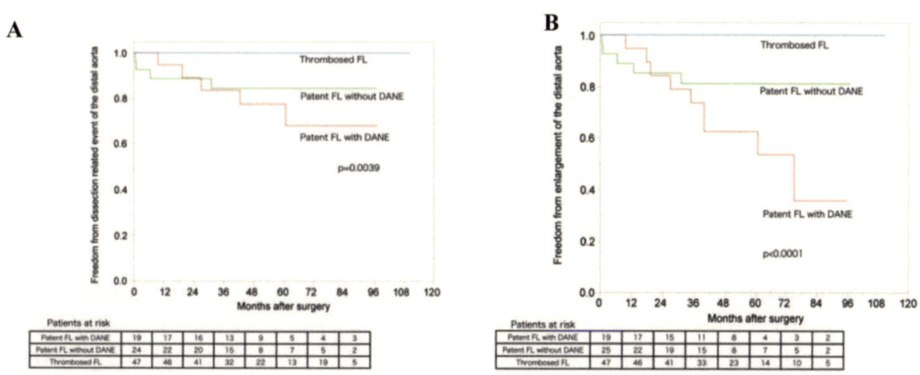

Figure 10.
Kaplan-Meier curves of freedom from the dissection-related event of the distal aorta between thrombosed FL, patent FL without DANE, and patent FL with DANE (A); Kaplan-Meier curves of overall survival rate between thrombosed FL, patent FL without DANE, and patent FL with DANE (B) [40].

a greater aortic growth rate of the descending aorta, and DANE was found to be a significant risk factor for distal aortic events, as we can see from the Kaplan-Meier curves of freedom from dissection-related events (**Figure 10**) [40].

5. Surgical and hybrid strategies

We describe below the most performed techniques for aortic arch management. We will not treat perfusion strategies because this is not a specific topic of this chapter and, moreover, they are dependent on each surgeon's preference. Furthermore, only the "distal procedures" will be described; the order of the anastomosis and the management of surgical times are strictly surgeon-dependent: some prefer to perform the "proximal procedure" before and during the cooling process; others support a distal-first approach just after cooling. In our center, we prefer the distal-first approach. Antegrade bilateral cerebral perfusion is preferred, with cannulation of the subclavian artery (for systemic perfusion as well) and selective cannulation of the left carotid artery.

5.1 Hemiarch replacement

Cerebral perfusion starts, supra-aortic vessels are clamped, and aortic clamp is removed. The distal ascending aorta is resected including the lesser curvature of the aortic arch in an oblong fashion, preserving the convexity of the aortic arch. A Dacron graft is cut in order to have a prosthesis tongue matching the distal aspect of the lesser curvature of the arch. A single polypropylene running suture is started with the first bite on the Dacron graft and then through the arch on the assistant side in the lower half of the lesser curvature; then the suture continues clockwise. When aortic tissue fragility is present, a PTFE strip could be included externally in the suture line. After completing the suture, the Dacron graft is de-aired and clamped, and cerebral perfusion is switched to systemic perfusion.

This technique is recommended when the intimal tear is located in the lesser curvature of the arch. Despite encouraging short- and long-term results are widely described, distal false lumen patency, as the result of a distal anastomosis new entry (DANE), is a common occurrence of hemiarch replacement, with an incidence between 39 and 70% [39].

5.2 Total arch replacement

Differently from the hemiarch technique, the total arch replacement is performed with an extended resection to the first tract of the descending aorta. Cooling, CPB, and cerebral perfusion setup do not differ between the two techniques. After cerebral perfusion starts, the aortic arch is opened, and a cannula is inserted in the left carotid artery to achieve bilateral perfusion. Then the resection is extended to the descending aorta. An appropriate 4-branched prosthesis is sutured to the descending aorta with a single polypropylene running suture, with or without Teflon reinforcement. Systemic perfusion is restarted from the side branch of the prosthesis together with cerebral perfusion, while supra-aortic prosthesis branches and the vascular prosthesis proximal to the reperfusion branch are clamped. Body temperature is progressively restored, and proximal anastomosis is performed at the desired level of the ascending aorta with a single polypropylene running suture, with or without PTFE reinforcement. Then supra-aortic vessels are selective anastomosed to the graft branches.

The described technique allows the surgeon to resect the full extension of the arch, but it is not free from technical difficulties due to the awkward position of the distal anastomosis.

5.3 Frozen elephant trunk

The Frozen Elephant Trunk (FET) technique represents an evolution of the Elephant Trunk technique, in which the ascending aorta and aortic arch are replaced with a Dacron prosthesis that is extended into the descending aorta. Since its first description in 2003 by the Hannover group [41], the FET has become the technique of choice for the treatment of complex arch lesions. It is performed with a hybrid prosthesis that has a covered stent portion to be released in the descending aorta and sutured with a special collar to the edge of the distal resection and a standard Dacron portion to replace the arch and the supra-aortic vessels.

The FET procedure allows to achieve a blood-tight seal in the descending aorta and permits to perform a dual treatment on the arch and the proximal descending aorta [42]. Furthermore, the stented portion of the prosthesis with its radial force facilitates the negative remodeling of the false lumen and allows the exclusion of small reentry tears in the descending aorta. Prosthesis supra-aortic branch configurations fit all the surgical strategies, allowing the surgeon to perform the distal anastomosis between the aorta and prosthesis collar in an arch zone more proximal than zone 3 or 4. Indeed, a trifurcated configuration is particularly indicated when a zone 0 or 1 distal anastomosis is preferred. This is a huge advantage for the surgeon who can perform a more comfortable distal anastomosis with fewer technical difficulties. Furthermore, a FET prosthesis can be easily relined for subsequent endovascular completion of descending and abdominal aorta treatment, offering a stable landing zone.

The resection of the dissected aortic arch is made according to the treatment strategy and the surgeon's preference because specific kinds of FET prosthesis are suitable for distal anastomosis from zone 0 to zone 3. Cooling and cerebral perfusion are achieved in a standard fashion. After aortic resection to the desired zone, the stented portion of the FET graft can be released in the arch/descending aorta and then the collar between stented and non-stented portions is sutured to the distal edge of the aorta. Once the distal anastomosis is completed, systemic perfusion can be restored through the reperfusion branch of the graft, after proximal prosthesis and supra-aortic branches clamping. During rewarming, supra-aortic vessels are anastomosed with each specific branch and proximal anastomosis can be performed.

The FET technique is particularly indicated when a hybrid approach is desired, as described previously, permitting at the same time to treat the arch, the descending aorta, and the abdominal aorta with an endovascular strategy.

In Europe, two hybrid prostheses are available: the E-vita Open Neo (Artivion, JOTEC GmbH, Hechingen, Germany) and the Thoraflex Hybrid (Terumo Aortic UK). Both prostheses have a distal stented portion and a proximal conventional Dacron portion, separated by a sewing collar that facilitates distal anastomosis.

Thoraflex Hybrid prosthesis is available in two configurations, with the distal stented portion that does not differ between the two variants:

- Straight configuration: different from the branched version, the straight configuration is made only with the reperfusion branch; it is chosen when supra-aortic vessels are reimplanted with the island technique.

- Branched configuration: the Dacron portion is made with four branches, three of which for supra-aortic vessels separate anastomoses. The fourth branch is used as a reperfusion branch at the end of the circulatory arrest surgical time (**Figure 11**).

This hybrid graft is particularly suitable when distal anastomosis in zone 2 or 3 is preferred.

E-vita Open Neo graft has three possible configurations, with the stented portion that does not differ from each other. As the Thoraflex prosthesis, the difference between each configuration in the supra-aortic branches:

- Straight configuration: only a reperfusion branch arises from the Dacron portion as a reperfusion line. This configuration is suitable for supra-aortic vessel reimplantation with island technique and distal collar anastomosis in zone 2 or 3.

- Branched configuration: as well as Thoraflex branched configuration, it has three branches for separated supra-aortic vessels and one reperfusion branch. This configuration allows distal collar anastomosis in zone 2 or 3 and, in specific situations, in zone 1.

- Trifurcated configuration: a single branch arises more proximally from the Dacron portion with a trifurcation for supra-aortic vessels separated anastomoses and a lateral reperfusion branch is still present. This configuration represents a great option for a more comfortable distal anastomosis because its more proximal trifurcated branch allows to perform collar anastomosis in zone 0 or 1 for the particular angulation of the head vessels branches, reducing technical problems related to a more distal anastomosis. Furthermore, zones 0–1 are better

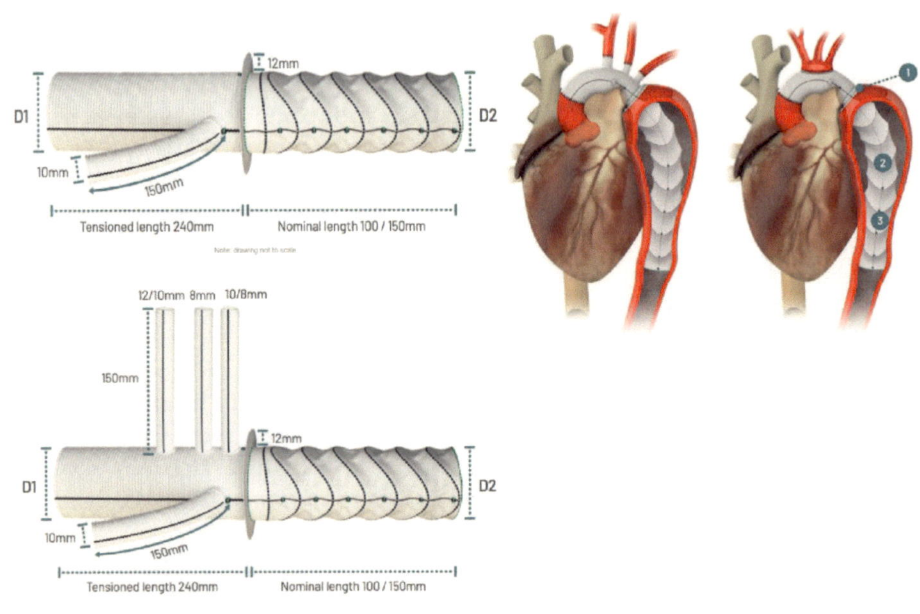

Figure 11.
Terumo Thoraflex configurations.

exposable, especially in minimally invasive accesses. It is also dutiful to consider that a less uncomfortable distal anastomosis could reduce circulatory arrest, cardiopulmonary bypass, and cross-clamp times (**Figure 12**) [43, 44].

5.4 AMDS device: a new paradigm?

As previously discussed, the primary target of aortic dissection treatment is the removal of the primary entry tear, the sealing of the false lumen at the distal anastomosis with false lumen, and pressurization of the true lumen to resolve and avoid further malperfusion. Unless the necessary treatment is FET/total arch replacement, with a more conservative treatment, the sealing of the false lumen at the distal anastomosis cannot be guaranteed, and this can lead to a distal anastomotic new entry. The DANE allows the antegrade flow in the false lumen leading to FL patency in 70% of cases and subsequent malperfusion, early mortality, reinterventions, and decreased long-term survival [45, 46].

Artivion AMDS is a novel, partially uncovered arch stent made with a proximal Teflon graft sewn to a tubular Nitinol stent with a low radial force, which aims to improve malperfusion and promote positive remodeling of the aortic arch and distal dissected aorta, by the active pressurization of the true lumen (**Figure 13**) [45, 47].

As previously described, this device has a proximal PTFE stent-supported cuff to strengthen the aortic tissue and reduce the tension on the suture during conventional graft to aorta anastomosis on a friable tissue, reducing the risk of DANE. The uncovered Nitinol wire braided stent expands and supports the true lumen across the aortic arch and descending aorta, thereby stabilizing the aortic wall and promoting remodeling, without compromising the supra-aortic vessels flow. Preliminary results by the Canadian group suggested that the AMDS is a safe and reproducible adjunct to current surgical strategies for acute DeBakey I aortic dissection repair [47]. The efficacy of the AMDS stent is supported by other studies in terms of clinical results, true lumen expansion, false lumen reduction, and aortic growth stabilization [45, 48, 49]. Furthermore, preliminary results from the DARTS trial seem to suggest that the AMDS device is promising as a technology that not only facilitates the repair of the arch or proximal descending aorta but also allows to achieve positive remodeling in the early to midterm period (**Figure 14**) [50].

AMDS device has a simple delivery system, with a pigtail tip. Sizing of the device (available in four different sizes) is very simple and does not require an advanced DICOM viewer: in a standard axial view, the first aortic measure must be taken

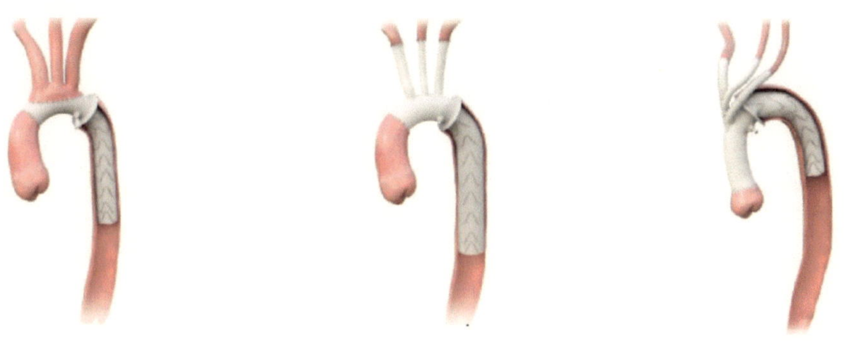

Figure 12.
Artivion e-vita open neo configurations.

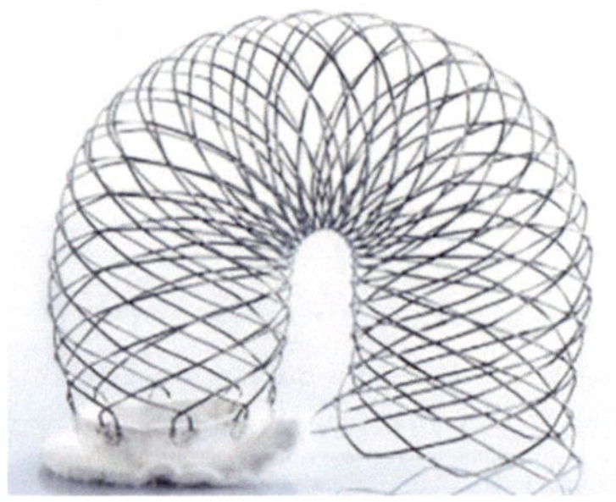

Figure 13.
The fully expanded ascyrus medical dissection stent outside of its delivery system [47].

A

Key Outcome Measures After AMDS	DARTS[1,2]	Berlin 100 Patient Series[4]
Presence of DANE	0%	NR
Malperfusion resolution	96%	80%
Average deployment time*	3 min	8 min
Early mortality	13%	18%
Reintervention	13%**	13%***
Spinal Cord Injury (SCI)	0%	NR

*Does not include suture time. **Average. 3 year follow up. *** 30 day follow up. NR = not reported

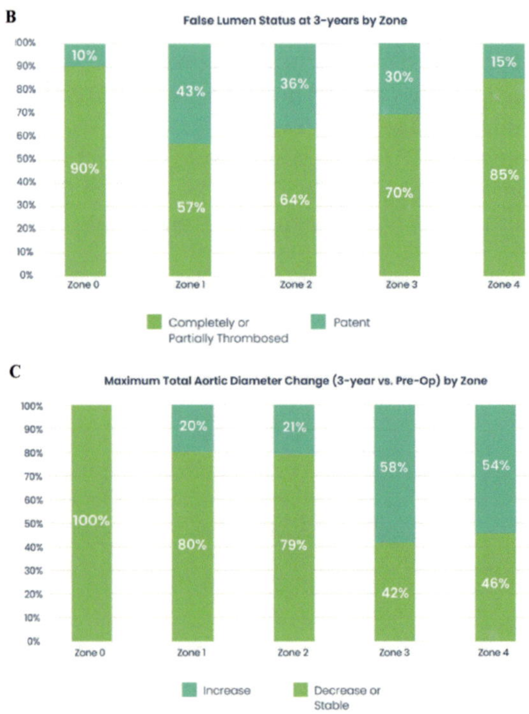

Figure 14.
Preliminary results of AMDS devices (derived from Artivion website). (A) Clinical results. (B) False lumen status at 3 years. (C) Aortic diameter changes at 3 years [45, 48–50].

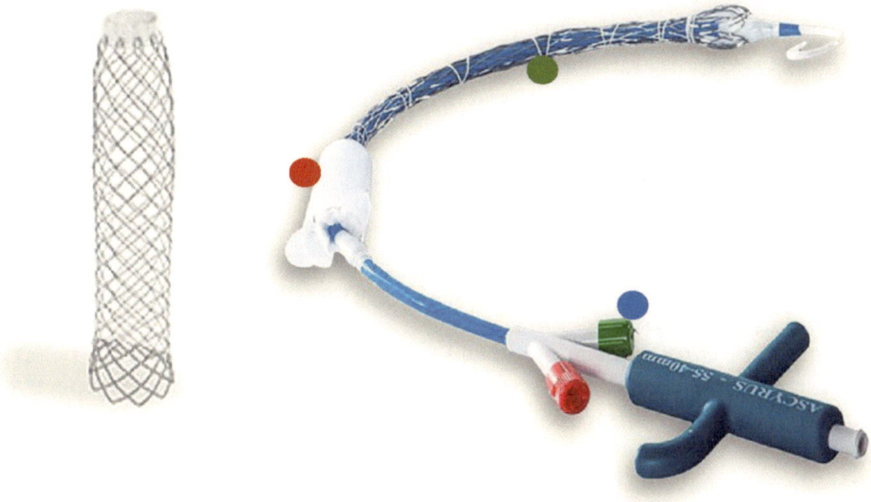

Figure 15.
AMDS device released (left) and on its delivery system (right). The red dot indicates the proximal protective sheath; the blue dot indicates the green cap to remove for stent releasing (green dot).

between the innominate artery and the left carotid artery; the second aortic measure must be taken at the level of the pulmonary artery bifurcation. Then, using a sizing table, the right device size can be easily identified. After the aortic arch resection (most commonly in zone 0) and circulatory arrest, the delivery system is inserted into the aorta, and the proximal protective sheath is removed to release the proximal stented cuff on the edge of the resected aorta; four stitches are placed at the four cardinal points to fix the stent to the aorta and then a continuous suture is performed to stabilize the aorta-cuff sealing. The green cap is removed to release the suture constraining the stent. The special Nitinol stent configuration facilitates the insertion of a cannula for the carotid artery through it. Distal conventional Dacron-aorta anastomosis can be performed in a standard fashion with the interposition of the AMDS cuff (**Figure 15**).

6. Discussion and outcomes

Aortic dissection with aortic arch involvement is still a challenging condition to deal with, especially if its systemic implications are considered. Outcomes of each kind of surgical treatment strictly depend not only on the immediate surgical result or the early mortality but on the "distal" effects of the treatment. Indeed, it is well known that a malperfusion syndrome represents an important cause of death before and after treatment [37]. Furthermore, even if the immediate results could seem satisfying, it has been noticed that a more conservative procedure may leave a residual pressurized false lumen with growth, rupture of the distal aorta, as well as pseudoaneurysms originating from fragile aortic tissue [51, 52].

Results about each surgical strategy suggest that appropriate surgical management should be found for each clinical presentation of type A dissection to achieve a satisfactory outcome, but the choice of optimal procedure is still controversial. Although some authors claim that both conservative and aggressive strategies have similar outcomes [35, 53], the incidence of a patent false lumen and its prognostic impact cannot be ignored [39, 40], if we consider the rate of reoperation for distal aortic events and its operative risk.

With the advent of new surgical and hybrid devices [45, 48–50, 54], aggressive strategies, despite their operative complexity, seem to have better long-term outcomes than a more conservative approach, in terms of survival rate and freedom from reintervention (**Figure 16**) [55, 56].

The lack of randomized studies could justify the controversies existing about the best surgical strategy to obtain good anatomical and clinical results, both on short- and long-term follow-up. The only data we have are derived from non-randomized studies and meta-analyses.

It seems to be clear that a standardized protocol is needed to choose the better surgical strategy for each clinical scenario. In our institution, we are retrospectively analyzing all the aortic dissection operated from 2013. Preliminary results, regarding 303 consecutive patients admitted to our Cardiac Surgery Department for acute type A aortic dissection from 2013 to 2021, seem to confirm that, despite a lower survival rate during the first 24 months, FET patients have better long-term survival if compared to hemiarch patients with a survival rate at 8 years of 75 versus 92% in the FET group. This could be related to the lower incidence of distal aortic events in FET patients, as previously discussed (**Figure 17**).

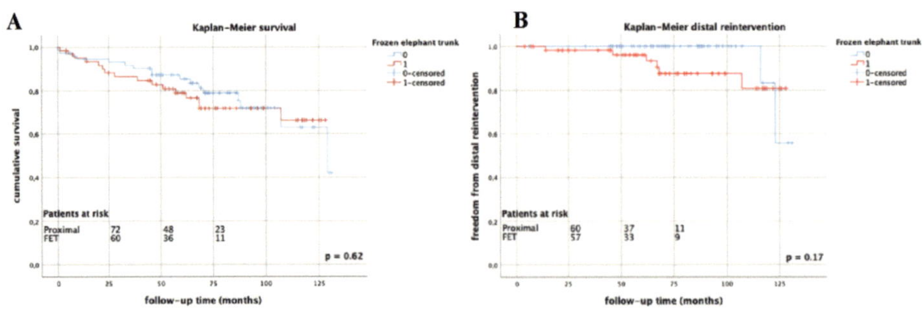

Figure 16.
(A) Kaplan-Meier survival curves comparing FET (red) vs. proximal repair (blue) at 10-year follow-up. (B) Kaplan-Meier curves for the need for reintervention comparing FET (red) vs. proximal repair (blue) at 10-year follow-up [54].

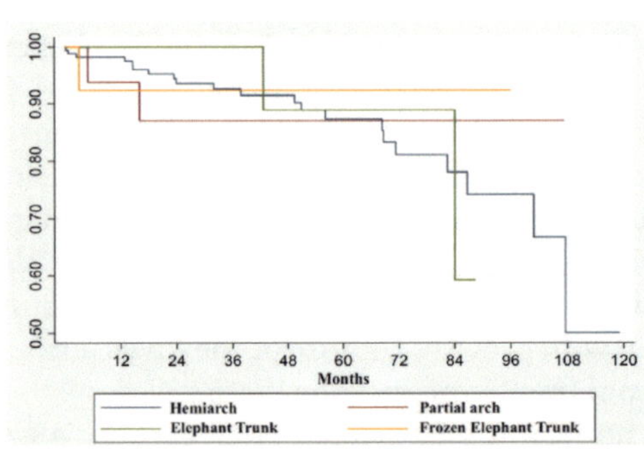

Figure 17.
Our institution (cardiac surgery unit AOU Careggi, Florence) Kaplan-Meier survival estimates comparing the FET group (orange) vs. hemiarch group (blue) vs. partial arch (purple) vs. elephant trunk (green).

As shown in **Table 1**, our preliminary results seem to confirm that a more complete procedure is associated to a lower rate of false lumen patency with a concomitant true lumen positive remodeling.

From March 2023, we implanted 23 AMDS devices. The small population cohort does not allow us to have statistically significant results, but our clinical evidence suggests that this new hybrid prosthesis can improve arch and abdominal aorta results. We had 13% postoperative mortality (2 patients with preoperative critical mesenteric malperfusion, 1 patient with an unknown secondary tear in the innominate artery) and 86.9% false lumen decompression with progressive true lumen positive remodeling. All the surviving patients were discharged in good clinical status. Recently, we

Parameters	Ascending aorta ± hemiarch (n = 234)	Partial arch (n = 23)	Elephant trunk (n = 25)	FET (n = 21)	p-value
FL thrombosis	60 (30.5%)	13 (59.1%)	7 (38.9%)	8 (50%)	<0.05 *
FL partial thrombosis	25 (12.7%)	2 (9.1%)	3 (16.7%)	5 (31.3%)	<0.05 *
FL patency	104 (52.8%)	7 (31.8%)	8 (44.4%)	3 (18.8%)	<0.05 *

*$p < 0.05$.

Table 1.
Our institution (cardiac surgery unit AOU Careggi, Florence) about false lumen fate at follow-up (mean 36 ± 32.95 months).

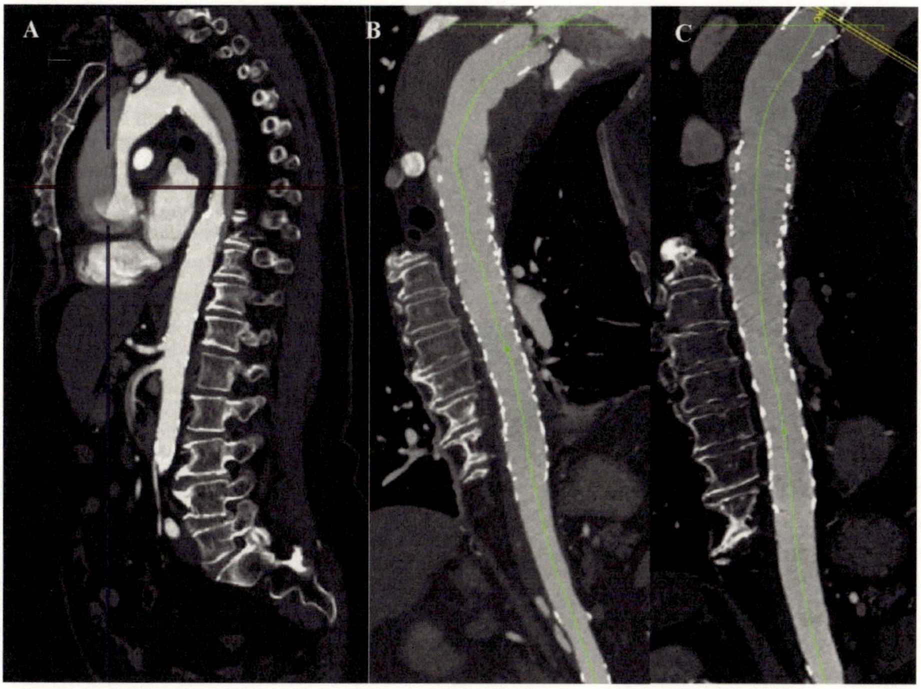

Figure 18.
A recent case admitted to our unit for aortic dissection (A) and treated with aortic valve replacement, ascending aorta replacement, and AMDS implantation. (B) 3-month follow-up CTA that shows a partial obliteration of false lumen. (C) 5-month follow-up CTA that shows a complete expansion of true lumen with the negative remodeling of false lumen.

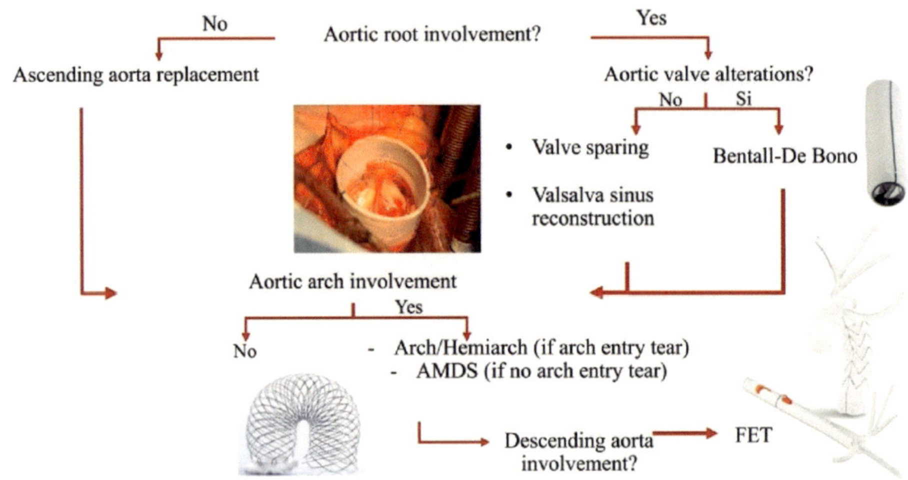

Figure 19.
Our institution (cardiac surgery unit AOU Careggi, Florence) protocol for the management of aortic dissection.

implanted 3 AMDS through IV intercostal space J ministernotomy, with no technical differences if compared to full sternotomy and with optimal results (see **Figure 18**).

On these bases, we elaborated an internal protocol that aims to standardize the surgical strategy, without any improvisation (**Figure 19**).

The advent of the new AMDS hybrid prosthesis, according to our direct experience and on the literature data, seems to offer a promising new surgical strategy to allow the surgeon, even without a deep expertise, to perform an arch procedure, with all its well-known advantages, without increasing procedural complexity and perioperative complication rate. In selected patients, when intimal tear is only proximal to the aortic arch but the intimal flap is extended distally, we suggest always using this aortic stent, considering it as an instrument to achieve the complete recovery from the dissecting pathology, as suggested by several studies reported above and by our results. Moreover, the superiority of an uncovered descending aorta stent over the covered stent of FET prosthesis should be mentioned and analyzed, in terms of risk for spinal cord ischemia. More studies are needed to clarify long-term outcomes of this new device, but as previously discussed, it could be, in the next future, a real change in the paradigm of aortic arch dissection treatment, bringing with it the "paradox" of a less invasive and complex procedure for a more complete, safe, and long-term durable treatment.

In conclusion, nowadays, we have new generation devices that could simplify a challenging procedure, lower the learning curve of young surgeons, and make aortic arch intervention more reproducible as possible.

DOI: http://dx.doi.org/10.5772/intechopen.1005781

Author details

Giulio Pellegrini*, Lorenzo Terzano and Pier Luigi Stefàno
University of Florence, Florence, Italy

*Address all correspondence to: giulio.pellegrini19@gmail.com

References

[1] Booth K, Hospital F, Ii KG. Acute aortic dissection (AAD)—A lethal disease: The epidemiology, pathophysiology and natural history. British Journal of Cardiology. 2023;**30**(1):16-20

[2] Merkle J et al. Impact of different aortic entry tear sites on early outcomes and long-term survival in patients with Stanford A acute aortic dissection. The Thoracic and Cardiovascular Surgeon. 2019;**67**(5):363-371

[3] Di Bartolomeo R, Leone A, Di Marco L, Pacini D. When and how to replace the aortic arch for type A dissection. Annals of Cardiothoracic Surgery. 2016;**5**(4):383-388

[4] Olsson C, Thelin S, Ståhle E, Ekbom A, Granath F. Thoracic aortic aneurysm and dissection: Increasing prevalence and improved outcomes reported in a nationwide population-based study of more than 14 000 cases from 1987 to 2002. Circulation. 2006;**114**(24):2611-2618

[5] Pacini D et al. Acute aortic dissection: Epidemiology and outcomes. International Journal of Cardiology. 2013;**167**(6):2806-2812

[6] Mollo F, Comino A, Passarino G. Incidence of acute aortic dissection at autopsy. Chest. 1983;**83**(4):712

[7] Harris KM et al. Early mortality in type A acute aortic dissection: Insights from the international registry of acute aortic dissection. JAMA Cardiology. 2022;**7**(10):1009-1015

[8] Czerny M et al. EACTS/STS guidelines for diagnosing and treating acute and chronic syndromes of the aortic organ. The Annals of Thoracic Surgery. 2024;**118**(1):5-115

[9] Pape LA et al. Presentation, diagnosis, and outcomes of acute aortic dissection: 17-year trends from the international registry of acute aortic dissection. Journal of the American College of Cardiology. 2015;**66**(4):350-358

[10] Debakey ME, Henly WS, Cooley DA, Morris GC, Crawford ES, beall AC. Surgical management of dissecting aneurysms of the aorta. The Journal of Thoracic and Cardiovascular Surgery. 1965;**49**:130-149

[11] Daily PO, Trueblood HW, Stinson EB, Wuerflein RD, Shumway NE. Management of acute aortic dissections. The Annals of Thoracic Surgery. 1970;**10**(3):237-247

[12] Nienaber CA, Clough RE. Management of acute aortic dissection. Lancet. 2015;**385**(9970):800-811

[13] Von Segesser LK et al. Dissection of the descending thoracic aorta extending into the ascending aorta: A therapeutic challenge. The Journal of Thoracic and Cardiovascular Surgery. 1994;**108**(4):755-761

[14] Okita Y et al. Surgery for aortic dissection with intimal tear in the transverse aortic arch. European Journal of Cardio-Thoracic Surgery. 1996;**10**(9):784-790

[15] Sievers HH et al. Aortic dissection reconsidered: Type, entry site, malperfusion classification adding clarity and enabling outcome prediction. Interactive Cardiovascular and Thoracic Surgery. 2020;**30**(3):451-457

[16] Sievers HH, Rylski B, Czerny M, Baier ALM, Kreibich M, Siepe M, et al. Aortic dissection reconsidered: Type, entry site, malperfusion classification adding clarity and enabling outcome prediction. Interdisciplinary CardioVascular and Thoracic Surgery. 1 Mar 2020;**30**(3):451-457. DOI: 10.1093/icvts/ivz281. PMID: 31755925

[17] Zhao Z, Chi H, Chen L, Wang J, Xiao C. Clinical outcome of a branch-first approach with a novel continuous whole-brain perfusion strategy for total arch surgery. Journal of Cardiothoracic Surgery. 2024;**19**(1):1-10

[18] Manoly I et al. Neuroprotective strategies with circulatory arrest in open aortic surgery—A meta-analysis. Asian Cardiovascular & Thoracic Annals. 2022;**30**(6):635-644

[19] Griepp RB, Stinson EB, Hollingsworth JF, Buehler D. Prosthetic replacement of the aortic arch. The Journal of Thoracic and Cardiovascular Surgery. 1975;**70**(6):1051-1063

[20] Kazui T et al. Aortic arch replacement using selective cerebral perfusion. The Annals of Thoracic Surgery. 2007;**83**(2):2006-2008

[21] Bachet J et al. Cold cerebroplegia: A new technique of cerebral protection during operations on the transverse aortic arch. The Journal of Thoracic and Cardiovascular Surgery. 1991;**102**(1):85-94

[22] Englum BR et al. Hypothermia and cerebral protection strategies in aortic arch surgery: A comparative effectiveness analysis from the STS adult cardiac surgery database. European Journal of Cardio-Thoracic Surgery. 2017;**52**(3):492-498

[23] Tian DH et al. A meta-analysis of deep hypothermic circulatory arrest versus moderate hypothermic circulatory arrest with selective antegrade cerebral perfusion. Annals of Cardiothoracic Surgery. 2013;**2**(2):148-158

[24] Apostolakis E, Shuhaiber JH. Antegrade or retrograde cerebral perfusion as an adjunct during hypothermic circulatory arrest for aortic arch surgery. Expert Review of Cardiovascular Therapy. 2007;**5**(6):1147-1161

[25] Gaudino M et al. Retrograde perfusion through superior vena cava reaches the brain during circulatory arrest. Journal of Thoracic Disease. 2018;**10**(3):1563-1568

[26] Bavaria JE, Pochettino A. Retrograde cerebral perfusion (RCP) in aortic arch surgery: Efficacy and possible mechanisms of brain protection. Seminars in Thoracic and Cardiovascular Surgery. 1997;**9**(3):222-232

[27] Ehrlich MP et al. Retrograde cerebral perfusion provides negligible flow through brain capillaries in the pig. The Journal of Thoracic and Cardiovascular Surgery. 2001;**122**(2):331-338

[28] Ghoreishi M et al. Factors associated with acute stroke after type A aortic dissection repair: An analysis of the society of thoracic surgeons national adult cardiac surgery database. The Journal of Thoracic and Cardiovascular Surgery. 2020;**159**(6):2143-2154.e3

[29] Sabashnikov A et al. Axillar or aortic cannulation for aortic repair in patients with Stanford A dissection? The Annals of Thoracic Surgery. 2016;**102**(3):787-794

[30] Sasaki M, Usui A, Yoshikawa M, Akita T, Ueda Y. Arch-first technique performed under hypothermic circulatory arrest with retrograde

cerebral perfusion improves neurological outcomes for total arch replacement. European Journal of Cardio-Thoracic Surgery. 2005;**27**(5):821-825

[31] Preventza O et al. Unilateral versus bilateral cerebral perfusion for acute type a aortic dissection. The Annals of Thoracic Surgery. 2015;**99**(1):80-87

[32] Zierer A, El-Sayed Ahmad A, Papadopoulos N, Moritz A, Diegeler A, Urbanski PP. Selective antegrade cerebral perfusion and mild (28°C-30°C) systemic hypothermic circulatory arrest for aortic arch replacement: Results from 1002 patients. The Journal of Thoracic and Cardiovascular Surgery. 2012;**144**(5):1042-1050

[33] Malvindi PG, Scrascia G, Vitale N. Is unilateral antegrade cerebral perfusion equivalent to bilateral cerebral perfusion for patients undergoing aortic arch surgery? Interactive Cardiovascular and Thoracic Surgery. 2008;**7**(5):891-897

[34] Westaby S, Saito S, Katsumata T. Acute type A dissection: Conservative methods provide consistently low mortality. The Annals of Thoracic Surgery. 2002;**73**(3):707-713. DOI: 10.1016/s0003-4975(01)03449-x

[35] Yang B et al. Late outcomes of strategic arch resection in acute type A aortic dissection. The Journal of Thoracic and Cardiovascular Surgery. 2019;**157**(4):1313-1321.e2

[36] Permanyer E, Ruyra X, Evangelista A. The aortic arch management for type A aortic dissection: Aggressive but experienced. Journal of Thoracic Disease. 2020;**12**(6): 3429-3432

[37] Crawford TC, Beaulieu RJ, Ehlert BA, Ratchford EV, Black JH. Malperfusion syndromes in aortic dissections. Vascular Medicine (United Kingdom). 2016;**21**(3):264-273

[38] Hagan PG et al. The international registry of acute aortic dissection (IRAD) new insights into an old disease. JAMA. 2000;**283**(7):897-903

[39] Rylski B et al. Fate of the dissected aortic arch after ascending replacement in type A aortic dissection. European Journal of Cardio-Thoracic Surgery. 2017;**51**(6):1127-1134

[40] Tamura K, Chikazawa G, Hiraoka A, Totsugawa T, Sakaguchi T, Yoshitaka H. The prognostic impact of distal anastomotic new entry after acute type I aortic dissection repair. European Journal of Cardio-Thoracic Surgery. 2017;**52**(5):867-873

[41] Karck M, Chavan A, Hagl C, Friedrich H, Galanski M, Haverich A. The frozen elephant trunk technique: A new treatment for thoracic aortic aneurysms. The Journal of Thoracic and Cardiovascular Surgery. 2003;**125**(6):1550-1553

[42] Harky A, Fok M, Bashir M. Which is the optimal frozen elephant trunk? A systematic review and meta-analysis of outcomes in 2161 patients undergoing thoracic aortic aneurysm surgery using e-vita open plus hybrid stent graft versus thoraflex™ hybrid prosthesis. Brazilian Society of Cardiovascular Surgery. 2020;**35**(4):427-436

[43] Rorris F-P, Antonopoulos CN, Gissis I, Tsagakis K, Kokotsakis J. E-Vita OPEN NEO hybrid stent graft: A new frontier for total arch replacement. Annals of Vascular Surgery. 2022;**84**:211-217

[44] El-Sayed Ahmad A et al. The frozen elephant technique using a novel hybrid prosthesis for extensive aortic arch

disease: A multicentre study. Advances in Therapy. 2023;**40**(3):1104-1113

[45] Bozso SJ et al. Midterm outcomes of the dissected aorta repair through stent implantation trial. The Annals of Thoracic Surgery. 2021;**111**(2):463-470

[46] Evangelista A et al. Long-term outcome of aortic dissection with patent false lumen: Predictive role of entry tear size and location. Circulation. 2012;**125**(25):3133-3141

[47] Bozso SJ et al. Dissected aorta repair through stent implantation trial: Canadian results. The Journal of Thoracic and Cardiovascular Surgery. 2019;**157**(5):1763-1771

[48] Montagner M et al. The arch remodelling stent for DeBakey I acute aortic dissection: Experience with 100 implantations. European Journal of Cardio-Thoracic Surgery. 2022;**62**(2):ezac384

[49] Bozso SJ et al. Three-year outcomes of the dissected aorta repair through stent implantation trial. The Journal of Thoracic and Cardiovascular Surgery. 2022;**167**(5):1661-1669.e3

[50] Brinkman WT. DARTS trial. The Annals of Thoracic Surgery. 2021;**111**(2):470-471

[51] Ma L et al. Outcomes of hemi- vs. total arch replacement in acute type A aortic dissection: A systematic review and meta-analysis. Frontiers in Cardiovascular Medicine. 2022;**9**(September):1-10

[52] Sun L, Qi R, Zhu J, Liu Y, Zheng J. Total arch replacement combined with stented elephant trunk implantation. Circulation. 2011;**123**(9):971-978

[53] Bassano C et al. Initial surgical strategy for the treatment of type a acute aortic dissection: Does proximal or distal extension of the aortic resection influence the outcomes? International Journal of Environmental Research and Public Health. 2022;**19**(14):8878

[54] Göbel N, Holder S, Hüther F, Anguelov Y, Bail D, Franke U. Frozen elephant trunk versus conventional proximal repair of acute aortic dissection type I. Frontiers in Cardiovascular Medicine. 2024;**11**(March):1-7

[55] Sun L, Qi R, Zhu J, Liu Y, Zheng J. Total arch replacement combined with stented elephant trunk implantation: A new standard therapy for type a dissection involving repair of the aortic arch? Circulation. 2011;**123**(9):971-978

[56] Tian DH, Ha H, Joshi Y, Yan TD. Long-term outcomes of the frozen elephant trunk procedure: A systematic review. Annals of Cardiothoracic Surgery. 2020;**9**(3):144-151

Chapter 8

Cerebral Protection during Repair of Type A Aortic Dissection

Thierry Carrel

Abstract

Surgical repair of type A aortic dissection includes most often a period of hypothermic circulatory arrest to allow inspection of the disease within the aortic arch and perform the most appropriate distal repair. Clinical methods of cerebral protection have considerably evolved during the last decades, starting with isolated hypothermic circulatory arrest without or with medicamentous protection and combined later with different methods of cerebral perfusion. One category aims at significantly reducing or suppressing the metabolic demands of the cerebral tissue. The second provides the brain with some metabolic requirements despite the exclusion of the supra-aortic branches from the aortic arch and can be summarized as perfusion of the brain through the arterial or venous network, in either an antegrade or a retrograde fashion. Numerous clinical studies have reported excellent results following antegrade perfusion of the brain. This represents most probably the best method to preserve the integrity of the senso-motoric functions and cognitive faculties, particularly in frail patients and in those requiring a more complex surgical procedure in the setting of acute type A dissection.

Keywords: aortic dissection, surgical repair, cerebral protection, selective antegrade cerebral perfusion, stroke

1. Introduction

The history of hypothermic circulatory arrest (HCA) started with the first attempts at surgical repair of the aortic arch by Cooley in 1955, while DeBakey described in 1957 a technique using cardiopulmonary bypass (CPB) and cerebral perfusion [1]. In addition to the usual CPB circuit, the system included four pumps and perfusion lines for both carotid and coronary arteries. Despite fair results, this technique did not receive much attention because of the complex configuration of the CPB. Later, Borst used deep hypothermia and circulatory arrest for the surgical repair of a rare pathology of the aortic arch, namely an arteriovenous fistula [2].

A complete resection of the total arch with consecutive prosthetic replacement was performed in 1966 in France [3]. In 1975, Griepp published four cases of aortic arch aneurysms successfully operated on using deep hypothermia associated with total circulatory arrest [4]. His technique represented a breakthrough in the concept of aortic arch surgery because it aimed at reducing as much as possible the need for oxygen and metabolites during the period of the circulatory arrest while the absence of clamps and blood in the operative field greatly simplified the procedure. The concept of cold cerebral perfusion of the brain combined with moderate hypothermia of the body was attempted by the group of Guilmet while Kazui published a similar method in which the cerebral perfusion and the main CPB were performed both at moderate hypothermia [5, 6]. At a pretty similar time, Ueda proposed a technique of retrograde perfusion of the brain through the superior vena cava and right jugular vein using deep hypothermia [7].

Since these first steps, a remarkable development has been made and HCA combined with cerebral perfusion can now be considered as a routine procedure with reliable and reproducible results in experienced institutions. A large scientific activity was necessary to understand the protective characteristics of hypothermia and the methods of cerebral protection to reduce the period during which the brain is not perfused [8–13].

Despite the growing research and clinical experience, there is still only scarce evidence for neuroprotective strategies yet. The most recent ACCF and EACTS guidelines recommend (class II) deep HCA and selective anterograde cerebral perfusion (SACP) as reasonable strategy while emphasizing the importance of institutional experience in selecting the most appropriate technique [14, 15].

2. Cerebral perfusion and autoregulation

The main goal of cerebral protection, whatever the technique is used, is to preserve the most physiological characteristics of cerebral function. In the adult, the brain weighs around 1400 g; this means 2–3% of the total body weight. In contrast, the mean cerebral flow is about 750 ml/min which represents about 15–16% of the total cardiac output. This relationship demonstrates the huge metabolic demand of the brain and the importance of preserving its metabolic activity. Along the cerebral circulation, there is a constant drop in intravascular pressure, with a mean pressure of 80 mmHg in the common carotid arteries, 60 mmHg in the intracranial carotid artery, and 20mmHg in the middle cerebral arteries. It is around 15 mmHg in the cortical veins and 5–7 mmHg in the longitudinal sinus.

Autoregulation of the cerebral blood flow plays a major role in preserving the integrity of the cerebral metabolism; in general, autoregulation is maintained for a spectrum mean arterial pressure values between 50 and 150 mmHg [16–18]. This means that there is no linear not exponential relationship between cerebral blood flow and the mean arterial pressure within these values. However, regulation of cerebral blood flow varies according to the central temperature, with a more or less constant reduction of flow of 7% for each degree Celsius of hypothermia. Cerebral autoregulation nearly disappears when the brain temperature is below 15°C [19]. Cerebral oxygen consumption is approximatively 2.9 ml/min/g at 37°C and reduced to 0.90 ml/min/g at 25°C while at 20°C, it is only 20% of its physiological value. At 8°C, metabolic status is still 10% of the normal value [20].

Any sudden interruption or major reduction of the cerebral blood flow occurring at normothermia results in a dramatic drop of the oxygen and glucose supply which results in a loss of active phosphorylation of the cells and rapidly empties the adenosine triphosphate (ATP) reserves indispensable to normal brain activity. The intracellular pH rapidly collapses, while the transmembrane exchanges are interrupted. The electrical polarity is rapidly reduced, and potassium gets out of the cells. At the same time, the calcium and natrium channels open widely and lead to a massive flow of both calcium and natrium into the intracellular space. Together with the ongoing tissue acidosis, several enzymes are activated and will accelerate degradation of proteins, while peroxynitrite acidotic radicals and endonucleases induce DNA fragmentation. Altogether, these biochemical processes rapidly lead to cellular death. This process of neuronal necrosis may be considerably increased in case of blood flow restoration and ends in additional reperfusion injuries.

Cooling and rewarming processes are also of major importance to avoid additional injury due to inhomogeneous temperatures within the brain. The relationship between cerebral blood flow and metabolism may be analyzed using transcranial Doppler sonography which is able to demonstrate peak flow velocity depending on the respective actual cranial temperature. At normothermia and mild hypothermia, the maintenance of coupling means that blood flow velocity and temperature remain in a linear relationship. However, when deep hypothermia is targeted, autoregulation will be lost. Cerebral blood flow becomes pressure-dependent [21]. In case of rapid cooling under the condition of alpha-stat acid–base management, transcranial Doppler ultrasound will demonstrate a significant drop of flow velocity. This may end in inhomogeneous thermal distribution which means that brain structures located deeper in the skull are less efficiently cooled than those located at the surface [22].

In the past, pH-stat acid–base management and slow cooling have been considered as the best strategy to obtain the most uniform cooling of the brain together with the maintenance of the most optimal perfusion [23]. Hypothermia-related disruption of the normal relationship between cerebral blood flow and metabolism is even more important during rewarming. Greeley described a phenomenon where a transient disruption of cerebral vascular reactivity occurs during rewarming following a period of deep hypothermia [24]. As a consequence, flow (and therefore also velocity) remains at a lower level, while the metabolic demand of the brain increases together with the brain temperature. Greeley used the wording 'cerebral vasoplegia' to describe the loss of the relationship between flow (velocity) and metabolism. This uncoupling may result in relative hypoperfusion and, more dramatically, in ischemic brain injury.

3. Physiology of hypothermic circulatory arrest

The metabolism of the brain is generated by adenosine triphosphate that is produced during aerobic glycolysis. The metabolic rate of the cerebral tissue is seven times higher than that of the body. Anaerobic glycolysis, unlike in liver or muscle, cannot sustain the required energy demands of the brain. Therefore, a short anaerobic period with consecutive rise in lactate concentration will rapidly be deleterious for the cerebral cells.

Since the brain does not have glucose reserves, a constant supply through a continuous blood flow is mandatory, although changes in metabolic demands can be met by appropriate changes of blood blow upon a certain limit (cerebral autoregulation).

Experimental and clinical research has demonstrated that cerebral blood flow autoregulation can be affected by patient's factors such as age, diabetes, and arterial hypertension but also by conditions associated with specific changes during such surgical procedures (anesthesiologic management, pressure changes during extracorporeal perfusion, hemodilution, loss of pulsatility, as well as hypothermia). Depending on how reduction of cerebral flow occurs, two different types of perioperative cerebral injury may happen during aortic and/or cardiac procedures. The most devastating one is the classical stroke which is caused by localized cerebral ischemia (through embolization of corpuscular or gaseous particles). The other type of injury may be the result of global ischemia and is related to interrupted or temporarily inadequate perfusion [25]. In contrary to the frank stroke that is usually easily detectable through CT-scan and MR-imaging, temporary neurological dysfunction is a much more subtle form of global ischemia that manifest clinically under various symptoms (disorientation, delirium, amnesia, restlessness, and others).

Since it is not possible to completely turn off the energy demands of the brain while maintaining cellular viability, the strategy of cerebral protection includes methods to prevent cerebral anoxia and acidosis during interruption of the cerebral blood flow or to provide some cerebral perfusion during a planned period of circulatory arrest while limiting its duration to a strict minimum.

Nevertheless, hypothermia (even at different temperature levels) remains the principal method of brain protection while additional strategies were developed later as a solution to avoid a "complete" circulatory arrest or to make the arrest safer (e.g., extending its duration without additional risks). Independently of these developments, the basic questions about circulatory arrest, namely how cold and how long is safe, remain crucial.

According to numerous experimental and clinical studies, a circulatory arrest period is considered to be safe for up to 30 minutes at 15°C and 40 minutes at 10°C [8, 10, 26, 27]. In the pediatric literature, there are sufficient data that hypothermic arrest over 40 minutes is associated with significantly poorer neuro-developmental outcomes. In adults, a decline in neurocognitive performance has been observed when the duration of arrest exceeds 25minutes in the absence of additional neuroprotective strategies.

3.1 Levels of hypothermia

With increasing surgical experience and rising numbers of procedures on the aortic arch, the concept of hypothermia has considerably developed. When referring to "hypothermia", some precisions may be necessary, namely the real level of temperature as well as the location where the temperature is assessed. Several papers have tried to define the different levels of hypothermia—they are summarized in **Table 1** [15, 29, 30]. These classifications differentiate between deep, moderate, and mild hypothermia and based on the belief that the reduction of the suppression of brain metabolism is the main determinant of a successful arrest temperature. Nasopharyngeal (alternatively esophageal) temperature was selected as the reference

Profound	< 14°C				
Deep	14–20°C	< 20°C		< 20°C	
			20–24°C		Moderate low
Moderate	20–28°C		20–25°C		
				24–28°C	Moderate high
Mild	> 28°C	> 25 °C		> 28°C	
	[28]	[29]		[15]	

Table 1.
Different classifications of hypothermia.

because it closely corresponds to the brain temperature during cooling and rewarming. However, no publication has studied in detail whether the spinal cord and the abdominal organs are sufficiently protected with moderate hypothermia, especially during prolonged HCA duration.

Whether or not repair of type A aortic dissection with either an open distal anastomosis at the level of the proximal arch or with total arch replacement can be performed under moderate hypothermia in patients receiving SACP is still a matter of actual clinical research. To be accepted and generalized into regular surgical practice, the resulting stroke and mortality rates should probably be less than 5–10%, respectively and 10–15% in the acute setting.

3.2 Deep hypothermic circulatory arrest (DHCA)

Lowering the temperature of the whole organism to 18°C has been considered in the past as a safe technique for complex aortic arch procedures, especially in dissection patients because of the uncertainty concerning the expected duration of circulatory arrest to safely perform the distal anastomosis will be performed.

To improve the safety of DHCA, additional points have been worked out to avoid gradients of temperature between different areas and organs as well as within the brain itself; smooth cooling and rewarming process and assessment of both the rectal (or urinary bladder) and nasopharyngeal temperatures while packing the patient's head in ice should help to maintain the most homogeneous level of cerebral hypothermia during the arrest duration.

DHCA is rather simple that does not require any special equipment other than the regular circuit with a high-performance heat exchanger. Its benefits include a bloodless field and no need for any cannula or additional aortic manipulation. However, it may be associated with some drawbacks. DHCA requires a long time to lower the patient's temperature to the targeted level and to rewarm as well, with all side-effects on the coagulation and inflammatory systems. The absence of clear criteria that indicate that circulatory arrest is safe—some consider that CPB can be discontinued as soon as the temperature reaches 18 or 20°C while others consider that the circulatory arrest can be initiated only when the electroencephalography (EEG) is completely flat or when oxygen saturation of the venous return in the jugular vein is higher than 95%.

The maximal duration of DHCA without neurological dysfunction remains unclear but the upper safe limit at 12–20°C is considered to be 25–30 minutes [31]. The risk of neurologic disturbance raises significantly when DHCA exceeds 40 minutes and the risk of mortality when it is over 65 minutes. DHCA without any additional protective adjuncts has been progressively abandoned by most groups in favor of more moderate hypothermia active cerebral perfusion methods. A meta-analysis by Manoly et al. with nearly 6000 patients showed significantly lower mortality and incidence of stroke with moderate hypothermia with SACP compared to deep hypothermia alone [32].

4. Institutional cannulation and perfusion technique

Different sites of cannulation (ascending aorta, iliac/femoral, or subclavian/axillary) have been used and successfully described as potential approaches for the arterial return of CPB during repair of acute type A aortic dissection. All of them have advantages and disadvantages that have been extensively described in the literature.

Therefore, I would like to focus on the technique we adopted more than 25years ago at the University Hospital in Bern, Switzerland and I would like to summarize the main principles in the following lines.

Although surgical preparation and access to the right subclavian artery need more time than exposure of the femoral artery, several publications have demonstrated excellent outcomes compared to the historical series in which arterial return was performed via femoral cannulation. Subclavian artery cannulation may attenuate the possibility of brain malperfusion which can occur at the beginning of CPB in case of pressurization of the false aortic channel, or when a cross-clamp is placed on the ascending aorta. Personally, I am not in favor of a routine direct aortic cannulation strategy, however, in case of any unexpected technical difficulty, I would accept it for rapid institution of CPB. Two additional smaller roller pumps are used, one for instillation of cardioplegia, the other, placed beyond the oxygenator for cerebral perfusion. Continuous running through a recirculation tubing is recommended during the period of systemic circulatory arrest.

Our strategy has been to avoid cross-clamping the aorta because this maneuver may lead to additional injuries of the already dissected aorta and the supra-aortic branches. This means that the procedure usually starts with distal repair once the target temperature has been reached and that proximal repair is performed during rewarming. This sequence has the additional advantage of shortening the time period the patient is kept cool. The logic for this approach has become evident at our institution with a yearly number of 50–60 type A aortic dissections.

Once the targeted temperature of 26–28°C has been obtained, CPB is interrupted, and the aortic arch is opened. Two flexible thin perfusion catheters (Le Maître, Burlington, MA, USA) are introduced in both common carotid arteries, and SACP is started with a flow between 10 and 15 ml/kg/min (total usually 500–800 ml/min) with a temperature of the perfusate between 22 and 24°C and a pressure around 50–70 mmHg. The balloons of these perfusion catheters are inflated smoothly once perfusion has started to de-air the supra-aortic branches. Another very important feature in patients with type A aortic dissection is to cannulate the true lumen after it has been clearly distinguished from the false lumen by visual inspection from within the aortic arch. Following cannulation, the balloons are gently inflated until backward pulling cannot displace the catheters (**Figures 1–3**).

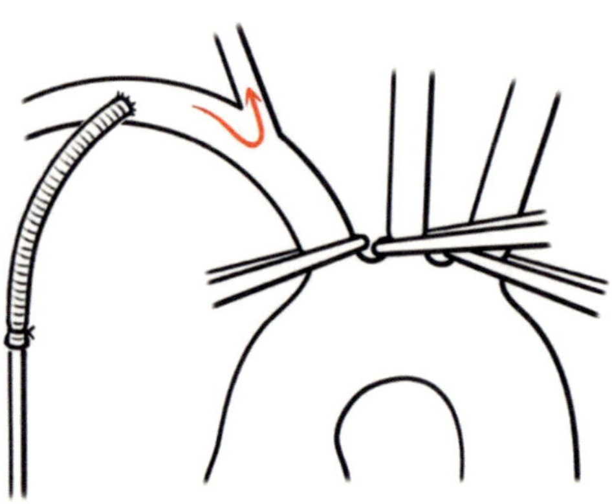

Figure 1.
Schematic drawing of unilateral antegrade cerebral perfusion through the right subclavian artery with clamping of the supra-aortic branches. (Reproduced with permission from Ref. [33]).

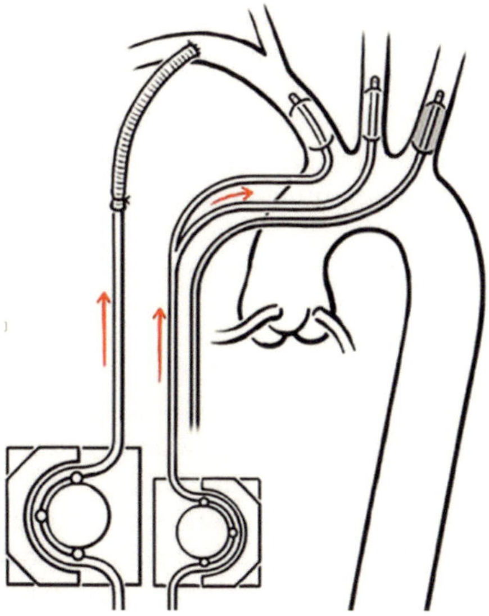

Figure 2.
Schematic drawing of bilateral antegrade cerebral perfusion through both common carotid artery with endovascular occlusion of the left subclavian artery using a Fogarty. (Reproduced with permission from Ref. [33]).

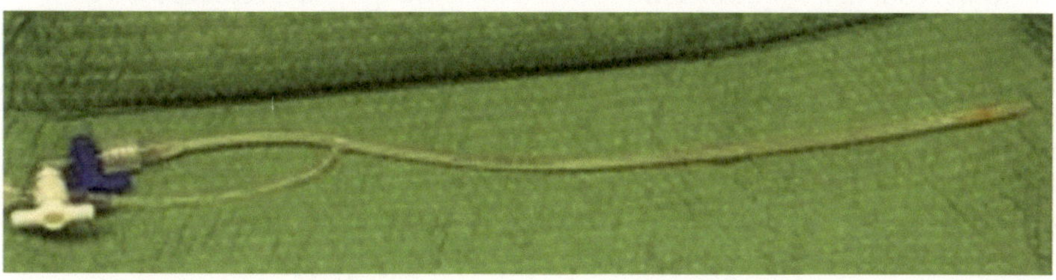

Figure 3.
Thin LeMaitre Vascular© perfusion catheter for selective antegrade cerebral perfusion with an inflatable balloon to block the backflow. (Reproduced with permission from Ref. [33]).

In the majority of cases, the left subclavian artery is occluded with a small Fogarty catheter from inside the vessel, except when the right vertebral artery is occluded. The right radial artery pressure as well as the pressure at the tip of both carotid catheters is maintained at 50 mm Hg.

To ensure true luminal perfusion after confection of the distal anastomosis and to minimize false luminal pressurization at all, reperfusion is started in an orthograde way via the side-arm graft of a Vascutek Anteflo prosthesis. During rewarming, proximal repair is performed while decannulation and reconstruction of the right subclavian artery can be performed safely.

5. Review of cerebral perfusion

The most optimal type of cerebral perfusion in the setting of acute type A aortic dissection repair remains a matter of preference/debate while different opinions are reported in the literature. Basically, there are several options:

- Unilateral antegrade cerebral perfusion via the right subclavian artery as it is cannulated for the arterial return of the CPB circuit,
- Bilateral SACP with two or three perfusion catheters introduced in the innominate artery (and pushed further into the right common carotid artery), the left common carotid artery, and eventually into the left subclavian artery,
- Retrograde cerebral perfusion (RCP) via the superior vena cava.

5.1 Antegrade cerebral perfusion (ACP)

The technique consists of perfusing one or several supra-aortic vessels with oxygenated blood in a physiological way at a flow and pressure compatible with the maintenance of a proper metabolic supply, providing equal distribution of the perfusate to both cerebral hemispheres while maintaining the core temperature at a moderate level. From the historical perspective, there are two different methods of ACP that differ regarding the temperature of the perfusate, the complexity of the CPB circuit, and the mode of cannulation of the supra-aortic branches.

The French technique uses perfusion with cold blood at a temperature of 10–12°C while the patient's core temperature is maintained at 25–28°C. The intention is to provide a homogeneous distribution of the cold perfusate to both hemispheres with significant reduction of the metabolic demand, although the cerebral blood flow regulation is not preserved. A regular circuit is modified through the addition of a heat exchanger beyond the oxygenator. The flow rate is maintained at 7–10 ml/min/kg, a pressure between 60 and 70 mmHg. No adjuncts are used to enhance cerebral protection [5].

The Japanese technique perfuses the brain and the body at the same temperature level. For this purpose, the CPB equipment is somewhat modified, with an additional arterial line that originates from the main arterial perfusion line. A separate pump is dedicated to brain perfusion. This technique has the advantage that a single heat exchanger is used because both, the CPB and the cerebral perfusion are performed at the same temperature. A total flow of 10 ml/kg is given through both cannulas. Because of its simplicity and the easy cannulation of the cerebral vessels, this technique of SACP has gained large acceptance [6].

Antegrade cerebral perfusion presents several advantages compared to hypothermic arrest alone or in combination with retrograde cerebral perfusion. It provides the most physiological type of perfusion - mimicking the normal blood flow to the brain, and obviates the need for deep hypothermia, thereby reducing the required time for cooling and rewarming and the risk of complications associated with a prolonged pump run like coagulopathy and pulmonary dysfunction. The suggested risks and drawbacks of antegrade perfusion include the risk of embolization of particles and air into the cerebral vessels during the introduction of the perfusion catheters, malperfusion through kinking of the catheters or false positioning, and finally the somewhat cumbersome procedure with additional manipulations of the supra-aortic branches. Nevertheless, these potential drawbacks can be rapidly eliminated with growing experience. Once the catheters have been introduced in the corresponding supra-aortic branches, they can be gently retracted to the head of the patient and do not obscure the view in the operative field.

5.1.1 Uni- or bilateral antegrade cerebral perfusion?

The rationale for one-, two-, or even three-vessel perfusion represents a matter of discussion. The debate was initiated following the publication of two clinical studies in which only unilateral perfusion from the right subclavian artery was used with excellent results regarding postoperative neurologic disorders [34, 35]. For this reason, unilateral perfusion technique has been adopted broadly in the clinical practice. In some studies, a decreased rate of permanent neurologic deficit following unilateral perfusion was observed, but not in the rate of transient neurologic disorders. Those in favor of unilateral perfusion concluded that the technique offers at least similar protection of the brain and the abdominal organs than bilateral SACP and that it may reduce the incidence of embolism arising from surgical manipulation on the supra-aortic branches [36].

However, equality of cerebral protection through unilateral or bilateral perfusion assumes that the circle of Willis provides enough blood flow on the contralateral brain hemisphere. Clinical studies have demonstrated that completeness of the circle can be expected in approximately 60% of patients. During unilateral cerebral perfusion, the flow velocity in the contralateral middle cerebral artery varies considerably, but the flow itself never disappears. From these observations, one can conclude that the anatomical particularities of the circle of Willis—with a broad range of variations—do not automatically correlate with its functional achievements when examined intra-operatively [37–39]. Meanwhile, both types of cerebral perfusion are largely accepted by the surgical community but it seems that bilateral SACP may be safer in case the circulatory arrest time is over 40 min [40–43]. In practice, the decision to use unilateral or bilateral perfusion is largely dependent on the institutional preference and experience, and the expected duration of the circulatory arrest plays a major role as well.

5.1.2 Clamping, snaring, or occlusion of supra-aortic branches with balloon catheters?

I personally consider the handling of the supra-aortic branches in the setting of a weakened arterial wall as it is the case in aortic dissection to be crucial [33]. For this purpose, we have used intraluminal occlusion with customized small and very smooth perfusion catheters with balloon occlusion (**Figure 1**). I see three potential advantages:

- Neither clamping nor snaring of any of the supra-aortic vessels is necessary. This is probably more important than generally considered, especially in the setting of a fragilized vessel wall through acute dissection. In this situation, there is an additional risk for a manipulative injury because of the dissection and this may cause obstruction or even complete occlusion is high.

- The introduction of a perfusion catheter into the true channel of the vessel with subsequent inflation of the balloon may favor the expansion of the dissected layers from inside and bring the dissected layers together, especially when they have been treated with biological glue.

- An additional benefit of balloon inflation may be the avoidance of downstream embolization of biological adhesive to glue the dissected layers of the vascular wall [44].

I had the privilege to recently work at another institution, where a strategy of unilateral ACP through the right subclavian artery was used routinely in patients operated on because of type A aortic dissection. All patients received an open distal anastomosis during which the innominate artery was clamped. In a consecutive series of 55 patients, I observed five cases of postoperative occlusion of the innominate artery, most probably due to a clamp injury. In four patients, the dissection process already involved the innominate artery on a preoperative CT scan. Postoperatively ipsilateral stroke was observed in all patients, in one patient it was associated with a lethal outcome. One patient underwent surgical revascularization with an interposition graft between the ascending aorta and the innominate artery and the other was treated with an endovascular stent of the innominate artery [33].

5.1.3 Should the left subclavian artery be perfused?

In the majority of reports of SACP, only the right subclavian and the left common carotid arteries have been perfused. No clinical consequences seem to be related to absence of left subclavian artery perfusion. Nevertheless, some groups, particularly in Japan perfuse systematically the left subclavian artery, especially in case the preoperative investigations have demonstrated occlusion of the right vertebral artery or a dominant/single left vertebral artery. In case of acute dissection without preoperative information, no or very weak backflow through the left subclavian artery may be considered as an indication to perfuse it antegradely. Independently of the previous considerations, it has been well demonstrated that the left subclavian artery may play an important role for the spinal cord perfusion through the anterior spinal artery [45, 46]. If the left subclavian artery is not selectively perfused, it may be important to occlude it to avoid steal syndrome and consecutive ischemia of the posterior cerebrum.

5.2 Retrograde perfusion

Retrograde cerebral perfusion has been first described by Mills and Ochsner in 1980 for another indication than aortic arch surgery, namely massive air embolism during CPB to flush out the arterial cerebral circulation on a retrograde way [47]. This technique was then described by Ueda as an adjunct to hypothermia during repair of aortic arch pathologies and is based on the idea that the brain could be perfused retrogradely through the venous and capillary systems on the analogy of retrograde cardioplegia [48]. The technique for retrograde cerebral perfusion may vary from institution to institution but the basics are similar; it includes a standard bi-caval cannulation with caval snaring. A simple modification to the normal CPB circuit is required with an additional connection between the arterial line and the superior vena cava line. This "shunt" remains closed during perfusion throughout CPB and once the targeted temperature is reached, the circulation is arrested. The arterial cannula is occluded, and the circuit is drained into the venous reservoir. The superior vena cava is snared at the entrance to the right atrium and the connection to the arterial line unclamped. Blood is then perfused retrogradely via the superior vena cava and returns to the opened aortic arch via the arterial system; this can be easily seen in the operative field when dark venous blood comes out of the supra-aortic branches (wash out of ischemic metabolites?) [49–51]. The latter can be returned into the circuit through cardiotomy suction. The perfusion pressure is kept around 20–25mmHg.

Among the most important potential benefits of RCP are maintaining cerebral hypothermia and flushing out atherosclerotic or gaseous emboli. However, this may not be the major problem in aortic dissection. On the other side, RCP may cause cerebral edema due to high venous flow rates and perfusion pressure.

Currently, there are no prospective randomized studies that show RCP has an advantage over HCA alone. Hagl analyzed the risk factors for stroke in a large collective of 700 patients [52]. RCP had no beneficial effects on outcome, but antegrade perfusion led to a decrease of temporary neurological events. Similar results were found by Okita who compared RCP to SACP in a prospective study [53]. Bonser has demonstrated that retrograde cerebral perfusion is unable to attenuate the metabolic changes induced in the brain by deep hypothermia [54].

From the current scientific evidence, it is actually not justified to support a strategy in favor of RCP. However, it is not excluded that RCP may somehow contribute to homogeneous cooling to the brain, and thereby makes prolonged duration of circulatory arrest safer than HCA alone.

6. Drugs

Several drugs have been used in the past and some of them are still administered today but the evidence to support this strategy is scarce. The most common substances used are lidocaine, thiopental and steroids, even though the mechanisms of protection are not fully elucidated. There is some evidence suggested that prophylactic use of dexmedetomidine for postoperative sedation reduced the rate and duration of postoperative delirium [55].

Diuretics like mannitol and furosemide are also interesting substances for adjuvant pharmacological protection during HCA—they work mainly through a reduction of cerebral edema [56]. Mannitol, besides reducing cerebral edema and intracranial pressure, has an important effect as a free radical scavenger and is administered both during the cooling and rewarming period. In Bern, our anesthesiologists have supported the use barbiturates 20years ago, but we have abandoned their use mainly because a net benefit could not be demonstrated so far. The results without barbiturates but instead with moderate hypothermia and SACP were even better. In addition, the potential myocardial depressant effect can be avoided. Others continue to incorporate high-dose thiopental in their protective regimen [57].

7. Intraoperative monitoring

Despite significant improvements in field of cardiovascular surgery (anesthesia, intensive care medicine, perfusion technology, and surgical technique itself), cerebral damage remains a fastidious complication of aortic dissection repair irrespective of the technique used for brain protection. Ideally, intraoperative monitoring should help to detect any global hypo- and hyperperfusion, significant regional perfusion deficits, and sudden changes in the perfusion characteristics. Nevertheless, there is no evidence so far that intraoperative monitoring reduces the risk of neurological injury. In the following, I will briefly review methods of intraoperative monitoring.

Classical electroencephalography (EEG) provides information on the whole cortical and subcortical structures in real time. EEG becomes totally flat when the cerebral temperature reaches a level below 20°C. Unfortunately, EEG does not give any information on deeper cerebral structures. The bi-spectral index (BIS) is a simpler surrogate of EEG. It provides reliable monitoring and is quite simple to use in any circumstance [58, 59].

Bilateral transcranial Doppler allows assessment of a symmetrical flow in the middle cerebral artery and detection of embolic phenomena but is limited to the anterior cerebral circulation [60]. Similarly to EEG, it requires a specialized technician in the operating theater. Transcranial Doppler is the only method to continuously assess changes in cerebral hemodynamics during CPB. It may be of particular interest during repair of acute ascending aortic dissection, for instance in case of malperfusion of the carotid arteries. This potentially catastrophic condition may be immediately recognized when sudden loss of Doppler signal may signify severe cerebral ischemia.

Serial determination of jugular venous bulb oxygen saturation allows continuous assessment of cerebral metabolism and may be used to detect intraoperative cerebral ischemia [61]. The method is easy to implement. A central venous catheter is used to cannulate the jugular bulb. Two punctures and two guidewires are necessary—the first is directed cephalad and the second is directed into the central circulation. A pulmonary artery catheter is placed in a standard fashion and the jugular bulb catheter is then advanced towards the jugular bulb using the Seldinger technique.

Near-infrared spectroscopy (NIRS)—also known as transcranial cerebral oximetry—is probably the most popular method of cerebral monitoring [62]. It is simple, noninvasive, and highly reproducible. It assesses regional cerebral oxygen saturation within the brain through the skull by absorption of infrared beams and may allow detection of cerebral hypoperfusion. It requires two or three adhesive electrodes to be placed on the forehead of the patient. The oxygen saturation of the underlying cortical structures appears directly on the monitor screen. A decrease in the regional saturation to values inferior to 60% of the baseline is a sign of severely altered brain perfusion, while a drop to 55% or less for of duration of 5 min means a high probability of a permanent neurologic lesion. Similarly to EEG, NIRS does not allow assessment of posterior and deeper structures of the brain.

A very simple method of monitoring is the recording of bilateral radial artery pressure that may give useful information about the perfusion pressure in the contralateral subclavian artery. Pressure should be maintained between 50 and 80 mmHg throughout the procedure.

In summary, monitoring of the brain function should be performed at least using BIS and regional NIRS of forehead even though there is few randomized evidence to support one technique over the other. A multimodal monitoring strategy may increase the sensitivity of detecting cerebral ischemia.

8. Clinical experience with cerebral protection in Europe: the result of a single survey

Because a definitive consensus has not yet been reached and many different approaches regarding site of cannulation, core and perfusate temperature, flow, monitoring methods as well as visceral protection, a survey was sent to 450 cardiac surgery units across Europe to evaluate the methods used for cerebral protection during aortic arch surgery and answered by 141 centers [63]. In the following, I will summarize the answers concerning the current handling of acute aortic dissection.

The right subclavian/axillary was the favorite site for arterial cannulation. Bilateral SACP was the most frequent method of brain protection in acute presentation. Unilateral perfusion was used in approximately 1/3 of the cases, while deep HCA and RCP are very rarely used in Europe and almost exclusively in patients with acute dissection.

In acute cases, 2/3 of centers perform distal anastomosis at a core temperature between 22 and 26°C, while 1/3 still use deeper temperature (down to 15°C in occasional cases). Only a few cardiac units use temperatures around 30–32°C. Flow and pressure of the are fairly similar among all centers (10–15 ml/kg), respectively around 60 mmHg, while average temperature of the perfusate is 22°C. At that time, barbiturates were used in 60% of centers, however, with a decreasing tendency since then.

The survey shows that the majority of the participating centers proceed within reasonable ranges published in the literature. Unilateral perfusion is still a broadly accepted method; however, if circulatory arrest duration is expected to be over 30–40 min, a bilateral SACP is preferred. Cerebral monitoring is part of the routine intraoperative strategy while NIRS associated with bilateral monitoring of perfusion pressure seems to be the preferred method of a majority of institutions. Hypothermia is always used, while circulatory arrest at warmer temperatures is being adopted more frequently.

9. Conclusion

Brain protection has been a major issue since the early period of aortic arch surgery [32, 64–69]. With improvements in surgical techniques, operative technology, and methods of blood management, the risk of stroke following repair of type A aortic dissection can be reduced to less than 5–10%, also with a mortality risk of less than 10%. This corresponds to the actual standard to which any innovation in the field of aortic dissection repair must be compared, including less invasive endovascular procedures.

Conflict of interest

"The authors declare no conflict of interest."

Author details

Thierry Carrel
Department of Cardiac Surgery, University of Zürich Consultant, University Hospital Basel, Switzerland

*Address all correspondence to: thierry.carrel@usb.ch

References

[1] De Bakey ME, Crawford ES, Cooley DA, Morris GC Jr. Successful resection of fusiform aneurysm of aortic arch with replacement by homograft. Surgery, Gynecology & Obstetrics. 1957;**105**:657-664

[2] Borst HG, Schaudig A, Rudolph W. Arterio-venous fistula of the aortic arch: Repair during deep hypothermia and circulatory arrest. The Journal of Thoracic and Cardiovascular Surgery. 1964;**48**:443-447

[3] Guilmet D, Scetbon V, Ricordeau G. Un cas d'anévrysme de la crosse aortique traité avec succès par résection-greffe. Mémoires Académie de Chirurgie. 1966;**92**:479-487

[4] Griepp RB, Stinson EB, Hollingsworth JF, Buehler D. Prosthetic replacement of the aortic arch. The Journal of Thoracic and Cardiovascular Surgery. 1975;**70**:1051-1063

[5] Bachet J, Guilmet D, Goudot B, Termignon JL, Dreyfus G, Teodori G, et al. A new technique of cerebral protection during surgery of the aortic arch. The Journal of Thoracic and Cardiovascular Surgery. 1991;**102**:85-94

[6] Kazui T, Inoue N, Yamada O, Komatsu S. Selective cerebral perfusion during operation for aneurysms of the aortic arch: A reassessment. The Annals of Thoracic Surgery. 1992;**53**:109-114

[7] Ueda Y, Miki S, Kusuhara OY, Tahata T, Yamanoka K. Deep hypothermic systemic circulatory arrest and continuous retrograde cerebral perfusion for surgery of aortic arch aneurysm. European Journal of Cardio-Thoracic Surgery. 1992;**6**:36-42

[8] Ergin AM, O'Connor J, Guinto R, Griepp RB. Experience with profound hypothermia and circulatory arrest in the treatment of aneurysm of the aortic arch. The Journal of Thoracic and Cardiovascular Surgery. 1982;**84**:649-654

[9] Livesay JJ, Cooley DA, Reul GJ, Walker WE, Frazier OH, Duncan JM. Resection of aortic arch aneurysms: A comparison of hypothermic techniques in 60 patients. The Annals of Thoracic Surgery. 1983;**36**:19-28

[10] Gega A, Rizzo JH, Johnson MH, Tranquilli M, Farkas EA, Elefteriades JA. Straight deep hypothermic arrest: Experience in 394 patients supports its effectiveness as a sole means of brain preservation. The Annals of Thoracic Surgery. 2007;**84**:759-767

[11] Shaikh FA, Khalil SI, Ander EH, Calvelli HR, Kashem MA, Mokashi S. Cerebral protection strategies for type A aortic dissection repair. Indian Journal of Thoracic and Cardiovascular Surgery. 2023;**39**(Suppl. 2):308-314

[12] Pitts L, Kofler M, Montagner M, Heck R, Iske J, Buz S, et al. Cerebral protection strategies and stroke in surgery for acute type A aortic dissection. Journal of Clinical Medicine. 2023;**12**:2271

[13] Hata M, Sezai A, Yoshitake I, Wakui S, Takasaka A, Minami K, et al. Clinical trends in optimal treatment strategy for type A acute aortic dissection. Annals of Thoracic and Cardiovascular Surgery. 2010;**16**:228-235

[14] Hiratzka LF, Bakris GL, Beckman JA, Bersin RM, Carr VF, Casey DE, et al. 2010 ACCF/AHA/AATS/ACR/ASA/SCA/SCAI/SIR/STS/SVM guidelines for the diagnosis and management of patients with thoracic aortic disease. Anesthesia and Analgesia. 2010;**111**:279-315

[15] Czerny M, Grabenwöger M, Berger T, Aboyans V, Della Corte A, Chen EP, et al. EACTS/STS guidelines for diagnosing and treating acute and chronic syndromes of the aortic organ. European Journal of Cardio-Thoracic Surgery. 1 Feb 2024;**65**(2):ezad426. DOI: 10.1093/ejcts/ezad426

[16] Peng L, Guo D, Shi Y, Yang J, Wei W. The incidence, risk factors and outcomes of impaired cerebral autoregulation in aortic arch surgery. Journal of Cardiothoracic Surgery. 2023;**18**:312

[17] Siddiqi AZ, Froese L, Gomez A, Sainbhi AS, Stein K, Park K, et al. The effect of burst suppression on cerebral blood flow and autoregulation: A scoping review of the human and animal literature. Frontiers in Physiology. 7 Jun 2023;**14**:1204874. DOI: 10.3389/fphys.2023.1204874. eCollection 2023

[18] Aguet J, Fakhari N, Nguyen M, Mertens L, Szabo E, Ertl-Wagner B. Impact of cardiopulmonary bypass on cerebrovascular autoregulation assessed by ultrafast ultrasound imaging. The Journal of Physiology. 2023;**60**:1077-1093

[19] Neri E, Sassi C, Barabesi L, Massetti M, Pula G, Buklas D, et al. Cerebral autoregulation after hypothermic circulatory arrest in operations on the aortic arch. The Annals of Thoracic Surgery. 2004;77:72-79

[20] Ehrlich MP, McCullough JN, Zhang N. Effect of hypothermia on cerebral blood flow and metabolism in the pig. The Annals of Thoracic Surgery. 2002;**73**:191-197

[21] Kern FH, Gieser WG, Farrell DM. Extracorporeal circulation and circulatory assist devices in the pediatric patient. In: Lake CL, editor. Pediatric Cardiac Anesthesia. 2nd ed. Norwalk, CN: Appleton & Lange; 1993. pp. 151-180

[22] Kern FH, Ungerleider RM, Quill TJ. Cerebral blood flow response to changes in PaCO2 during hypothermic cardiopulmonary bypass in children. The Journal of Thoracic and Cardiovascular Surgery. 1991;**101**:618-622

[23] Sakamoto T, Zurakowski D, Duebener LF, Lidov HG, Holmes GL, Hurley RJ, et al. Interaction of temperature with hematocrit level and pH determines safe duration of hypothermic circulatory arrest. The Journal of Thoracic and Cardiovascular Surgery. 2004;**128**:220-232

[24] Greeley WJ, Underleider RM, Kern FH, Brusino FG, Smith LR, Reves JG. Effects of cardiopulmonary bypass on cerebral blood flow in neonates, infants and children. Circulation. 1989;**80**:I209-I215

[25] Ergin MA, Galla JD, Lansmans SL, Quintana C, Bodian C, Griepp RB. Hypothermic circulatory arrest in operations on the thoracic aorta. Determinants of operative mortality and neurologic outcome. The Journal of Thoracic and Cardiovascular Surgery. 1994;**107**:788-797

[26] O'Connor JV, Wilding T, Farmer P, Sher J, Ergin MA, Griepp RB. The protective effect of profound hypothermia on the canine central nervous system in surgery of the ascending aorta and the aortic arch. The Annals of Thoracic Surgery. 1986;**41**:255-259

[27] Griepp RB, Di Luozzo G. Hypothermia for aortic surgery. The Journal of Thoracic and Cardiovascular Surgery. 2013;**145**:S56-S58

[28] Yan TD, Bannon PG, Bavaria J, Coselli JS, Elefteriades JA, Griepp RB, et al. Consensus on hypothermia in aortic arch surgery. Annals of Cardiothoracic Surgery. 2013;**2**:163-168

[29] Abjigitova D, Notenboom ML, Veen KM, van Tussenbroek G, Bekkers JA, Mokhles MM, et al. Optimal temperature management in aortic arch surgery: A systematic review and network meta-analysis. Journal of Cardiac Surgery. 2022;**37**:5379-5387

[30] Preventza O, Coselli JS, Akvan S, Kashyap SA, Garcia A, Simpson KH, et al. The impact of temperature in aortic arch surgery patients receiving antegrade cerebral perfusion for >30 minutes: How relevant is it really? The Journal of Thoracic and Cardiovascular Surgery. 2017;**153**:767-776

[31] Reich DL, Uysal S, Sliwinski M, Ergin MA, Kahn RA, Konstadt SN, et al. Neuropsychologic outcome after deep hypothermic circulatory arrest in adults. The Journal of Thoracic and Cardiovascular Surgery. 1999;**117**:156-163

[32] Manoly I, Uzzaman M, Karangelis D, Kuduvalli M, Georgakarakos E, Quarto C, et al. Neuroprotective strategies with circulatory arrest in open aortic surgery - A meta-analysis. Asian Cardiovascular & Thoracic Annals. 2022;**30**:635-644

[33] Carrel T, Schmiady M, Ouda A, Vogt PR. Uni-versus bilateral antegrade cerebral perfusion during repair of acute aortic dissection: Still a discussed matter! JTCVS Techniques. 2023;**17**:18-22

[34] Reutebuch O, Schurr U, Hellermann J, Prêtre R, Künzli A, Lachat M, et al. Advantages of subclavian artery perfusion for repair of acute type A dissection. European Journal of Cardio-Thoracic Surgery. 2004;**26**:592-598

[35] Tasdemir O, Saritas A, Kucuker S, Ozatik MA, Sener E. Aortic arch repair with right brachial artery perfusion. The Annals of Thoracic Surgery. 2002;**73**:1837-1841

[36] Zierer A, El-Sayed Ahmad A, Papadopoulos N, Moritz A, Diegeler A, Urbanski PP. Selective antegrade cerebral perfusion and mild systemic hypothermic circulatory arrest for aortic arch replacement: Results from 1002 patients. The Journal of Thoracic and Cardiovascular Surgery. 2012;**144**:1042-1049

[37] Urbanski PP, Lenos A, Blume JC, Ziegler V, Griewing B, Schmitt R, et al. Does anatomical completeness of the circle of Willis correlate with sufficient cross-perfusion during unilateral cerebral perfusion? European Journal of Cardio-Thoracic Surgery. 2008;**33**:402-408

[38] Macchi C, Catini C, Federico C, Gulisano M, Pacini P, Cecchi F, et al. Magnetic resonance angiographic evaluation of circulus arteriosus cerebri (circle of Willis) (a morphologic study in 100 human healthy subjects). Italian Journal of Anatomy and Embryology. 1996;**101**:115-123

[39] Krabbe-Hartkamp MJ, van der Grond J, de Leeuw FE, de Groot JC, Algra A, Hillen B. Circle of Willis (morphologic variation on three-dimensional time-of-flight MR angiograms). Radiology. 1998;**207**:103-111

[40] Olsson C, Thelin S. Antegrade cerebral perfusion with a simplified technique: Unilateral versus bilateral perfusion. The Annals of Thoracic Surgery. 2006;**81**:868-874

[41] Krähenbühl ES, Clément M, Reineke D, Czerny M, Stalder M, Ayamard T, et al. Antegrade cerebral protection in thoracic aortic surgery: Lessons from the past decade. European Journal of Cardio-Thoracic Surgery. 2010;**38**:46-51

[42] Angeloni E, Melina G, Refice SK, Roscitano A, Capuano F, Comito C, et al. Unilateral versus bilateral antegrade cerebral protection during aortic surgery: An updated meta-analysis. The Annals of Thoracic Surgery. 2015;**99**:2024-2031

[43] Spielvogel D, Kai M, Tang GH, Malekan R, Lansman SL. Selective cerebral perfusion: A review of the evidence. The Journal of Thoracic and Cardiovascular Surgery. 2013;**145**(Suppl. 3):S59-S62

[44] Carrel T, Maurer M, Tkebuchava T, Niederhäuser U, Schneider J, Turina M. Embolization of biologic glue during repair of aortic dissection. The Annals of Thoracic Surgery. 1995;**60**:1118-1120

[45] Griepp RB, Griepp EB. Spinal cord perfusion and protection during descending thoracic and thoracoabdominal aortic surgery: The collateral network concept. The Annals of Thoracic Surgery. 2007;**83**:S865-S869

[46] Biglioli P, Roberto M, Cannata A, Paroalri A, Fumero A, Grillo F, et al. Upper and lower spinal cord blood supply: The continuity of the anterior spinal artery and the relevance of the lumbar arteries. The Journal of Thoracic and Cardiovascular Surgery. 2004;**127**:1188-1192

[47] Mills NL, Ochsner JL. Massive air embolism during cardiopulmonary bypass. Causes, prevention, and management. The Journal of Thoracic and Cardiovascular Surgery. 1980;**80**:708-717

[48] Ueda Y, Miki S, Kusuhara K, Okita Y, Tahata T, Yamanaka K. Surgical treatment of aneurysm or dissection involving the ascending aorta and aortic arch, utilizing circulatory arrest and retrograde cerebral perfusion. The Journal of Cardiovascular Surgery. 1990;**31**:553-558

[49] Reich DL, Uysal S, Ergin MA, Bodian CA, Hossain S, Griepp RB. Retrograde cerebral perfusion during thoracic aortic surgery and late neuropsychological dysfunction. European Journal of Cardio-Thoracic Surgery. 2001;**19**:594-600

[50] Okita Y, Takamoto S, Ando M, Morota T, Matsukawa R, Kawashima Y. Mortality and cerebral outcome in patients who underwent aortic arch operations using deep hypothermic circulatory arrest with retrograde cerebral perfusion: No relation of early death, stroke, and delirium to the duration of circulatory arrest. The Journal of Thoracic and Cardiovascular Surgery. 1998;**115**:129-138

[51] Girardi LN, Shavladze N, Sedrakyan A, Neragi-Miandoab S. Safety and efficacy of retrograde cerebral perfusion as an adjunct for cerebral protection during surgery on the aortic arch. The Journal of Thoracic and Cardiovascular Surgery. 2014;**148**:2927-2933

[52] Hagl C, Ergin MA, Galla JD, Lansman SL, McCullough JN, Spielvogel D, et al. Neurologic outcome after ascending aorta-aortic arch operations: Effect of brain protection technique in high-risk patients. The Journal of Thoracic and Cardiovascular Surgery. 2001;**121**:1107-1121

[53] Okita Y, Miyata H, Motomura N, Takamoto S. A study of brain protection during total arch replacement comparing antegrade cerebral perfusion versus hypothermic circulatory arrest with or without retrograde cerebral perfusion: Analysis based on the Japan adult cardiovascular surgery database. The Journal of Thoracic and Cardiovascular Surgery. 2015;**149**:S65-S73

[54] Bonser RS, Wong CH, Harrington D, Pagano D, Wilkes M, Clutton T, et al.

Failure of retrograde cerebral perfusion to attenuate metabolic changes associated with hypothermic circulatory arrest. The Journal of Thoracic and Cardiovascular Surgery. 2002;**123**:943-950

[55] Djaiani G, Silverton N, Fedorko L, Carroll J, Styra R, Rao V, et al. Dexmedetomidine versus propofol sedation reduces delirium after cardiac surgery: A randomized controlled trial. Anesthesiology. 2016;**124**:362-368

[56] Hirotani T, Kameda T, Kumamoto T, Shirota S. Aortic arch repair using hypothermic circulatory arrest technique associated with pharmacological brain protection. European Journal of Cardio-Thoracic Surgery. 2000;**18**:545-549

[57] Al-Hashimi S, Zaman M, Waterworth P, Bilal H. Does the use of thiopenthal provide added cerebral protection during deep hypothermic circulatory arrest? Interactive Cardiovascular and Thoracic Surgery. 2013;**17**:392-397

[58] Myles PS, Leslie K, McNeil J, Forbes A, Chan MT. Bispectral index monitoring to prevent awareness during anaesthesia: The B-aware randomised controlled trial. Lancet. 2004;**363**:1757-1763

[59] Mathew JP, Weatherwax KJ, East CJ, White WD, Reves JG. Bispectral analysis during cardiopulmonary bypass: The effects of hypothermia on the hypnotic state. Journal of Clinical Anesthesia. 2001;**13**:301-305

[60] DeVries AJ. Transcranial Doppler technique for monitoring the efficacy of selective antegrade cerebral perfusion. Anesthesia and Analgesia. 1999;**89**:1587-1588

[61] McCullough JN. Monitoring the brain: Jugular venous oxygen saturation. In: Coselly JS, Lemaire SA, editors. Aortic Arch Surgery: Principles, Strategies and Outcome, Blackwell Publishing Ltd. Oxford: UK; 2008. pp. 125-127

[62] Orihashi K, Sueda T, Okada K, Imai K. Near-infrared spectroscopy for monitoring cerebral ischemia during selective cerebral perfusion. European Journal of Cardio-Thoracic Surgery. 2004;**26**:907-911

[63] De Paulis R, Czerny M, Weltert L, Bavaria J, Borger MA, Carrel TP, et al. Current trends in cannulation and neuroprotection during surgery of the aortic arch in Europe. European Journal of Cardio-Thoracic Surgery. 2015;**47**:917-923

[64] Abjigitova D, Veen KM, van Tussenbroek G, Mokhles MM, Bekkers JA, Takkenberg JJM, et al. Cerebral protection in aortic arch surgery: Systematic review and meta-analysis. Interactive Cardiovascular and Thoracic Surgery. 2022;**35**:ivac128

[65] Bonser RS, Ranasinghe AM, Loubani M, Evans JD, Thalji N, Bachet E, et al. Evidence, lack of evidence, controversy, and debate in the provision and performance of the surgery of acute type A aortic dissection. Journal of the American College of Cardiology. 2011;**58**:2455-2474

[66] Seese L, Chen EP, Badhwar V, Thibault D, Habib RH, Jacobs JP, et al. Optimal circulatory arrest temperature for aortic hemiarch replacement with antegrade brain perfusion. The Journal of Thoracic and Cardiovascular Surgery. 2023;**165**:1759-70.e3

[67] Fan S, Wang D, Wu C, Pan Z, Li Y, An Y, et al. Effects of 4 major brain protection strategies during aortic arch surgery: A protocol for a systematic review and network meta-analysis using Stata. Medicine (Baltimore). 2018;**97**:e11448

[68] Tian DH, Wilson-Smith A, Koo SK, Forrest P, Kiat H, Yan TD. Unilateral versus bilateral antegrade cerebral perfusion: A meta-analysis of comparative studies. Heart, Lung & Circulation. 2019;**28**:844-849

[69] Tian DH, Weller J, Hasmat S, Preventza O, Forrest P, Kiat H, et al. Temperature selection in antegrade cerebral perfusion for aortic arch surgery: A meta-analysis. The Annals of Thoracic Surgery. 2019;**108**:283

Chapter 9

Unilateral Antegrade Cerebral Perfusion during Aortic Arch Repair

Boris Kozlov and Dmitri Panfilov

Abstract

Circulatory arrest is one of the most crucial timeframes during aortic arch surgery due to the increased ischemic risk for inner organs, including the brain. In this regard, the issue of intraoperative cerebral protection is of great importance. Despite the fact that antegrade cerebral perfusion is the preferred neuroprotective strategy during aortic arch surgery, including the frozen elephant trunk procedure, the choice of the best perfusion technique for cerebral protection is still a matter of debate. We conducted a comprehensive analysis of cerebral status in 97 patients who underwent total arch repair using the frozen elephant trunk technique under moderate hypothermia and unilateral cerebral perfusion via an innominate artery. Our analysis, including intraoperative monitoring of cerebral oximetry, the incidence of postoperative neurological deficit and cognitive impairment, and added assessment of a neuronal injury marker level (neuron-specific enolase), demonstrates the high efficacy and safety of unilateral antegrade cerebral perfusion via an innominate artery.

Keywords: unilateral cerebral perfusion, innominate artery, neurological deficit, neuron-specific enolase, cognitive impairment

1. Introduction

It is known that aortic arch surgery requires temporary interruption of cerebral circulation [1]. However, the safe period of such a maneuver is only 4–5 minutes, which is not enough to perform an adequate aortic arch reconstruction. Therefore, certain measures are required to ensure cerebral protection during aortic arch surgery. The main components of neuroprotection include systemic hypothermia leading to a decrease of cerebral metabolism, and cerebral perfusion during circulatory arrest (CA), allowing the delivery of energy substrates, oxygen, and, at the same time, the removal of metabolites.

1.1 Hypothermic circulatory arrest

Systemic hypothermia is distinguished into several degrees with the following temperature ranges: mild (28.1–34°C), moderate (20.1–28°C), severe (20–14°C), and deep (≤ 14°C) [2]. The degree of hypothermic protection is still a highly controversial issue. In fact, with a hypothermia level deeper by 10°C, cellular metabolism slows down by 5–7% [3]. Consequently, neuronal activity decreases proportionally to body temperature. Thus, with hypothermia at 15–17°C, cellular metabolism decreases approximately by six times (to 12–25% of the metabolic rate at normothermia), and at a temperature of 10–12°C, it shows electrocerebral silence. However, numerous studies found that the absence of electrical cerebral activity can also be observed at higher temperatures (up to 27°C) [3, 4].

Despite all the advantages, including cerebral protection, avoidance of clamping, a bloodless and motionless operative field, and no need for additional perfusion equipment, the safe time provided by hypothermia is limited [5]. Thus, deep hypothermia protects from cerebral ischemia for a period of up to 30–40 minutes [2, 3, 6]. Hypothermia of longer than 40 minutes was found to lead to increased neurological complications, and in cases of over 65 minutes, the risk of mortality was significantly higher [7, 8]. Additionally, with deep hypothermia, there is an increased risk of bleeding, as well as cardiac, respiratory, and renal complications due to the development of endothelial dysfunction caused by prolonged cardiopulmonary bypass (CPB) [4–6].

The necessity to reduce complications required altering the strategy for protecting from ischemia. Di Eusanio et al. [9] analyzed their own surgical experience performed under deep and moderate hypothermia amplified with antegrade cerebral perfusion (ACP). The authors noted that the postoperative rate of deaths and strokes decreased in moderate hypothermia. Vallabhajosyula et al. and Gong et al. made similar conclusions [10, 11]. Thus, increasing body temperature during aortic arch surgery was found to reduce the number of complications related to deep hypothermia. However, moderate hypothermia alone does not provide safety due to the time limit, which does not exceed 10–20 minutes, because of increased cerebral oxygen consumption. As a result, there is a need for additional perfusion support during aortic arch operations [2].

1.2 Cerebral perfusion

To date, there are several neuroprotective strategies during aortic arch repair: retrograde cerebral perfusion (RCP) as well as uni- and bilateral antegrade cerebral perfusion [5, 6, 12].

1.2.1 Retrograde cerebral perfusion

Retrograde cerebral perfusion provides cerebral protection by perfusing cold oxygenated blood into the superior vena cava, maintaining a flow rate of 500 ml/min and a pressure of no lower than 25–30 mm Hg. The opening of internal jugular vein valves, which are the primary venous drain for the human brain, is ensured only under these conditions [13, 14]. There is compelling evidence that retrograde cerebral perfusion may provide neuroprotection not only through the support of cerebral metabolism but also by expelling emboli from the cerebral vasculature [15, 16]. According to Rylski et al. [15], retrograde cerebral perfusion is superior in the prevention of focal neurological deficits during "short" aortic arch procedures (<40 min). However, some data demonstrate opposite outcome. Thus, temporary neurological deficit (agitation, delirium) with retrograde cerebral perfusion has been reported in

12.8–25.1% and the incidence of permanent neurological events (stroke) was observed in 2.8–13.5% of cases [17, 18]. Moreover, a number of papers did not reveal significant differences in neurological complication rates between isolated hypothermic circulatory arrest and retrograde cerebral perfusion [19, 20].

The relatively low degree of cerebral protection during RCP is due to some of its peculiarities. Thus, up to 90% of blood is shunted through arterio-venous and veno-venous shunts into the inferior vena cava, the functionality of which increases during hypothermia [5, 21]. Cerebral edema is another negative factor resulting from conditions of high perfusion pressure [6, 16, 17]. Fluid extravasation due to high hydrostatic pressure leads to increased perivascular pressure and compressed parenchymal arterioles, causing cerebral edema followed by delirium development [13, 14]. Attempts to reduce perfusion pressure in the experiment have demonstrated the ineffectiveness of such perfusion. It has been shown that in primates, RCP for up to 60 minutes duration with the maintenance of perfusion pressure around 20 mm Hg provides only 1% of the cerebral flow from antegrade values [13].

Additionally providing of RCP is limited in patients with occlusive disease of supra-aortic vessels. This entity causes cerebral edema development due to positive (even residual) pressure in the arterial system. For this reason, RCP is less effective and even dangerous in these patients [22].

Thus, the role of retrograde perfusion in cerebral protection during aortic arch repair is still controversial, mostly due to the high risk of neurocognitive disorders (up to 40%) [1, 23]. To date, most clinics have abandoned the use of this type of cerebral protection and have focused their efforts on antegrade cerebral perfusion [24, 25].

1.2.2 Antegrade cerebral perfusion

Antegrade cerebral perfusion was popularized by Bachet and Guilmet in Europe and Kazui in Asia. The fundamental difference between ACP from RCP is in the cerebral blood supply via a physiological route, namely through supra-aortic vessels instead of the superior vena cava. A significant advantage of ACP is a longer safe period of circulatory arrest (up to 90 minutes) at a higher body temperature. Antegrade cerebral perfusion allows for better elimination of metabolites as well as lower biomarker levels of cerebral damage [5, 7, 26], consequently reducing hospital mortality and stroke rate [27]. To date, uni- and bilateral approaches are proposed for ACP during aortic arch surgery.

Bilateral antegrade cerebral perfusion is the most physiological approach, providing blood supply to the brain through both carotid arteries. On the other side, unilateral ACP possibility is based on cerebral multiple ways of cross-perfusion. An important role in collateral cerebral circulation is played by the ophthalmic artery, leptomeningeal vessels, and external carotid arteries [28–31]. Alongside this, the role of the Circle of Willis remains unclear. Thus, Urbanski et al. [32] revealed that up to 40% of patients have abnormalities in the Circle of Willis. However, in these cohorts, flow velocity was recorded in the contralateral middle cerebral artery during unilateral ACP. This indicates collateral pathways function that ensures adequate perfusion of both cerebral hemispheres.

Taking these circumstances into account, the choice of the best strategy is still debated. Malvindi et al. [33] analyzed the results of 3548 patients and concluded that bilateral perfusion provides greater safety during prolonged circulatory arrest (> 50 minutes) compared to unilateral perfusion. Others consider it mandatory to provide bilateral ACP during complex aortic arch repair, ensuring the most physiological cerebral perfusion [34, 35].

Meanwhile, a meta-analysis (6788 patients) conducted by Angeloni et al. [36] demonstrated the superiority of unilateral perfusion over bilateral perfusion in terms of the incidence of postoperative neurological complications (5.8 versus 6.9%, $p = 0.53$) and mortality (7.6 versus 9.8%; $p = 0.19$). A possible explanation of the increase of temporary and permanent neurologic deficit in patients with bilateral ACP related to additional manipulations with supra-aortic vessels that lead to increased risk of embolism. At the same time, unilateral ACP may prevent neurological complications by high-velocity retrograde flow from the supra-aortic vessels.

Zierer et al. [37] showed a comparable 30-day mortality rate and two times higher stroke rate after bilateral ACP compared to unilateral cerebral perfusion (4 versus 2%, $p = 0.06$). Supporting the theory of unilateral ACP superiority, Özatik et al. [31] showed that the levels of cerebral damage markers (S-100 protein and neuron-specific enolase), as well as lactate, pH, glucose, and blood oxygen, do not differ significantly between different hemispheres with unilateral cerebral perfusion. Moreover, it has been shown that prolonged unilateral perfusion, even more than 60 minutes, is not accompanied by a significant increase either in early mortality or cerebral complications [38, 39].

However, Tong et al. [40], comparing outcomes of bilateral and unilateral ACP, did not reveal any advantages of one technique over the other regarding 30-day mortality and neurologic complications. Moreover, the findings of a meta-analysis conducted by Tian et al. [41] served as additional evidence for the adequacy of unilateral perfusion. They found that both unilateral and bilateral cerebral perfusion techniques do not significantly differ in neurological outcomes or mortality.

To sum up, currently, the effects of uni- and bilateral ACP remain controversial and require further investigations.

1.2.3 Arterial cannulation

A number of arterial cannulation sites for antegrade cerebral perfusion have been described in the literature. The optimal site depends on thoracic aortic pathology, including anatomical features of the patient, surgical conditions, and the experience of the surgical team.

In the mid-90s, Sabik et al. [42] were the first who suggested subclavian artery for arterial cannulation site during thoracic aortic surgery. Subclavian artery cannulation allows to provide antegrade flow during cardiopulmonary bypass, as well as adequate antegrade cerebral perfusion within circulatory arrest [43, 44]. The disadvantages of this approach include the impossibility of initiating cardiopulmonary bypass if the artery diameter is too small or has subclavian stenosis or thrombosis [15, 43, 45]. Overall, the incidence of complications related to inadequate perfusion, vascular complications, and brachial plexus injuries is up to 14%. Moreover, the need to replace the arterial cannula with an alternative site is required in 11% of cases [46].

Cannulation of the common carotid artery is considered another option, especially in emergency cases. According to Rylski et al. [15], the common carotid artery has an advantage over the subclavian artery, primarily due to its larger diameter and convenient anatomy. In addition, a cannula placed into the carotid artery allows for lower pressure from the pump of the heart-lung machine. On the other hand, obstacles in the aortic arch lead to an increase in blood flow and pressure in the arterial system. This, in turn, can cause over-perfusion and cerebral damage. Hence, it necessitates additional cannulation, which eliminates all the advantages of common carotid artery cannulation.

An alternative option to central aortic cannulation is the cannulation of the innominate artery (IA), which allows for antegrade cerebral perfusion within circulatory arrest, avoiding high pump pressure due to the larger size of the vessel [47–49]. IA cannulation does not require an additional skin incision, which enables good visual control of the cannulation site. Additionally, there is no risk of neural plexus injuries [50]. Nevertheless, the IA is not suitable for cannulation when dissected or if its arterial wall is severe atheromatous [51].

The body of evidence regarding the efficacy and safety of cerebral perfusion via the innominate artery is sparse. Thus, we conducted a comprehensive analysis of cerebral status in 97 patients who underwent total arch repair using the frozen elephant trunk (FET) technique under moderate hypothermia and unilateral cerebral perfusion via the innominate artery.

2. Surgical techniques

2.1 Technique of unilateral cerebral perfusion via innominate artery

After median sternotomy IA up to its bifurcation is mobilized. After the administration of a 1 mg/kg heparin dose, the artery is side-clamped. The IA is opened to decrease the arterial pressure in the right radial artery by no more than 50% and to decrease the right hemisphere cerebral oximetry not lower than 20% compared to the baseline values. Then, an anastomosis is performed using a continuous 5–0 Prolene suture with an 8–10 mm vascular graft in an end-to-side fashion. After washing off possible debris and eliminating air from the vascular graft, it is connected to the arterial line of the CPB circuit (**Figures 1** and **2**).

Very rarely, when the side clamp of the IA is considered technically impossible or unsafe, IA was cross-clamped with flow interruption.

During the entire procedure, cerebral oximetry is carefully monitored using the near-infrared spectroscopy (NIRS), while maintaining mean arterial pressure at 50–60 mmHg in both radial arteries.

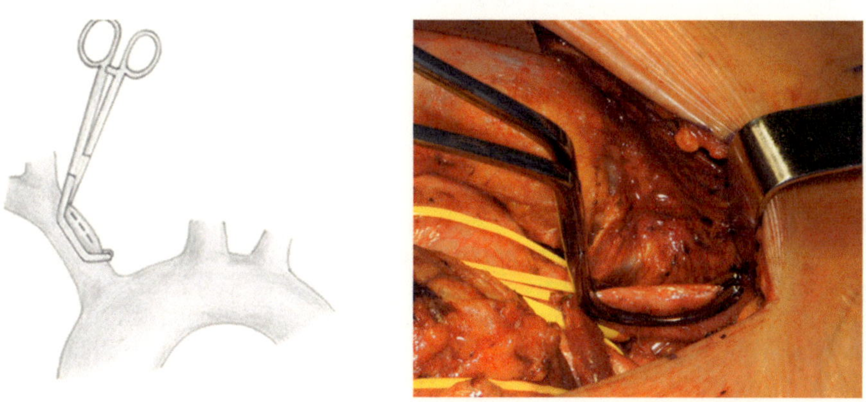

Figure 1.
Side clamp of the IA in a schematic diagram (left image) and intraoperative image (right image).

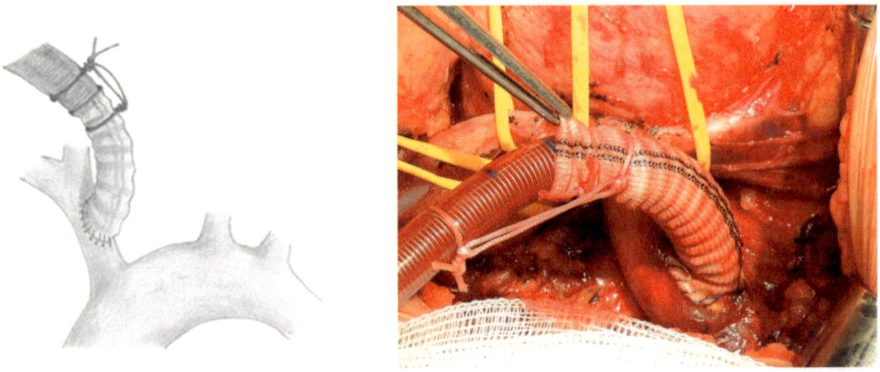

Figure 2.
The arterial line of the CPB circuit connecting to the innominate artery in a schematic diagram (left image) and intraoperative image (right image).

Mannitol and hydrocortisone are administered intraoperatively to prevent cerebral edema, which can ensue due to temperature gradient.

Unilateral cerebral perfusion is carried out through the IA while the left common carotid artery and left subclavian artery are clamped. The flow rate is 8–10 ml/kg/min maintaining the mean blood pressure at 50–70 mm Hg under 25–28°C degrees. Based on an experimental study of cerebral metabolism and histopathologic findings in dogs, Tanaka et al. [52] assumed that the aforementioned values provide about 50% of the physiologic flow rate, which is sufficient for intraoperative cerebral protection.

However, taking into account the unilateral cerebral perfusion, which directly supplies blood to only one hemisphere, a decrease in the NIRS values in the opposite hemisphere of more than 10% from the baseline forced us to increase the flow to 13–15 ml/kg/min.

Technically, connecting the arterial line to the IA using a side graft has several advantages: (i) no additional arterial cannulation site for CPB; (ii) visual control of the graft inside the surgical field promotes bleeding control from the anastomosis; (iii) ensuring the correct measurement of arterial pressure in the right radial artery since there is no cannula in the lumen of the vessel.

The strategy of IA cannulation for aortic arch pathology has always been used in our practice and is considered to be safe and effective since no serious complication has been encountered when using the IA as an arterial port for either CPB or ACP. Cannulation of the IA with a side graft allows for eliminating artery lumen occlusion with a cannula, turbulent flow around the cannula, as well as reducing unnecessary trauma to the fragile wall of the IA.

Other groups have also obtained excellent results with IA cannulation. Huang et al. [53] used cannulation of the IA with a side graft. The authors reported five (10.9%) patients with diagnosed temporal neurological deficit (TND) in the early postoperative period, without any stroke. Di Eusanio et al. [54] used a similar technique for IA cannulation for either CPB or ACP. In 55 patients, only 1 (1.8%) patient had TND. Preventza et al. [55] analyzed the results of aortic arch procedures, including those performed with IA cannulation with a graft sewn in an end-to-side fashion. Postoperatively, 3 (4.4%) patients had a stroke. It is worth noting that only one patient had an irreversible neurological deficit; the other two patients underwent partial neurological recovery. Additionally, 7 (10.3%) patients had postoperative delirium.

Meanwhile, Ji et al. [56] cannulated the innominate artery directly in 68 patients. The cannula tip was oriented toward the aortic arch during the period of CPB, and it was turned cranially during lower body circulatory arrest with ACP. The authors reported no neurologic events after the surgery.

Svensson et al. [23], analyzing results of 1336 operations, diagnosed only 1 (4.2%) case of stroke using direct IA cannulation. The authors noted that IA cannulation with a side graft can be considered a more preferable option for preventing neurologic complications compared to direct arterial cannulation. Moreover, this technique is considered easier and safer to use than direct artery cannulation.

Taking into account the aforementioned features of different arterial cannulation sites for uACP, we adopted IA cannulation on a regular basis during aortic arch surgery, regardless of the condition of alternative arteries. From our point of view, IA cannulation is more advantageous compared to other arterial sites in light of the benefit-risk ratio. Specifically, the innominate artery, as a relatively large brachiocephalic vessel, provides a higher volumetric blood flow rate without high blood pressure compared to other arterial cannulation sites (subclavian, carotid artery, or axillary artery) additionally to the technical advantages listed above.

2.2 FET implantation technique

The FET procedure was performed according to a surgical management procedure adopted in our clinic [57]. The sequence of the surgical steps during the operation was the same for all patients. In brief, surgical repair is conducted under moderate lower body circulatory arrest (25–28°C) and unilateral ACP via the innominate artery. A hybrid graft with a diameter of 24–30 mm is implanted in all cases. The length of the stent graft was 150 mm only. After establishing CPB, body cooling is started. Once the target temperature is achieved, lower body circulatory arrest with ACP is initiated. Then the aortic arch is opened and resected. The stent graft is implanted in the descending aorta, and fixed to the aortic tissue by continuous Prolene 4/0 suture without oversizing. Cerebrospinal fluid drainage and pressure monitoring are not performed. The distal aortic anastomosis is performed in Z2 or Z3 and depends on the patients' anatomical features and the technical possibilities encountered during the operation. Subsequently, re-implantation of the supra-aortic vessels is performed using one of the known techniques. After ACP is stopped, the CPB is reinstituted with warming of the patient's body. The proximal aorta is reconstructed during rewarming, and, if necessary, concomitant cardiac procedures are performed.

3. Study population

A retrospective single-center study was conducted. Between March 2012 and December 2022, a total of 311 aortic arch repairs were performed in our center. In this cohort, 97 patients underwent the FET procedure using the E-vita Open Plus hybrid graft (Jotec GmbH, Hechingen, Germany) and MedEng (MedEng, Penza, Russia). Detailed demographics and comorbidities of analyzed patients are shown in **Table 1**.

Variable	Patients (n = 97)
Age, years	54.5 [51; 63]
Male, n (%)	68 (70.1%)
Height, cm	173 [166; 178]
Weight, kg	94 [64.5; 101]
BMI, kg/m^2	29.3 [21.9; 33.1]
BSA, m^2	2.1 [1.8; 2.2]
Aortic dissection, n (%)	80 (82.5%)
Degenerative aneurysm, n (%)	17 (17.5%)
Hypertension, n (%)	65 (67%)
Diabetes mellitus, n (%)	7 (7.2%)
COPD, n (%)	10 (10.2%)
Creatinine, mg/dl	10 [8.9; 12.2]
CAD, n (%)	15 (15.5%)
LVEF, %	61 [57.5; 66]
Redo surgery, n (%)	9 (9.3%)

BMI – body mass index, BSA – body surface area, COPD – chronic obstructive pulmonary disease, CAD – coronary artery disease, LVEF – left ventricle ejection fraction. Categorical variables are presented as n (%). Continuous data are described as median with the [25th; 75th] percentiles.

Table 1.
Demographics and comorbidities.

4. Neurological results of antegrade unilateral cerebral perfusion via an innominate artery

4.1 Cerebral oximetry

As known, regional cerebral oximetry (rSO_2) is a safe, robust, and operator-independent method for assessing the adequacy of cerebral oxygen balance [58]. The method is based on a local measurement of the oxygemoglobin/deoxyhemoglobin ratio (according to the modification of Beer-Lambert law) mainly in venous blood [59]. Cerebral oximetry values in normothermic settings ranged from 60 to 80%.

Changes in rSO_2 in the range of 5–15% were found to correlate with changes in transcranial Doppler-measured cerebral blood flow velocity, electroencephalogram, and somatosensory evoked potentials [59]. A drop in saturation values during CPB below 40–50% (or 65–85% of the baseline) is known to be associated with high neurological complications, a rate confirmed by laboratory, instrumental, and histological findings [59, 60]. Hence, rSO_2 is considered as a simple alternative to complex methods for assessing cerebral perfusion during aortic arch surgery.

According to aforementioned statements, we use intraoperative cerebral neuromonitoring of the right and left hemispheres with near-infrared spectroscopy (Invos 5100, Somanetics Corp, USA). Cerebral oximetry values were recorded

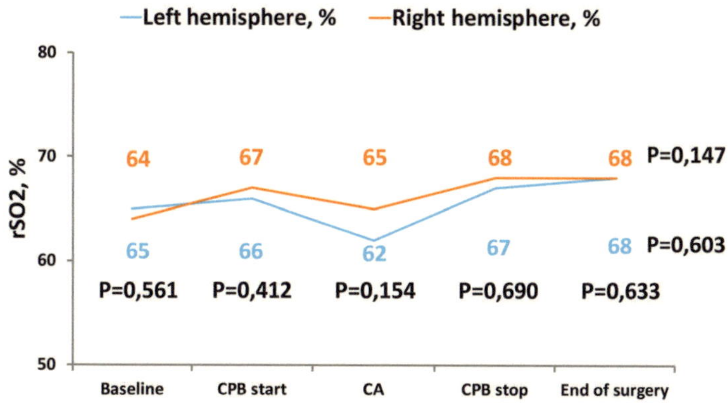

Figure 3.
Intraoperative regional cerebral oximetry of the right and left hemispheres.

throughout the entire surgical procedure: (1) at anesthesia induction, (2) at the initiation of CPB, (3) during CA, (4) after weaning from CPB, and (5) at the end of the surgery.

Our analysis showed that the range of intraoperative rSO_2 values was from 60 to 70% in both hemispheres during surgery in normal arterial blood gas settings (**Figure 3**). At different stages of the operation, the difference in rSO_2 between the cerebral hemispheres did not exceed 3%. The maximum asymmetry was revealed during circulatory arrest. Moreover, rSO_2 values of each hemisphere were stable during the operation without significant differences.

In addition, mean blood pressure was monitored in both radial arteries throughout the surgery (**Table 2**). It is worth emphasizing that blood pressure in the left radial artery as a possible surrogate of efficacy assessment of cerebral perfusion indirectly reflected the blood supply of the left hemisphere, which was derived from cross-hemispheric extra- and intracranial cerebral blood flow during right-sided cerebral perfusion.

Right-left asymmetry of intraoperative mean blood pressure (MBP) ranged from 1.4 to 46.3%. MBP asymmetry increasing was observed at the initiation of CPB (13%) and reached a maximum during CA (46.3%).

Variable	Baseline	CPB start	CA	CPB stop	End of surgery	p-value
MBP right RA, mm Hg	72 [67;80]	46 [44;51]	47.5 [41;51]	64 [60;67]	70 [64;73]	<0.001
MBP left RA, mm Hg	71 [68;79]	40 [37;44]	25.5 [22;30]	63 [60;66]	69 [63;72]	<0.001
Δ, %	1.4	13	46.3	1.6	1.4	
p-value	0.74	0.01	<0.001	0.90	0.94	

CPB – cardiopulmonary bypass, CA – circulatory arrest, MBP – mean blood pressure, RA – radial artery.

Table 2.
Intraoperative mean blood pressure values.

Comparing rSO_2 values and blood pressure asymmetry, there were differences between analyzed parameters at different stages of the operation. During CA, the difference in MBP values was 9.8 times higher (46.3%) than the difference in cerebral oximetry (3%). Nevertheless, despite the MBP in the left radial artery being as low as 25.5 mm Hg, left cerebral hemisphere oxygenation was within the normal range due to adequate cerebral cross-perfusion. Our data are in line with Urbanski et al. [61]. They observed that the MBP value in the radial arteries around 30 mm Hg is considered sufficient for cerebral cross-perfusion during unilateral antegrade cerebral perfusion.

4.2 Neurological deficit

A total of 10 (10.3%) patients had a neurological deficit postoperatively. Of these, 8 (8.2%) cases were reversible: 4 (4.2%) patients had delirium with manifestation within 14 days, and 2 (2.1%) other patients had a transient ischemic attack, which resolved within 12 hours without residual focal neurological deficit. In 2 (2.1%) patients, a non-fatal minor stroke (with a reversible neurological deficit) was recorded; additionally, in 2 (2.1%) patients, a hemorrhagic stroke was observed.

Our findings are consistent with other studies. The incidence of permanent neurological deficit (PND) after innominate cannulation during thoracic aortic surgery varies from 2.4 to 4.5%, and TND is in the range of 3–13.4% [48, 62, 63].

It is known that the duration of CPB, CA, and ACP negatively affects neurological status. However, according to our data, there were no significant differences in ischemic periods in patients with and without neurological deficits (**Table 3**). In an attempt to elucidate the impact of the duration of CPB, circulatory arrest, and ACP on neurological outcomes, we performed a Persons's correlation analysis. This analysis found weak correlations between the incidence of neurological deficit and the duration of CPB (0.073, $p = 0.4782$), CA (−0.146, $p = 0.1560$), and ACP (0.15, $p = 0.1456$). Thus, in our patients, these variables did not influence the neurological status.

4.3 Neuron-specific enolase

As known any conventional instrumental methods for evaluating postoperative cerebral damage are widely used due to their reproducibility but not accuracy. Thus, to overcome this issue, an analysis of neuron-specific markers has been proposed [64]. In contrast to well-known S100 and S100B proteins, the most reliable and specific marker reflecting cerebral damage is a neuron-specific enolase (NSE) [65].

Duration	Without neurological deficit (n = 87)	Neurological deficit (n = 10)		p-value
		PND	TND	
CPB, min	216 [180; 308]	230 [212; 270]	230 [215; 280]	0.144
Lower body CA, min	44 [25; 53]	47.3 [44; 53]	51.5 [45; 57]	0.475
uACP	55 [47;69]	47.3 [44; 53]	51.5 [45; 57]	0.155

ACP – unilateral antegrade cerebral perfusion; CA – circulatory arrest; CPB – cardiopulmonary bypass; TND – temporary neurological deficit (including transient ischemic attack, delirium), PND – permanent neurological deficit (stroke).

Table 3.
Duration of ischemic periods in patients with or without neurological deficit.

One study [66] showed that serum NSE level within 24 hours after surgery is a useful predictor of neurologic injury onset and severity. It has been demonstrated that NSE level significantly correlated with the extent of stroke, which is in line with our results. However, to date, there is a lack of data regarding the changes of NSE values during thoracic aortic surgery in different grade of neurological deficit.

Striving to assess the cerebral damage grade in patients who underwent the frozen elephant trunk procedure, we assessed NSE serum levels by measuring an enzyme immunoassay before and after surgery in every patient. Venous blood assays were collected in the operating room before skin incision and 24 hours after surgery. Blood serum was centrifuged at 3000 rpm for 60 minutes to prevent the leakage of NSE from blood cells, with subsequent evaluation of results. NSE values between 0 and 9.9 μg/L were considered normal.

Pre- and postoperative NSE serum levels in patients without neurological deficit, with TND and PND, are presented in **Figure 4**.

Patients without postoperative neurological deficit based on clinical assessment showed a 1.9-fold increase in NSE level (from 1.8 to 3.4 μg/L) after surgery compared to the baseline. However, despite statistically significant increase in postoperative NSE value ($p < 0.001$), its level did not exceed the normal range.

NSE levels in patients with postoperative TND increased by 5.6 times compared to the baseline and amounted to 6.2 [5.2; 6.6] μg/l. The difference between pre-and postoperative results was statistically significant ($p < 0.001$); however, NSE values were within the normal range.

In contrast to our aforementioned results, the NSE value in patients with post-operative PND was 10.74 [9.9; 11.8] μg/l, which exceeded the normal range. In this group of patients, a 6.7-fold increase in NSE value from baseline was recorded with a statistically significant difference ($p < 0.001$).

Our results suggested that NSE level might correlate with the severity of postoperative neurological deficit in patients who underwent aortic arch surgery. Our findings are supported by Kimura et al. [66] who demonstrated a similar correlation.

4.4 Cognitive assessment

To date, there is a focus on strong cerebral damage such as TND (i.e., delirium) and PND (i.e., stroke) when assessing postoperative neurological outcomes after

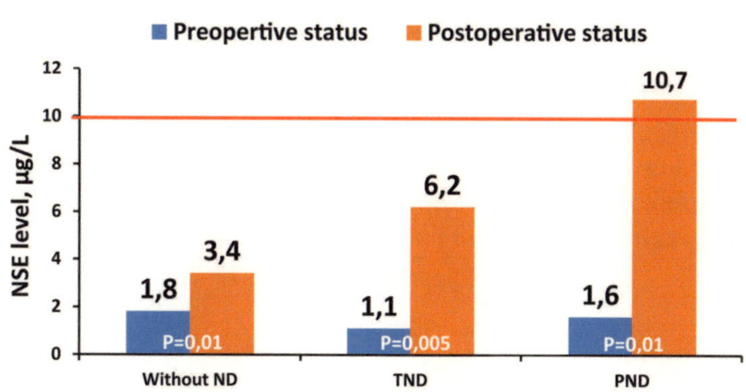

Figure 4.
Pre- and postoperative NSE serum levels in patients without neurological deficit (ND), with TND and PND.

thoracic aortic surgery. However, it is not the one manifestation that could worsen the quality of life. Recently, postoperative cognitive dysfunction, characterized as a mild neurological disorder, has become a paramount concern [67]. This kind of neurological deficit can manifest with poor attention, memory, speech, and other cognitive impairments, diagnosed by validated neurological screening tests [68, 69].

At present, the Montreal Cognitive Assessment (MoCA) has been proposed as one of the best tools for detecting the mild cognitive impairments compared to other tests [70]. Hence, it has been successfully used in patients who have suffered a stroke or underwent cardiac surgery [71]. This test assesses abstraction, language, memory, attention, and orientation abilities.

The test takes into account the patient's initial level of education, as it adds value when comparing patients with initially different levels of cognitive reserve, which serves to maintain functional and structural properties of the brain to compensate and minimize cognitive failure after strokes, injuries, chronic cerebrovascular, neurodegenerative diseases or due to age-related changes [72].

All of the patients scheduled for surgery passed the MoCA test preoperatively. After the surgery, 10 (10.3%) patients with documented TND or PND were excluded from the assessment of cognitive function. In total, data from 87 (89.7%) patients were analyzed. The score of every patient was recorded. Evaluating the severity of cognitive postoperative cognitive dysfunction the 'normal' cutoff was 26 points: scores > 26 indicated no cognitive impairment (normal test), and scores < 26 indicated mild cognitive impairment [73].

In the analyzed patients with complete data, mean preoperative MoCA score was 24 [21, 25]. The "normal" cutoff was attained by 53 (60.9%) of 87 patients.

The postoperative MoCA score in the analyzed patients was 26 [1, 26]. The "normal" cutoff was reached by 57 (65.5%) out of 87 patients. According to our analysis, postoperative patients' cognitive function was comparable to preoperative parameters, i.e., without an increasing rate of cognitive impairment.

In detail, there was an increase in attention ($p = 0.012$) and orientation ($p = 0.009$) abilities, as well as improvements in both short-term ($p = 0.491$) and long-term ($p < 0.001$) memory after surgery compared to the preoperative status. Simultaneously, we observed non-inferior postoperative values of language and abstraction abilities. Taking these results into account, we assume that ACP via innominate artery during aortic arch surgery is not associated with a decline of cognitive function or additional postoperative mental disorders.

5. Conclusion

Unilateral cerebral perfusion via the innominate artery during aortic arch repair is associated with a low incidence and severity of neurological deficit, minor changes in intraoperative cerebral oximetry in both hemispheres, and the absence of significant cerebral damage without a decline in postoperative cognitive function.

Acknowledgements

The authors would like to thank Elena Kim for her contribution to the manuscript editing.

Conflict of interest

The authors declare no conflict of interest.

Author details

Boris Kozlov and Dmitri Panfilov*
Cardiovascular Department, Cardiology Research Institute, Tomsk National Research Medical Centre, Russian Academy of Sciences, Tomsk, Russian Federation

*Address all correspondence to: pand2006@yandex.ru

References

[1] Apostolakis E, Koletsis EN, Dedeilias P, Kokotsakis JN, Sakellaropoulos G, Psevdi A, et al. Antegrade versus retrograde cerebral perfusion in relation to postoperative complications following aortic arch surgery for acute aortic dissection type A. Journal of Cardiac Surgery. 2008;**23**:480-487. DOI: 10.1111/j.1540-8191.2008.00587.x

[2] Yan TD, Bannon PG, Bavaria J, Coselli JS, Elefteriades JA, Griepp RB, et al. Consensus on hypothermia in aortic arch surgery. Annals of Cardiothoracic Surgery. 2013;**2**(2):163-168. DOI: 10.3978/j.issn.2225-319X.2013.03.03

[3] Ziganshin BA, Elefteriades JA. Deep hypothermic circulatory arrest. Annals of Cardiothoracic Surgery. 2013;**2**(3):303-315. DOI: 10.3978/j.issn.2225-319X.2013.01.05

[4] Englum BR, Andersen ND, Husain AM, Mathew JP, Hughes GC. Degree of hypothermia in aortic arch surgery – Optimal temperature for cerebral and spinal protection: Deep hypothermia remains the gold standard in the absence of randomized data. Annals of Cardiothoracic Surgery. 2013;**2**(2):184-193. DOI: 10.3978/j.issn.2225-319X.2013.03.01

[5] Bashir M, Shaw M, Desmond M, Kuduvalli M, Field M, Oo A. Cerebral protection in hemi-aortic arch surgery. Annals of Cardiothoracic Surgery. 2013;**2**(2):239-244. DOI: 10.3978/j.issn.2225-319X.2013.02.04

[6] Misfeld M, Mohr FW, Etz CD. Best strategy for cerebral protection in arch surgery - antegrade selective cerebral perfusion and adequate hypothermia. Annals of Cardiothoracic Surgery. 2013;**2**(3):331-338. DOI: 10.3978/j.issn.2225-319X.2013.02.05

[7] Luehr M, Bachet J, Mohr FW, Etz CD. Modern temperature management in aortic arch surgery: The dilemma of moderate hypothermia. European Journal of Cardio-Thoracic Surgery. 2014;**45**(1):27-39. DOI: 10.1093/ejcts/ezt154

[8] Bachet J. Open repair techniques in the aortic arch are still superior. Annals of Cardiothoracic Surgery. 2018;**7**(3):328-344. DOI: 10.21037/acs.2018.05.05

[9] Di Eusanio M, Wesselink RMJ, Morshuis WJ, Dossche KM, Schepens MAAM. Deep hypothermic circulatory arrest and antegrade selective cerebral perfusion during ascending aorta – Hemiarch replacement: A retrospective comparative study. The Journal of Thoracic and Cardiovascular Surgery. 2003;**125**:849-854. DOI: 10.1067/mtc.2003.8

[10] Vallabhajosyula P, Jassar AS, Menon RS, Komlo C, Gutsche J, Desai ND, et al. Moderate versus deep hypothermic circulatory arrest for elective aortic transverse hemiarch reconstruction. The Annals of Thoracic Surgery. 2015;**99**:1511-1517. DOI: 10.1016/j.athoracsur.2014.12.067

[11] Gong M, Ma W-G, Guan X-L, Wang L-F, Li J-C, Lan F, et al. Moderate hypothermic circulatory arrest in total arch repair for acute type A aortic dissection: Clinical safety and efficacy. Journal of Thoracic Disease. 2016;**8**(5):925-933. DOI: 10.21037/jtd.2016.02.75

[12] Englum BR, He X, Gulack DC, Ganapathi AM, Mathew JP, Brennan JM, et al. Hypothermia and cerebral

protection strategies in aortic arch surgery: A comparative effectiveness analysis from the STS adult cardiac surgery database. European Journal of Cardio-Thoracic Surgery. 2017;**52**(3):492-498. DOI: 10.1093/ejcts/ezx133

[13] Ueda Y. A reappraisal of retrograde cerebral perfusion. Annals of Cardiothoracic Surgery. 2013;**2**(3):316-325. DOI: 10.3978/j.issn.2225-319X.2013.01.02

[14] Kin N, Ono N, Mori Y, Ninagawa J, Yamada Y. Increased cerebrovascular resistance after retrograde cerebral perfusion: A Doppler study. BioScience Trends. 2012;**6**(5):276-282. DOI: 10.5582/bst.2012.v6.5.276

[15] Rylski B, Urbanski PP, Siepe M, Beyersdorf F, Bachet J, Gleason TG, et al. Operative techniques in patients with type a dissection complicated by cerebral malperfusion. European Journal of Cardio-Thoracic Surgery. 2014;**46**:156-166. DOI: 10.1093/ejcts/ezu251

[16] Girardi LN, Shavladze N, Sedrakyan A, Neragi-Miandoab S. Safety and efficacy of retrograde cerebral perfusion as an adjunct for cerebral protection during surgery on the aortic arch. The Journal of Thoracic and Cardiovascular Surgery. 2014;**148**:2927-2935. DOI: 10.1016/j.jtcvs.2014.07.024

[17] Estrera AL, Miller CC III, Lee T-Y, Shah P, Safi HJ. Ascending and transverse aortic arch repair. The impact of retrograde cerebral perfusion. Circulation. 2008;**118**(Suppl. 1):S160-S166. DOI: 10.1161/circulationaha.107.757419

[18] Perreas K, Samanidis G, Dimitriou S, Kalogris P, Balanika M, Antzaka C, et al. Outcomes after ascending aorta and proximal aortic arch repair using deep hypothermic circulatory arrest with retrograde cerebral perfusion: Analysis of 207 patients. Interactive Cardiovascular and Thoracic Surgery. 2012;**15**:456-461. DOI: 10.1093/icvts/ivs252

[19] Reich DL, Uysal S. Con: Retrograde cerebral perfusion is not an optimal method of neuroprotection in thoracic aortic surgery. Journal of Cardiothoracic and Vascular Anesthesia. 2003;**17**(6):768-769. DOI: 10.1053/j.jvca.2003.09.021

[20] Aziz SA. Total circulatory arrest and retrograde cerebral perfusion during ascending aorta and arch surgery. The Journal of Egyptian Society of Cardiothoracic Surgery. 2005;**13**(1-2):39-43

[21] Griepp RB, Griepp EB. Perfusion and cannulation strategies for neurological protection in aortic arch surgery. Annals of Cardiothoracic Surgery. 2013;**2**(2):159-162. DOI: 10.3978/j.issn.2225-319X.2013.03.12

[22] Pochettino A, Cheung AT. Pro: Retrograde cerebral perfusion is useful for deep hypothermic circulatory arrest. Journal of Cardiothoracic and Vascular Anesthesia. 2003;**17**(6):764-767. DOI: 10.1053/j.jvca.2003.09.020

[23] Svensson LG, Blackstone EH, Rajeswaran J, Sabik JF III, Lytle BW, Gonzalez-Stawinski G, et al. Does the arterial cannulation site for circulatory arrest influence stroke risk? The Annals of Thoracic Surgery. 2004;**78**:1274-1284. DOI: 10.1016/j.athoracsur.2004.04.063

[24] Gutsche JT, Feinman J, Silvay G, Patel PA, Ghadimi K, Landoni G, et al. Practice variations in the conduct of hypothermic circulatory arrest for adult aortic arch repair: Focus on an emerging European paradigm. Heart, Lung and Vessels. 2014;**6**(1):43-51

[25] Augoustides JGT, Patel P, Ghadimi K, Choi J, Yue Y, Silvay G. Current conduct

of deep hypothermic circulatory arrest in China. HSR Proceedings in Intensive Care & Cardiovascular Anesthesia. 2013;**5**(1):25-32

[26] Li B, Zhu Y, Liu A, Lu W, Su J, Zhang J, et al. Selective antegrade cerebral perfusion reduces brain injury following deep hypothermic circulatory arrest in the piglets' model by decreasing the levels of protein SUMO2/3-ylation. International Journal of Clinical and Experimental Medicine. 2014;**7**(11):4562-4571

[27] Leontyev S, Davierwala PM, Semenov M, von Aspern K, Krog G, Noack T, et al. Antegrade selective cerebral perfusion reduced in-hospital mortality and permanent focal neurological deficit in patients with elective aortic arch surgery. European Journal of Cardio-Thoracic Surgery. 2019;**56**(5):1001-1008. DOI: 10.1093/ejcts/ezz091

[28] Urbanski PP, Lenos A, Zacher M, Diegeler A. Unilateral cerebral perfusion: Right versus left. European Journal of Cardio-Thoracic Surgery. 2010;**37**:1332-1337. DOI: 10.1016/j.ejcts.2010.01.006

[29] Akamatsu Y, Nishijima Y, Lee CC, Yang SY, Shi L, An L, et al. Impaired leptomeningeal collateral flow contributes to the poor outcome following experimental stroke in the type 2 diabetic mice. The Journal of Neuroscience. 2015;**35**(9):3851-3864. DOI: 10.1523/jneurosci.3838-14.2015

[30] Spielvogel D, Tang GHL. Selective cerebral perfusion for cerebral protection: What we do know. Annals of Cardiothoracic Surgery. 2013;**2**(3):326-330. DOI: 10.3978/j.issn.2225-319X.2013.03.02

[31] Özatik MA, Kocabeyoglu S, Kücüker SA, Saritas A, Altintas A, Kervan Ü, et al. Neurochemical markers during selective cerebral perfusion via the right brachial artery. Interactive Cardiovascular and Thoracic Surgery. 2010;**10**:948-952. DOI: 10.1510/icvts.2009.228858

[32] Urbanski PP, Lenos A, Blume JC, Ziegler V, Griewing B, Schmitt R, et al. Does anatomical completeness of the circle of Willis correlate with sufficient cross-perfusion during unilateral cerebral perfusion? European Journal of Cardio-Thoracic Surgery. 2008;**33**:402-408. DOI: 10.1016/j.ejcts.2007.12.021

[33] Malvindi PG, Scrascia G, Vitale N. Is unilateral antegrade cerebral perfusion equivalent to bilateral cerebral perfusion for patients undergoing aortic arch surgery? Interactive Cardiovascular and Thoracic Surgery. 2008;**7**:891-897. DOI: 10.1510/icvts.2008.184184

[34] Bachet J. I have only 1 brain but 2 hemispheres: Please perfuse both adequately! The Journal of Thoracic and Cardiovascular Surgery. 2017;**154**:765-766. DOI: 10.1016/j.jtcvs.2017.03.032

[35] Takayama H, Borger MA. Bilateral antegrade cerebral perfusion during aortic dissection surgery: If no harm, then why not? The Journal of Thoracic and Cardiovascular Surgery. 2017;**154**:776-777. DOI: 10.1016/j.jtcvs.2017.04.030

[36] Angeloni E, Melina G, Refice SK, Roscitano A, Capuano F, Comito C, et al. Unilateral versus bilateral antegrade cerebral protection during aortic surgery: An updated meta-analysis. The Annals of Thoracic Surgery. 2015;**99**:2024-2031. DOI: 10.1016/j.athoracsur.2015.01.070

[37] Zierer A, Ahmad AE-S, Papadopoulos N, Moritz A, Diegeler A, Urbanski PP. Selective antegrade cerebral perfusion and mild (280°C-300°C)

systemic hypothermic circulatory arrest for aortic arch replacement: Results from 1002 patients. The Journal of Thoracic and Cardiovascular Surgery. 2012;**144**:1042-1050. DOI: 10.1016/j.jtcvs.2012.07.063

[38] Fukunaga N, Saji Y, Kanemitsu H, Koyama T. Prolonged antegrade cerebral perfusion via right axillary artery (≥60 min) does not affect early outcomes in a repair of type a acute aortic dissection. Annals of Thoracic and Cardiovascular Surgery. 2015;**21**:557-563. DOI: 10.5761/atcs.oa.15-00057

[39] Verhoye J-P, Soulami RB, Fouquet O, Ruggieri VG, Kaladji A, Tomasi J, et al. Elective frozen elephant trunk procedure using the E-Vita open. Plus prosthesis in 94 patients: A multicentre French registry. European Journal of Cardio-Thoracic Surgery. 2017;**52**(4):733-739. DOI: 10.1093/ejcts/ezx159

[40] Tong G, Zhang B, Zhou X, Tao Y, Yan T, Wang X, et al. Bilateral versus unilateral antegrade cerebral perfusion in total arch replacement for type a aortic dissection. The Journal of Thoracic and Cardiovascular Surgery. 2017;**154**:767-775. DOI: 10.1016/j.jtcvs.2017.02.053

[41] Tian DH, Wilson-Smith A, Koo SK, Forrest P, Kiat H, Yan TD. Unilateral versus bilateral antegrade cerebral perfusion: A meta-analysis of comparative studies. Heart, Lung & Circulation. 2019;**28**:844-849. DOI: 10.1016/j.hlc.2019.01.010

[42] Sabik JF, Lytle BW, McCarthy PM, Cosgrove DM. Axillary artery: An alternative site of arterial cannulation for patients with extensive aortic and peripheral vascular disease. The Journal of Thoracic and Cardiovascular Surgery. 1995;**109**:885-891

[43] Apostolakis EE, Baikoussis NG, Katsanos K, Karanikolas M. Postoperative peri-axillary seroma following axillary artery cannulation for surgical treatment of acute type A aortic dissection. Journal of Cardiothoracic Surgery. 2010;**5**:43. DOI: 10.1186/1749-8090-5-43

[44] Garg V, Tsirigotis DN, Dickson J, Dalamagas C, Latter DA, Verma S, et al. Direct innominate artery cannulation for selective antegrade cerebral perfusion during deep hypothermic circulatory arrest in aortic surgery. The Journal of Thoracic and Cardiovascular Surgery. 2014;**148**:2920-2924. DOI: 10.1016/j.jtcvs.2014.07.021

[45] Sabik JF, Nemeh H, Lytle BW, Blackstone EH, Gillinov AM, Rajeswaran J, et al. Cannulation of the axillary artery with a side graft reduces morbidity. The Annals of Thoracic Surgery. 2004;**77**:1315-1320. DOI: 10.1016/j.athoracsur.2003.08.056

[46] Ayyash B, Tranquilli M, Elefteriades JA. Femoral artery cannulation for thoracic aortic surgery: Safe under transesophageal echocardiographic control. The Thoracic and Cardiovascular Surgeon. 2011;**142**:1478-1481. DOI: 10.1016/j.jtcvs.2011.04.005

[47] Preventza O, Garcia A, Tuluca A, Henry M, Cooley DA, Simpson K, et al. Innominate artery cannulation for proximal aortic surgery: Outcomes and neurological events in 263 patients. European Journal of Cardio-Thoracic Surgery. 2015;**48**:937-942. DOI: 10.1093/ejcts/ezu534

[48] Uchino G, Yunoki K, Sakoda N, Saiki M, Hisamochi K, Yoshida H. Innominate artery cannulation for arterial perfusion during aortic arch surgery. Journal of Cardiac Surgery. 2017;**32**:110-113. DOI: 10.1111/jocs.13091

[49] Kashani A, Doyle M, Horton M. Direct innominate artery cannulation as

a sole systemic and cerebral perfusion technique in aortic surgery. Heart, Lung & Circulation. 2019;**28**(4):67-70. DOI: 10.1016/j.hlc.2018.08.001

[50] Banbury MK, Cosgrove DM. Arterial cannulation of the innominate artery. The Annals of Thoracic Surgery. 2000;**69**:957. Bachet, 2018

[51] Unal M, Yilmaz O, Akar I, Ince I, Aslan C, Koc F, et al. Brachiocephalic artery cannulation in proximal aortic surgery that requires circulatory arrest. Texas Heart Institute Journal. 2014;**41**(6):596-600. DOI: 10.14503/THIJ-13-3947

[52] Tanaka H, Kazui T, Sato H, Inoue N, Yamada O, Komatsu S. Experimental study on the optimum flow rate and pressure for selective cerebral perfusion. The Annals of Thoracic Surgery. 1995;**59**(3):651-657

[53] Huang FJ, Wu Q, Ren CW, Lai YQ, Yang S, Rui QJ, et al. Cannulation of the innominate artery with a side graft in arch surgery. The Annals of Thoracic Surgery. 2010;**89**:800-803. DOI: 10.1016/j.athoracsur.2009.12.005

[54] Di Eusanio M, Ciano M, Labriola G, Lionetti G, Di Eusanio G. Cannulation of the innominate artery during surgery of the thoracic aorta: Our experience in 55 patients. European Journal of Cardio-Thoracic Surgery. 2007;**32**:270-273. DOI: 10.1016/j.ejcts.2007.03.050

[55] Preventza O, Bakaeen FG, Stephens EH, Trocciola SM, de la Cruz KI, Coselli JS. Innominate artery cannulation: An alternative to femoral or axillary cannulation for arterial inflow in proximal aortic surgery. The Journal of Thoracic and Cardiovascular Surgery. 2013;**145**:S191-S196. DOI: 10.1016/j.jtcvs.2012.11.061

[56] Ji S, Yang J, Ye X, Wang X. Brain protection by using innominate artery cannulation during aortic arch surgery. The Annals of Thoracic Surgery. 2008;**86**:1030-1032. DOI: 10.1016/j.athoracsur.2008.03.044

[57] Kozlov BN, Panfilov DS. False lumen thrombosis after frozen elephant trunk procedure in acute and chronic aortic dissection. The Journal of Cardiovascular Surgery. 2022;**63**(2):195-201. DOI: 10.23736/S0021-9509.21.11800-2

[58] Bergeron EJ, Mosca MS, Aftab M, Justison G, Reece TB. Neuroprotection strategies in aortic surgery. Cardiology Clinics. 2017;**35**(3):453-465. DOI: 10.1016/j.ccl.2017.03.011

[59] Zheng F, Sheinberg R, Yee M-S, Ono M, Zheng Y, Hogue CW. Cerebral near-infrared spectroscopy monitoring and neurologic outcomes in adult cardiac surgery patients: A systematic review. Anesthesia and Analgesia. 2013;**116**:663-676. DOI: 10.1213/ane.0b013e318277a255

[60] Urbanski PP, Lenos A, Kolowca M, Bougioukakis P, Keller G, Zacher M, et al. Near-infrared spectroscopy for neuromonitoring of unilateral cerebral perfusion. European Journal of Cardio-Thoracic Surgery. 2013;**43**(6):1140-1144. DOI: 10.1093/ejcts/ezs557

[61] Urbanski PP, Lenos A, Lindemann Y, Weigang E, Zacher M, Diegeler A. Carotid artery cannulation in aortic surgery. The Journal of Thoracic and Cardiovascular Surgery. 2006;**132**:1398-1403. DOI: 10.1016/j.jtcvs.2006.07.024

[62] Harky A, Wong CHM, Chan JSK, Zaki S, Froghi S, Bashir M. Innominate artery cannulation in aortic surgery: A systematic review. Journal of Cardiac Surgery. 2018;**33**:818-825. DOI: 10.1111/jocs.13962

[63] Preventza O, Price MD, Spiliotopoulos K, Amarasekara HS, Cornwell LD, Omer S, et al. In elective arch surgery with circulatory arrest, does the arterial cannulation site really matter? A propensity score analysis of right axillary and innominate artery cannulation. The Journal of Thoracic and Cardiovascular Surgery. 2018;**155**(5):1953-1960. DOI: 10.1016/j.jtcvs.2017.11.095

[64] Yuan S-M. Biomarkers of cerebral injury in cardiac surgery. Anadolu Kardiyoloji Dergisi. 2014;**14**:638-645. DOI: 10.5152/akd.2014.5321

[65] Schaefer ST, Koenigsperger S, Olotu C, Saller T. Biomarkers and postoperative cognitive function: Could it be that easy? Current Opinion in Anaesthesiology. 2019;**32**(1):92-100. DOI: 10.1097/ACO.0000000000000676

[66] Kimura F, Kadohama T, Kitahara H, Ise H, Nakanishi S, Akasaka N, et al. Serum neuron-specific enolase level as predictor of neurologic outcome after aortic surgery. The Thoracic and Cardiovascular Surgeon. 2020;**68**(04):282-290. DOI: 10.1055/s-0038-1677511

[67] Newman MF, Grocott HP, Mathew JP, White WD, Landolfo K, Reves JG, et al. Report of the substudy assessing the impact of neurocognitive function on quality of life 5 years after cardiac surgery. Stroke. 2001;**32**(12):2874-2881

[68] Cumming TB, Bernhardt J, Linden T. The Montreal cognitive assessment short cognitive evaluation in a large stroke trial. Stroke. 2011;**42**:2642-2644. DOI: 10.1161/Strokeaha.111.619486

[69] Jabagi H, Wells G, Boodhwani M. Commence trial (comparing hypothermic temperatures during hemiarch surgery): A randomized controlled trial of mild vs moderate hypothermia on patient outcomes in aortic hemiarch surgery with anterograde cerebral perfusion. Trials. 2019;**20**(1):691. DOI: 10.1186/s13063-019-3713-9

[70] Chun CT, Seward K, Patterson A, Melton A, MacDonald-Wicks L. Evaluation of available cognitive tools used to measure mild cognitive decline: A scoping review. Nutrients. 2021;**13**(11):3974. DOI: 10.3390/nu13113974

[71] Naito Y, Hiraoka A, Himeno M, Chikazawa G, Arimichi M, Yuguchi S, et al. Clinically optimal neuropsychological tests for postoperative cognitive dysfunction in heart valve surgeries. Circulation Journal. 2022;**86**(11):1719-1724. DOI: 10.1253/circj.CJ-22-0390

[72] Hachinski V, Iadecola C, Petersen RC, Breteler MM, Nyenhuis DL, Black SE, et al. National institute of neurological disorders and stroke–Canadian stroke network vascular cognitive impairment harmonization standards. Stroke. 2006;**37**:2220-2241. DOI: 10.1161/01.STR.0000237236.88823.47

[73] Fu C, Jin X, Chen B, et al. Comparison of the mini-mental state examination and Montreal cognitive assessment executive subtests in detecting post-stroke cognitive impairment. Geriatrics & Gerontology International. 2017;**17**:2329-2335. DOI: 10.1111/ggi.13069

Chapter 10

Immediate Perioperative Results and Early Survival in Patients Undergoing Aortic Repair for Thoracic Acute Aortic Dissection: Risk Factors Analysis and Surgical Implications

Paolo Nardi, Alessandro Cristian Salvati, Mattia Scognamiglio, Valentina Ajello, Marzia Flaminio, Manuela Moresco, Laura De Felice and Claudia Altieri

Abstract

Emergent surgical repair of thoracic acute aortic dissection (TAAD) aims to prevent potentially lethal complications including cardiac tamponade, neurological damage, acute aortic valve dysfunction, rupture of the aortic wall into the pericardial space, or myocardial infarction due to the dissection of the coronary ostia. Furthermore, the progression of the dissection involving peripheral arteries with, consequently, a possible preoperative multiple-organ malperfusion can lead to a drastic increase in operative risk. In fact, even with prompt surgical treatment, TAAD continues to be associated with an in-hospital mortality rate of 20–30%, and malperfusion of various organ systems can dramatically increase the operative mortality. From the analysis of the various pre- and perioperative risk factors, it is possible to evaluate the real operative risk and establish in which patients emergency surgery continues to offer a substantial prognostic benefit in comparison with medical therapy only and in which surgery, on the contrary, may not offer any prognostic advantage.

Keywords: acute aortic dissection, aortic complications, aortic repair, malperfusion, risk factors analysis

1. Introduction

Thoracic acute aortic dissection (TAAD) is a disease with a catastrophic impact on the patient's life. Its incidence is about 30 cases/million/year; the natural history of this serious disease if surgically untreated, is associated with a mortality rate of

56% according to the International Registry of Acute Aortic Dissections (IRAD) [1], with a risk of death that increases by 1% per hour in the first 48 hours from the onset of symptoms [1, 2]. Despite numerous diagnostic innovations, development of new surgical techniques, and advances in postoperative therapies, that is, percutaneous tracheostomy, renal replacement therapy, it remains a disease with a high operative mortality. Emergent surgical repair of De Bakey type I and II TAAD has the aim to prevent potentially lethal complications including serious ischemic neurological damage, that is, stroke and coma, acute aortic valve dysfunction, complete rupture of the aortic wall into the pericardium, or myocardial infarction due to acute hypoperfusion of the coronary artery ostia. The involvement of the peripheral arteries due to the progression of the dissection and, consequently, the preoperative multiple-organ malperfusion can lead to a drastic increase in operative mortality. In fact, even with prompt surgical repair, TAAD continues to be associated with an in-hospital mortality rate of 20–30%; moreover, preoperative malperfusion of various organ systems can dramatically increase the operative mortality. In fact, preoperative malperfusion has been identified as one of the independent predictive factors of significantly increased operative risk and still remains the most evaluated clinical variable for the therapeutic management to be adopted in such patients. Other risk factors have also been analyzed in several registries and retrospective published analyses to evaluate in-hospital outcomes and to establish which TAAD patient populations are at the most risk of adverse early outcomes [3–8].

The aim of the chapter is to analyze the most important risk factors influencing the postoperative outcomes, in light of both the data present in the literature and our long experience. From the analysis of the data, it is possible to identify patients for whom surgery is still confirmed to offer a notable prognostic benefit, or, on the contrary, patients for whom the very high perioperative risk may not lead to any prognostic benefit after surgery. On this way, we have evaluated the impact of perioperative risk factors and intraoperative variables on the immediate outcome, and at early and mid-term follow-up period. Further considerations will be made on the type of surgical strategy to be adopted in emergency setting, and the possible risk of late reoperation.

2. Our experience and early outcomes

Between January 2005 and December 2021, 393 patients (mean age 63.4 ± 12.5 years, range 16–88 years; males/females 286:107) underwent aortic repair for TAAD at the referred center for TAAD surgery at the Tor Vergata University Hospital.

Diagnosis of preoperative coronary arteries, visceral, or peripheral arterial malperfusion was based on clinical symptoms and/or imaging features, that is, absence or reduction of organ perfusion detected by computed tomography-scan angiography and/or increase of enzymes and creatinine serum levels, electrocardiographic changes suggestive of acute ischemia or myocardial infarction, alterations of cardiac contractile function detected at the trans-esophageal echocardiography. Malperfusion was classified as renal, in presence of impairment of renal function, that is, oliguria or anuria; as visceral, if there was evidence of abdominal tension and pain, intestinal dysfunction, increased serum levels of liver and/or pancreatic enzymes; as myocardial or coronary, in presence, CK-MB/CK total ratio > 10% and troponin I value above 20 ng/mL. In particular, the effect of these different types of malperfusion was accurately examined on the early and at 1-year outcomes, given their higher incidence in comparison with other risk factors, at the time of the admission at our center.

In the operating room, prior to surgical procedures, all patients were monitored by means of venous central cannulation, arterial cannulations, that is, both radial or radial and femoral arteries, measurements of corporeal temperature, that is, rectal, esophageal, or tympanic. Cerebral monitoring was performed with near-infrared spectroscopy (INVOS System, Somanetics Corp., Troy, MI, US). Trans-cranial Doppler was used to assess blood flow velocities in the anterior and middle cerebral arteries of the Willis circle during hypothermia and antegrade selective cerebral perfusion. Arterial access for cardiopulmonary by-pass in two-third of cases was through the right axillary artery, in the other one third of patients through the femoral artery; central cannulation was rarely performed.

In-hospital mortality included both intraoperative and postoperative mortality within 30 days after surgery. In this report, we have also collected data of patients up to 1 year of follow-up in order to evaluate the impact of the most important risk factors on short-term survival.

Statistical analysis was performed using Stat View 4.5 program (SAS Institute Inc., Abacus Concepts, Berkeley, CA, USA). To evaluate continuous variables and categorical variables, the Fisher's exact test and the Chi-squared or Fisher's exact tests were used. To identify independent predictors of in-hospital mortality, logistic regression analysis was performed. All the variables that reached statistical significance by univariate analysis at a P-value <0.1 were inserted into the multivariate regression model. Preoperative analyzed variables included gender, age, hypertension, diabetes mellitus, smoking status, body mass index, body surface area, previous cardiac surgery, left ventricular function, extent of the dissection, that is, De Bakey types I and II, presence and types of malperfusion, cardiac tamponade/pericardial effusion, and site of the entry tear. Intraoperative analyzed variables included the site of arterial cannulation, circulatory techniques to obtain brain perfusion, surgical times, whether there was a need for circulatory arrest, and type of operation, that is, ascending aorta replacement with or without the replacement of the hemi-arch, aortic root replacement with Bentall operation, the arch replacement, and the need of coronary artery bypass grafting. Short-term survival, including in-hospital mortality, was expressed as a mean of the values plus or minus 1 standard deviation. Survival analyses were computed using the Kaplan-Meier method; Mantel-Cox log-rank test was used to compare survival estimates between subgroups. Cox regression analysis was used to evaluate the influence of the analyzed variables on time to death. In particular, we have analyzed the impact of patient age groups ant the presence and type of malperfusion, separately and in combination on the short-term survival. The variables with a statistical significance by linear Cox analysis at a P-value <0.1 were entered into the Cox regression model. All P values less than 0.05 were considered statistically significant.

Results. Coronary malperfusion was present in 48 patients (12.2%), visceral malperfusion (renal with or without liver-mesenteric) in 90 (23%), and peripheral arterial malperfusion in 89 (22.6%) patients. Patients aged <65 years were 192 (group 1, 48.9%), aged 65–69 years, 60 (group 2, 15.3%), aged 70–74 years, 56 (group 3, 14.2%), with age 75–79 years, 58 (group 4, 14.7%), +80 years, 27 (group 5, 6.9%). Intraoperative death occurred in 39 patients (9.9%), and in-hospital mortality, including intraoperative, was 32.5% (n = 128 patients). Operative mortality including intraoperative deaths due to all postoperative malperfusions was 17.6% (69 cases /393).

Tables 1 and **2** show the risk factors and independent predictors of intraoperative and in-hospital mortality. The main causes of intraoperative deaths were the massive

	Univariate analysis	Multivariate analysis		
Variables	***P*-value**	**Exp.(Coef)**	**95% CI**	***P*-value**
Cardiopulmonary by-pass time ↑ (284 vs. 169 min.)	<0.0001	1.02	1.01–1.05	<0.0001
T°C cardiopulmonary by-pass ↓ (26 vs. 27 °C)	0.036	1.34	1.02–1.76	0.034
Aortic cross-clamp time ↑ (141 vs. 97 min.)	<0.0001	0.99	0.97–1.00	0.179
Re-do operation	0.021	3.79	0.88–16.3	0.074
Cardiac tamponade/pericardial effusion	0.092	1.69	0.61–4.65	0.305
Coronary artery malperfusion	0.007	0.81	0.22–2.92	0.744
Visceral malperfusion	0.015	6.49	0.86–48.9	0.069
Peripheral arterial malperfusion	0.048	0.47	0.61–3.62	0.472
Arch replacement	0.0002	2.05	0.69–6.07	0.193
Coronary ostia re-implantation	0.096	2.68	0.93–7.75	0.067
CABG	0.021	1.97	0.31–12.4	0.469

CABG: Coronary artery bypass grafting.

Table 1.
Risk factors and independent predictors of intraoperative mortality (univariate and logistic regression analyses).

	Univariate analysis	Multivariate analysis		
Variables	***P*-value**	**Exp. (Coef)**	**95% CI**	***P*-value**
Age ↑ (66 vs. 62 years)	0.005	1.06	1.02–1.09	0.0007
Age, groups 2–5	<0.05	0.59 4.49 7.13 17.4	0.18–1.93 1.44–14.1 2.14–23.7 3.84–79.5	0.382 0.01 0.0014 0.0002
BMI ↑ (28 vs. 27)	0.024	1.03	0.97–1.11	0.342
De Bakey type-I dissection	0.088	1.82	0.89–4.76	0.089
Coronary artery malperfusion	0.002	4.45	0.70–8.47	0.018
Visceral malperfusion	0.003	5.06	0.79–32.4	0.087
Peripheral arterial malperfusion	0.021	0.27	0.39–1.86	0.184
Arch replacement	<0.0001	4.12	1.59–10.7	0.004
Cardiopulmonary by-pass time ↑ (223 vs. 162 min.)	<0.0001	1.01	1.00–1.02	0.0001
Cerebral perfusion time ↑ (42 vs. 32 min.)	0.023	0.99	0.98–1.01	0.269
Need for CABG	0.007	1.29	0.19–8.48	0.791
Postop. neurological dysfunction	0.004	0.96	0.09–1.03	0.05
Postop. dialysis requirement	<0.0001	7.95	3.68–31.0	<0.0001

Groups of age: 2 = 65–69 years; 3 = 70–74 years; 4 = 75–79 years; 5 = +80 years. BMI: body mass index. CABG: coronary artery bypass grafting.

Table 2.
Risk factors and independent predictors of operative (30-day) mortality (univariate and logistic regression analyses).

			Regression analysis	
Variables	**Chi-square value**	**Exp. (Coef)**	**95% CI**	***P*-value**
Age, groups 2–5	0.76	1.01	1.00–1.01	0.384
	5.19	3.04	1.17–7.89	0.022
	11.8	5.06	2.01–12.7	0.0006
	17.8	13.3	3.99–44.0	<0.0001
Coronary artery malperfusion	0.98	0.99	0.35–2.81	0.983
Visceral malperfusion	0.01	1.03	0.25–4.28	0.971
Peripheral arterial malperfusion	0.021	0.27	0.39–1.86	0.184
Arch replacement	2.36	2.02	0.83–4.39	0.124
Coronary ostia reimplantation	0.22	0.84	0.41–1.71	0.635
Cardiopulmonary by-pass time ↑	13.9	1.01	1.00–1.01	0.0002
CABG	5.14	7.33	1.31–41.0	0.023
Postop. neurological dysfunction	0.17	0.21	0.04–1.23	0.683
Postop. dialysis requirement	40.1	18.3	7.44–45.0	<0.0001

Groups of age: 2 = 65–69 years; 3 = 70–74 years; 4 = 75–79 years; 5 = +80 years. CABG: coronary artery bypass grafting.

Table 3.
Independent predictors of 1-year survival (Cox-regression analysis).

bleeding following aortic repair and heart failure (especially, of the right heart). Intraoperative mortality was strictly related, from a statistical point of view, with the greater length and complexity of the surgical intervention (**Table 1**).

Higher age groups, preoperative malperfusions, and neurological (disabling stroke) and renal complications had a dramatic impact on the 30-day mortality risk (**Table 2**) and on the 1-year survival (**Table 3**). Specifically, in relation to the age of the patients, 1-year mortality was 29% for group 1, 38% for group 2, 32% for group 3, and 40% and 63% in groups 4 and 5, respectively.

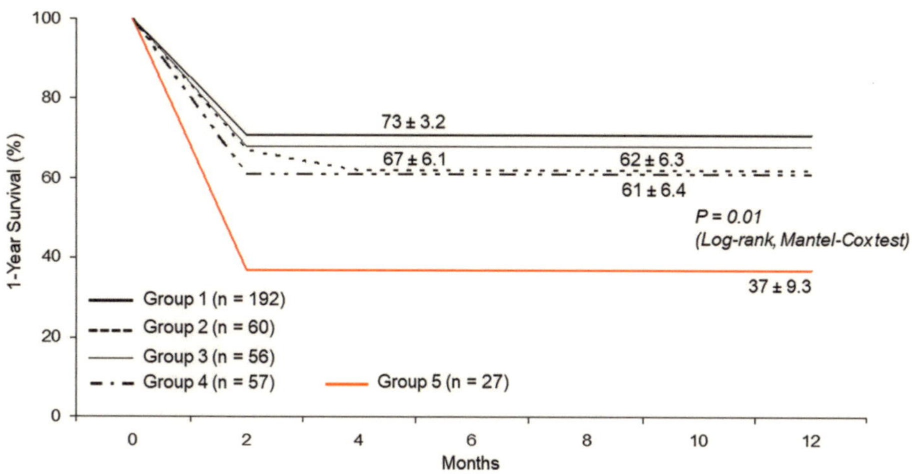

Figure 1.
Short-term survival in relation to the division of patients by age group.

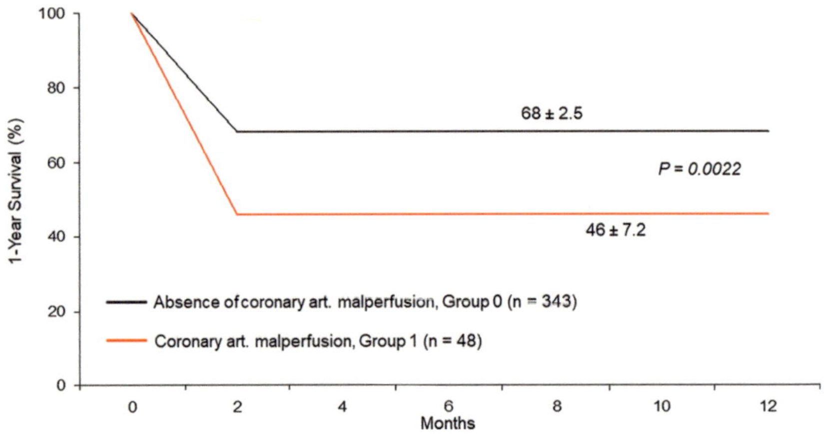

Figure 2.
Short-term survival in relation to presence or absence of preoperative coronary artery malperfusion.

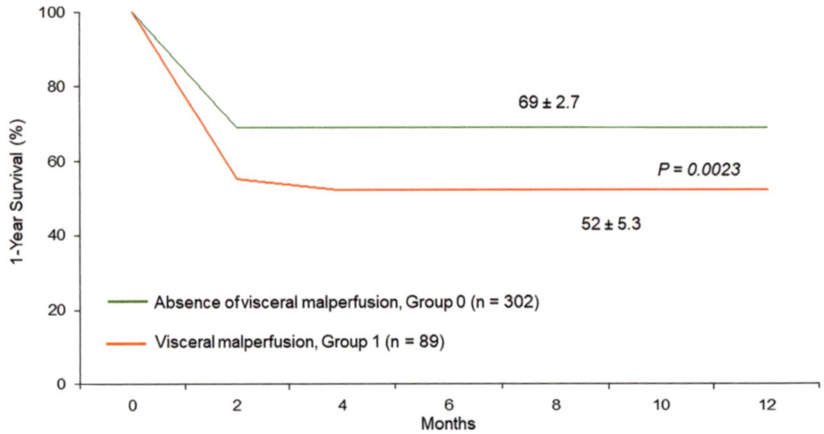

Figure 3.
Short-term survival in relation to presence or absence of preoperative visceral malperfusion.

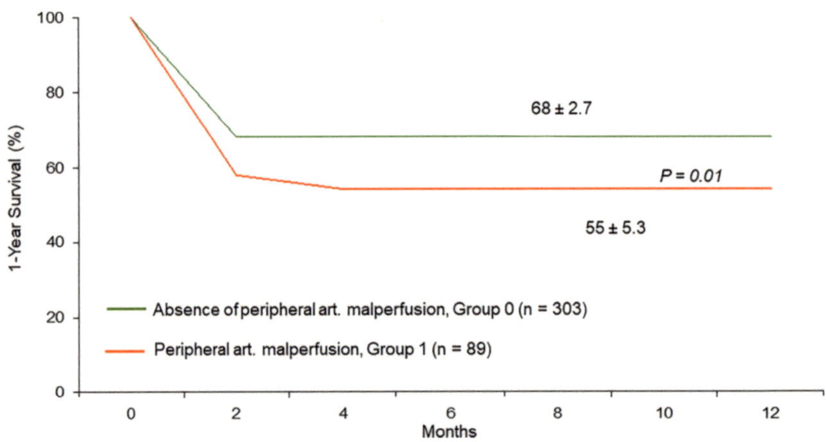

Figure 4.
Short-term survival in relation with presence or absence of preoperative peripheral arterial malperfusion.

At 1 year of follow-up, overall survival was 65.2 ± 2.4%. **Figures 1–4** show the survival at 1 year of follow-up based on the age groups of the patients and the presence or absence of coronary, visceral, and peripheral arterial malperfusion, respectively.

3. Discussion and early clinical results

Various preoperative and perioperative variables have been identified over the years as risk factors and predictors of operative mortality, especially by the International Registry of Acute Aortic Dissection (IRAD) [1]: age > 70 years, cardiac tamponade, pulse deficit, hypotension, and different forms and localizations of malperfusion. The initially reported operative mortality of 32.5% has tended to decrease in subsequent years, but is still estimated to be high, between 17 and 26% [9], depending on the different clinical presentation of patients: in certain cases, in the presence of localized or generalized malperfusion, it even exceeds 80%. Among the perioperative risk factors, the most important to include as predictive are the increased operation time, the combined coronary artery bypass graft, the replacement of the aortic arch. Data from IRAD [2] showed that surgical mortality significantly increases with increased age, that is, 38% in patients ≥70 years vs. 26% of younger patients; data similar to what we observed: 29% in younger patients vs. ≥38% in older patients ($P < 0.05$). Given the 60% mortality with medical therapy alone, it has been proposed that, in general, a surgical approach should not be denied on the basis of advanced age alone. Again in agreement with the previous study, Hemli and collaborators [10] report from the IRAD database of 5553 patients observed in the period 1996–2018 an operative mortality of octogenarians similar to that observed in septuagenarians (25 vs. 21%), confirming again how age alone should not contraindicate the surgical indication. It should be noted, however, that only 68% of patients aged +80 years underwent surgery compared to septuagenarian patients (86%) ($P < 0.0001$), suggesting that the remaining 1/3 of non-operated eighty-year-old patients presented a preoperative clinical picture such as to be considered at prohibitive operative risk, for whom mortality would probably have reached or even exceeded that expected with medical treatment alone.

Similar indication rationale was proposed in the IRAD also with regards to the presence of malperfusion, especially visceral-mesenteric malperfusion, given that the mortality observed without intervention was 95 vs. 42% with aortic repair ($P < 0.001$) [9]. The mortality rate remains high because, as pointed out in literature [7], clinical presentation of the patients affected by TAAD in recent years has become increasingly serious, with a higher incidence of one or multi-organ malperfusion. In our previous publication, we found that the mortality rate in the presence of malperfusion was 47 vs. 23% without malperfusion ($P < 0.0001$) [11]. Augoustides and coworkers [12] on 221 patients affected by TAAD and undergoing aortic repair, reported a 8.3-fold difference on in-hospital mortality for no compared with any ischemia (3.1 vs. 25.8%, $P = 0.0001$). Ischemic presentation of more than one district accounted for 85.7% of all deaths. In the same way, we performed a retrospective analysis of data of our center with enough experience in the treatment of TAAD, paying particular attention to preoperative malperfusion involving specific organs, that is, myocardial, renal, and visceral, and the influence of this complication on the outcome in the short and in the medium term. In our experience, preoperative peripheral malperfusion of all types, that is, renal, visceral, others, and cardiac malperfusion, whether associated or not, occurred in 227 patients or in more than 57% of cases, and it correlated significantly with the postoperative development of malperfusive syndrome. The incidence of postoperative malperfusion was 20%, and it was the main cause of death intraoperatively and after surgery at 30 days (17.6%). Therefore, the surgery allowed the resolution of the malperfusion in about 2/3 of the cases, but in the other 1/3 of cases, proximal aortic replacement surgery does not provide a prognostic benefit in such patients. Peripheral malperfusion of any kind obviously correlates with the extent of the dissection [13]. In De Bakey type II TAAD, it can only be observed a coronary malperfusion and not distal. In fact, the minor extension of the type II acute dissection at the logistic regression analysis was identified as an independent protective factor of operative mortality.

Given the non-negligible incidence of preoperative onset of organ or multi-organ malperfusion and, consequently, the high mortality that this condition entail, in the last years, there is an open debate on the choice of therapeutic strategy to be adopted [14–24]. That is, if aortic surgical repair is always in any case promptly indicated, or if it may be better to carry out interventional procedures on the false lumen of the aorta to treat immediately, at least in part, the malperfusion syndrome and to improve the organs perfusion before surgery [25–28]. Coselli et al. [29] emphasize that the primary purpose of the treatment, in the acute setting, is to save the patient, with an intervention on the proximal aorta that should be as short as possible, thus confirming the guidelines that place the replacement of the ascending aorta segment in class I of indication. Undoubtedly, it should be considered that the severity of preoperative malperfusion is not always well known, and that any delay in evaluation may increase the risk of death. Based on these clinical aspects, the authors, when the dissection affects the left main stem or the right coronary ostium, recommend to by-pass the left anterior descending and/or the right coronary artery to prevent myocardial ischemia or infarction. While, in presence of a dissection involving the superior mesenteric artery with a dynamic or static malperfusion, the authors suggest to do immediately endovascular aortic fenestration/stenting followed by surgical repair. If after mesenteric arterial reperfusion, patients develop acute respiratory failure, septic shock, multi-organ failure; in those cases, the authors suggest to wait for 2–4 weeks for a possible restoration of clinical conditions suitable for undergoing surgery. On the contrary, if isolated renal malperfusion is present, the authors agree for immediate surgery. Lawton et al. [30], Narayan et al. [31], Feier et al. [32], Yang et al. [26, 27], and their coworkers, analyzing data from over 1200 patients affected by TAAD, underline that, in patients with preoperative lactic acidosis and mesenteric ischemia, surgical treatment can lead to unacceptable mortality, with a ten-fold rise of mortality. Therefore, also in this study, the authors suggest the absolute necessity of a two-stage treatment, in order to restore in the first-stage intestinal adequate perfusion. Then, after reaching the improvement of the patient's general condition, in the second stage, they confirm the indication for surgical repair. Furthermore, as we have assessed, it is important to consider both risk factors, that is, very advanced age and the concomitant presence of malperfusion. Vinholo et al. [33], in a recent review addressing which patients with TAAD surgery may not be indicated, underlines how the older age associated with frailty, preexisting neurological degenerative disease like dementia, malperfusion, and redo operation makes these patients at very high operative risk high or even prohibitive, also taking into consideration the type of postoperative complications that may occur, such as immobilization, severe chronic renal failure, prolonged intubation, and cognitive worsening. So much as to suggest that patients and family members should be well informed of the risks of surgery and suitable octogenarians selected for surgical treatment [34]. From the analysis of our data, as reported in **Tables 4** and **5**, we can see that at 1 year, the impact of age over 75 and over 80 associated with coronary or visceral malperfusion determines a dramatic reduction in survival, even to 16% only or 0% in patients over 80 associated with coronary or visceral malperfusion.

	Deaths	Censored	Survival (%)
No malperfusion/age, group 1	47	125	72.7
No malperfusion/age, group 2	17	33	66.0
No malperfusion/age, group 3	15	35	70.0
No malperfusion/age, group 4	19	32	62.7
No malperfusion/age, group 5	12	8	40.0
No malperfusion/age, all groups	110	233	67.9*
Malperfusion/age, group 1	9	11	55.0
Malperfusion/age, group 2	6	4	40.0
Malperfusion/age, group 3	3	3	50.0
Malperfusion/age, group 4	3	3	50.0
Malperfusion/age, group 5	5	1	16.7
Malperfusion/age, all groups	26	22	45.8*

*Groups of age: group 1 = < 65 years; group 2 = 65–69 years; group 3 = 70–74 years; group 4 = 75–79 years; group 5 = +80 years. *P = 0.012 (log rank, Mantel-Cox test).*

Table 4.
Correlation between age groups of patients and coronary artery malperfusion on the 1-year actuarial survival (including in-hospital deaths).

	Deaths	Censored	Survival (%)
No malperfusion/age, group 1	36	107	74.8
No malperfusion/age, group 2	14	29	67.4
No malperfusion/age, group 3	9	35	79.5
No malperfusion/age, group 4	19	29	60.4
No malperfusion/age, group 5	15	9	37.5
No malperfusion/age, all groups	93	209	69.2**
Malperfusion/age, group 1	20	29	59.2
Malperfusion/age, group 2	9	8	47.1
Malperfusion/age, group 3	9	3	25.0
Malperfusion/age, group 4	3	6	66.7
Malperfusion/age, group 5	2	0	00.0
Malperfusion/age, all groups	43	46	51.7**

*Groups of age: group 1 = < 65 years; group 2 = 65–69 years; group 3 = 70–74 years; group 4 = 75–79 years; group 5 = +80 years. **P = 0.001 (log rank, Mantel-Cox test).*

Table 5.
Correlation between age groups of patients and visceral malperfusion on the 1-year actuarial survival (including in-hospital deaths).

In Sievers' study [35], in which the new TEM classification of TAAD has been proposed (T: type Stanford A, non-A non-B, and B; E: entry tear - E0 = tear non-visible, E1 = ascending aorta, E2 = arch, E3 = descending aorta - M: malperfusion - M0, M1 coronary, M2 supra-aortic vessels, M3 visceral-renal and/or lower extremity), it is reported an operative mortality of 40% for E2 and 22% for E0, respectively, vs. 14% for E1 ($P = 0.023$), highlighting a significantly higher risk when arch surgery is performed. Nappi et al. [36] in a multicenter registry including a total of 601 patients affected by TAAD undergoing aortic repair reported a higher rate of cerebrovascular complications after arch replacement (21.7 vs. 7.6%, $P = 0.01$). Rylski et al. [37] in a study conducted in 197 TAAD patients showed that, limiting the extent of surgery for type A aortic dissection to ascending aortic replacement was associated with low perioperative mortality (9.8% for isolated ascending aorta replacement; 21.6% for hemi-arch replacement; 28.6% for total arch replacement). Thus, aortic arch repair can be deferred because it can be performed electively with a lower mortality risk. Age > 80 years, malperfusion syndrome and arch replacement were identified as independent predictors of perioperative mortality (P-values ≤ 0.01). In fact, the guidelines on the treatment of TAAD do not routinely recommend the replacement of the aorta extended to the arch in all cases, but rather to be as conservative as possible given the severity of the condition of the patients who arrive in the operating room [38, 39]. In class I of indication, the main following indications are given in TAAD. (1) Aortic valve resuspension is recommended over its replacement. (2) In the presence of extensive destruction of the aortic root, of an aortic root aneurysm or a known genetic disorder, aortic root replacement with a mechanical or a biological valved conduit, that is, Bentall operation, is recommended. (3) An open distal anastomosis is recommended to improve survival and increase false-lumen thrombosis rates. (4) In patients without an intimal tear in the arch or a significant arch aneurysm, hemi-arch repair is recommended over more extensive arch replacement. Class 2b: in patients with dissection flap extending through the arch into the descending aorta, an extended aortic repair with antegrade stenting of the proximal segment of the descending aorta, that is, elephant trunk operation, may be considered to reduce the risk during the follow-up of distal aorta complications.

4. Discussion of the early and mid-term outcomes

In other ways, however, once the high risk of operative mortality has been overcome, short and medium-long term survival appears to be quite satisfactory: at 5 years in one previously performed study, we observed a late survival rate of 90.8% [11]. Cox regression and log-rank tests analyses identified that independent predictors of mid-term survival were age > 75 years (65 vs. 92%) (P-values <=0.05) and postoperative renal malperfusion (79 vs. 94%) (P-values <= 0.01). In another published study, we observed a 5-year late survival rate of 74%, with independent predictors of reduced survival being preoperative coronary malperfusion and greater extension toward the distal aorta of the De Bakey type I dissection (RR 5.78 and 5.37, respectively; P-values <0.05) [13]. Sievers et al. [35] reported a 2-year survival rate of 83% for Stanford A surgically treated dissections. Eranki et al. [34] on a total of 16,641 patients collected in a review analysis, reported a 5-year survival rate of 76% in the non-octogenarians patients vs. 54% in the octogenarians ($P < 0.001$). Freedom from aortic events appears to be conditioned by the extent of the aortic dissection, that is, type I De Bakey, by the presence of the false lumen with progression of the aneurysmal pathology, by the need for re-intervention due to progression of the aortic pathology at the level of the root and distal to the first aortic repair surgery. In our analysis, 5-year freedom from cardiac death and new vascular procedures to treat the distal aorta were 92 and 81%, respectively. Extension of the De Bakey type I TAAD into the thoracic-abdominal aorta was a predictor for the need for new vascular procedures (RR 1.66) [13]. Moreover, we have observed that patients in whom only replacement of the supra-junctional ascending aorta with or without hemi-arch was performed at the first operation, the incidence of reoperation on the proximal aorta, that is, Bentall re-do, during long-term follow-up, was significantly higher (13.2 vs. 2.9%, $P < 0.05$) [40].

5. Conclusions

Acute aortic dissection still is one of the most challenging diseases faced by cardiac surgeons, and despite preventative measures including early surgical referrals for patients, preoperative and postoperative care, and improved surgical techniques, in-hospital mortality remains high. Malperfusion syndromes and very advanced age, that is, > 75 and > 80 years, undoubtedly heavily influence the short-term outcome of these patients and are still today associated with a very high operative risk. Replacement of the proximal portion of the aorta is able to reduce the incidence of postoperative malperfusion in more than half of patients. However, in particular conditions, such as in the presence of an age over 80 years in association with concomitant presence of malperfusion syndromes and particular preoperative comorbidity conditions, surgical treatment, considering the observed risk of death and mortality within the first year of over 80%, should be weighed very carefully.

Conflict of interest

The authors declare no conflict of interest.

Author details

Paolo Nardi[1*], Alessandro Cristian Salvati[1], Mattia Scognamiglio[1], Valentina Ajello[2], Marzia Flaminio[2], Manuela Moresco[2], Laura De Felice[2] and Claudia Altieri[3]

1 Cardiac Surgery Division, Tor Vergata University Hospital, Tor Vergata University, Rome, Italy

2 Cardio-Thoracic Anesthesia Unit, Tor Vergata University Hospital, Tor Vergata University, Italy

3 Cardiology Unit of the Cardiac Surgery Division, Tor Vergata University Hospital, Tor Vergata University, Italy

*Address all correspondence to: pa.nardi4@libero.it

References

[1] Mehta RH, Suzuki T, Hagan PG, Bossone E, Gilon D, Llovet A, et al. International registry of acute aortic dissection (IRAD) Investigators. Predicting death in patients with acute type A aortic dissection. Circulation. 2002;**105**(2):200-206. DOI: 10.1161/hc0202.102246

[2] Trimarchi S, Eagle KA, Nienaber CA, Rampoldi V, FHW J, De Vincentiis C, et al. Role of age in acute type A aortic dissection outcome: Report from the international registry of acute aortic dissection (IRAD). The Journal of Thoracic and Cardiovascular Surgery. 2010;**140**(4):784-789. DOI: 10.1016/j.jtcvs.2009.11.014

[3] Conzelmann LO, Weigang E, Mehlhorn U, Abugameh A, Hoffmann I, Blettner M, et al. Mortality in patients with acute aortic dissection type A: Analysis of pre- and intraoperative risk factors from the German registry for acute aortic dissection type A (GERAADA). European Journal of Cardio-Thoracic Surgery. 2015;**49**(2):e44-e52. DOI: 10.1093/ejcts/ezv356

[4] Rampoldi V, Trimarchi S, Eagle KA, et al. Simple risk models to predict surgical mortality in acute type A aortic dissection: The international registry of acute aortic dissection (IRAD) investigators. The Annals of Thoracic Surgery. 2007;**83**(1):55-61. DOI: 10.1016/j.athoracsur.2006.08.007

[5] Orihashi K. Malperfusion in acute type A aortic dissection: Unsolved problem. The Annals of Thoracic Surgery. 2013;**95**(5):1570-1576. DOI: 10.1016/j.athoracsur.2013.02.025

[6] Nardi P, Scafuri A, Pellegrino A, Bassano C, Zeitani J, Bertoldo F, et al. Surgery for type A aortic dissection: Long-term results and risk factor analysis. Giornale Italiano di Cardiologia. 2007;**8**(9):580-585

[7] Wang TK, Wei D, Evans T, Ramanathan T, Haydock D. Surgery for type A aortic dissection: 14-year contemporary cohort study. Heart, Lung & Circulation. 2020;**29**(8):1210-1216. DOI: 10.1016/j.hlc.2020.01.008

[8] Zhu X, Wang J, Chong H, Jiang Y, Fan F, Pan J, et al. Analysis of risk factors for postoperative mortality in acute type A aortic dissection patients under different critical levels. Scientific Reports. 2023;**13**(1):8107. DOI: 10.1038/s41598-023-35351-w

[9] Berretta P, Patel HJ, Gleason TG, Sundt TM, Myrmel T, Desai N, et al. IRAD experience on surgical type A acute dissection patients: Results and predictors of mortality. Annals of Cardiothoracic Surgery. 2016;**5**(4):346-351. DOI: 10.21037/acs.2016.05.10

[10] Hemli JM, Pupovac SS, Gleason TG, Sundt TM, Desai ND, Pacini D, et al. Management of acute type A aortic dissection in the elderly: An analysis from IRAD. European Journal of Cardio-Thoracic Surgery. 2022;**61**(4):838-846. DOI: 10.1093/ejcts/ezab546

[11] Nardi P, Olevano C, Bassano C, Bovio E, Cecchetti L, Forlani S, et al. The effect of postoperative malperfusion after surgical treatment of type A acute aortic dissection on early and mid-term survival. Vessel Plus. 2017;**1**:77-83

[12] Augoustides JG, Geirsson A, Szeto WY, Walsh EK, Cornelius B, Pochettino A, et al. Observational study of mortality risk stratification by ischemic

presentation in patients with acute type A aortic dissection: The Penn classification. Nature Clinical Practice. Cardiovascular Medicine. 2009;**6**(2): 140-146. DOI: 10.1038/ncpcardio1417

[13] Nardi P, Bassano C, Pisano C, Altieri C, Ferrante M, Greci M, et al. The effects of DeBakey type acute aortic dissection and preoperative peripheral and cardiac malperfusion on the outcomes after surgical repair. Kardiochir Torakochirurgia Pol. 2021;**18**(1):1-7. DOI: 10.5114/kitp.2021.105187

[14] Immer FF, Grobéti V, Lauten A, Carrel TP. Does malperfusion syndrome affect early and mid-term outcome in patients suffering from acute type A aortic dissection? Interactive Cardiovascular and Thoracic Surgery. 2006;**5**(2):187-190. DOI: 10.1510/icvts.2005.125484

[15] Kimura N, Ohnuma T, Itoh S, Sasabuch Y, Asaka K, Shiotsuka J, et al. Utility of the Penn classification in predicting outcomes of surgery for acute type A aortic dissection. The American Journal of Cardiology. 2014;**113**(4):724-730. DOI: 10.1016/j.amjcard.2013.11.017

[16] Zindovic I, Sjögren J, Bjursten H, Danielsson E, Ingemansson R, Nozohoor S. Impact of hemodynamic instability and organ Malperfusion in elderly surgical patients treated for acute type A aortic dissection. Journal of Cardiac Surgery. 2015;**30**(11):822-829. DOI: 10.1111/jocs.12633

[17] Böning A, Kretzer J, Arif R, Etz CD, Pöling J, Rylski B, et al. Risk factors for long-term mortality after acute aortic dissection-results of the german registry for acute aortic dissection type A long-term follow-up. European Journal of Cardio-Thoracic Surgery. 2024;**26**:ezae116. DOI: 10.1093/ejcts/ezae116

[18] Geirsson A, Szeto WY, Pochettino A, McGarvey ML, Keane MG, Woo YJ, et al. Significance of malperfusion syndromes prior to contemporary surgical repair for acute type A dissection: Outcomes and need for additional revascularization. European Journal of Cardio-Thoracic Surgery. 2007;**32**(2):255-262. DOI: 10.1016/j.ejcts.2007.04.012

[19] Girdauskas E, Kuntze T, Borger MA, Falk V, Mohr FW. Surgical risk of preoperative malperfusion in acute type A aortic dissection. The Journal of Thoracic and Cardiovascular Surgery. 2009;**138**(6):1363-1369. DOI: 10.1016/j.jtcvs.2009.04.059

[20] Kawahito K, Kimura N, Yamaguchi A, Aizawa K. Malperfusion in type A aortic dissection: Results of emergency central aortic repair. General Thoracic and Cardiovascular Surgery. 2019;**67**(7):594-601. DOI: 10.1007/s11748-019-01072-z

[21] Velayudhan BV, Idhrees AM, Mukesh K, Kannan RN. Mesenteric Malperfusion in acute aortic dissection: Challenges and Frontiers. Seminars in Thoracic and Cardiovascular Surgery. 2019;**31**(4):668-673. DOI: 10.1053/j.semtcvs.2019.03.012

[22] Zindovic I, Gudbjartsson T, Ahlsson A, Fuglsang S, Gunn J, Hansson EC, et al. Malperfusion in acute type A aortic dissection: An update from the Nordic consortium for acute type A aortic dissection. The Journal of Thoracic and Cardiovascular Surgery. 2019;**157**(4):1324-1333.e6. DOI: 10.1016/j.jtcvs.2018.10.134

[23] Uchida K, Karube N, Kasama K, Minami T, Yasuda S, Goda M, et al. Early reperfusion strategy improves the outcomes of surgery for type A acute aortic dissection with malperfusion. The Journal of Thoracic and Cardiovascular

Surgery. 2018;**156**(2):483-489. DOI: 10.1016/j.jtcvs.2018.02.007

[24] Ong CS, Nam L, Yesantharao P, Dong J, Canner JK, Teuben RJ, et al. The strongest risk factor for operative mortality in acute type A aortic dissection is acidosis: Validation of risk model. Seminars in Thoracic and Cardiovascular Surgery. 2020;**32**(4):674-680. DOI: 10.1053/j.semtcvs.2020.02.023

[25] Goldberg JB, Lansman SL, Kai M, Tang GHL, Malekan R, Spielvogel D. Malperfusion in type A dissection: Consider reperfusion first. Seminars in Thoracic and Cardiovascular Surgery. 2017;**29**(2):181-185. DOI: 10.1053/j.semtcvs.2016.10.017

[26] Yang B, Norton EL, Rosati CM, Wu X, Kim KM, Khaja MS, et al. Managing patients with acute type A aortic dissection and mesenteric malperfusion syndrome: A 20-year experience. The Journal of Thoracic and Cardiovascular Surgery. 2019;**158**(3):675-687.e4. DOI: 10.1016/j.jtcvs.2018.11.127

[27] Yang B, Rosati CM, Norton EL, Kim KM, Khaja MS, Dasika N, et al. Endovascular fenestration/stenting first followed by delayed open aortic repair for acute type A aortic dissection with malperfusion syndrome. Circulation. 2018;**138**(19):2091-2103. DOI: 10.1161/CIRCULATIONAHA.118.036328

[28] Leshnower BG, Keeling WB, Duwayri YM, Jordan WD, Chen EP. The "thoracic endovascular aortic repair-first" strategy for acute type A dissection with mesenteric malperfusion: Initial results compared with conventional algorithms. The Journal of Thoracic and Cardiovascular Surgery. 2019;**158**(6):1516-1524. DOI: 10.1016/j.jtcvs.2019.01.116

[29] Chen E, Gleason T, Yang B, Coselli J, Shrestha M. Discussions in cardiothoracic treatment and care: The contemporary management of acute type A aortic dissection. Seminars in Thoracic and Cardiovascular Surgery. 2020;**32**(2):202-210. DOI: 10.1053/j.semtcvs.2020.02.011

[30] Lawton JS, Moon MR, Liu J, Koerner DJ, Kulshrestha K, Damiano RJ Jr, et al. The profound impact of combined severe acidosis and malperfusion on operative mortality in the surgical treatment of type A aortic dissection. The Journal of Thoracic and Cardiovascular Surgery. 2018;**155**(3):897-904. DOI: 10.1016/j.jtcvs.2017.11.002

[31] Narayan P, Rogers CA, Benedetto U, Caputo M, Angelini GD, Bryan AJ. Malperfusion rather than merely timing of operative repair determines early and late outcome in type A aortic dissection. The Journal of Thoracic and Cardiovascular Surgery. 2017;**154**(1):81-86. DOI: 10.1016/j.jtcvs.2017.03.041

[32] Feier H, Cozma D, Sintean M, Deutsch P, Ursoniu S, Gaspar M, et al. How much Malperfusion is too much in acute type A aortic dissections? Journal of Clinical Medicine. 2019;**8**:304. DOI: 10.3390/jcm8030304

[33] Vinholo TF, Awtry J, Semco R, Newell P, Sabe AA. Acute type A aortic dissection: When not to operate, a review. Vessel Plus. 2024;**8**:11. DOI: 10.20517/2574-1209.2023.150

[34] Eranki A, Merakis M, Williams ML, Flynn CD, Villanueva C, Wilson-Smith A, et al. Outcomes of surgery for acute type A dissection in octogenarians versus non-octogenarians: A systematic review and meta analysis. Journal of Cardiothoracic Surgery. 2022;**17**:22. DOI: 10.1186/s13019-022-01980-x

[35] Sievers HH, Rylski B, Czerny M, Baier ALM, Kreibich M, Siepe M, et al. Aortic dissection reconsidered: Type, entry site, malperfusion classification adding clarity and enabling outcome prediction. Interactive Cardiovascular and Thoracic Surgery. 2020;**30**(3): 451-457. DOI: 10.1093/icvts/ivz281

[36] Nappi F, Gambardella I, Avtaar Singh SS, Salsano A, Santini F, Spadaccio C, et al. Survival following acute type A aortic dissection: A multicenter study. Journal of Thoracic Disease. 2023;**15**(12):6604-6622. DOI: 10.21037/jtd-23-1137

[37] Rylski B, Beyersdorf F, Kari FA, Schlosser J, Blanke P, Siepe M. Acute type A aortic dissection extending beyond ascending aorta: Limited or extensive distal repair. The Journal of Thoracic and Cardiovascular Surgery. 2014;**148**(3):949-954; discussion 954. DOI: 10.1016/j.jtcvs.2014.05.051

[38] Members WC, Isselbacher EM, Preventza O, Hamilton Black J, Augoustides JG, Beck AW, et al. 2022 ACC/AHA guideline for the diagnosis and management of aortic disease: A report of the American Heart Association/American College of Cardiology Joint Committee on clinical practice guidelines. The Journal of Thoracic and Cardiovascular Surgery. 2023;**166**(5):e182-e331. DOI: 10.1016/j.jtcvs.2023.04.023

[39] Czerny M, Grabenwöger M, Berger T, Aboyans V, Della Corte A, Chen EP, et al. EACTS/STS scientific document group. EACTS/STS guidelines for diagnosing and treating acute and chronic syndromes of the aortic organ. European Journal of Cardio-Thoracic Surgery. 2024;**65**(2):ezad426. DOI: 10.1093/ejcts/ezad426

[40] Bassano C, Pugliese M, Mve Mvondo C, Pisano C, Nardi P, Buioni D, et al. Initial surgical strategy for the treatment of type A acute aortic dissection: Does proximal or distal extension of the aortic resection influence the outcomes? International Journal of Environmental Research and Public Health. 2022;**19**(14):8878. DOI: 10.3390/ijerph19148878

Chapter 11

Endovascular Strategies for Addressing Acute Malperfusion in Aortic Dissection

Nicola Habash, Jin Park, Natalie Lukasik and Babak Abai

Abstract

Aortic dissection (AD) involves a tear in the intimal layer of the aorta that creates a false lumen within the aortic wall and can result in malperfusion of distal branch vessels. Herein, a comprehensive examination of malperfusion in the context of acute AD is provided, with a focus on the mechanisms underlying dynamic and static obstructions, their effects on branch vessel perfusion, and the diagnostic challenges they present. The use of endovascular strategies such as thoracic endovascular aortic repair (TEVAR), branch vessel stenting, and aortic flap fenestration are presented. We also discuss the importance of timely intervention through staged aortic repair to optimize organ perfusion and minimize adverse outcomes in high-risk patients. Additionally, hybrid repair highlights the complex pathology of AD with malperfusion. By integrating scientific evidence with clinical expertise, this chapter intends to serve as a valuable resource for clinicians seeking to improve the management of acute malperfusion in AD using endovascular techniques.

Keywords: aortic dissection, malperfusion, malperfusion syndrome, TEVAR, dynamic obstruction, static obstruction, endovascular fenestration, endovascular-first

1. Introduction

1.1 Overview of aortic dissection

Aortic dissection (AD) is an acute condition characterized by a tear in the intimal layer of the aorta, allowing blood to flow through an entry tear into a false lumen (FL) between the intimal and medial layers. The FL is separated from the true lumen (TL) by the intimal-medial septum. The FL can originate throughout the aorta with the location of the entry tear determining the dissection classification [1, 2]. Accordingly, the anatomical pathology of a specific AD can influence the presenting symptoms depending on its propagation along the length of the aorta to include branch vessels. The disruption of blood flow to branch vessels can lead to a range of complications, including acute malperfusion syndromes (MPS).

The traditional treatments of AD have mainly involved open operations that have a high morbidity and mortality and are invasive. Along with an increasing favor for endovascular treatment, there has been a change in the way we treat malperfusion in patients with AD. Many endovascular techniques have been adapted to address this issue with improved outcomes.

1.2 Epidemiology

The incidence of AD is estimated to range from 5 to 30 cases per million person-years, predominantly affecting males aged 50–65 years [1, 2]. Prompt diagnosis and management are critical due to the high mortality associated with untreated dissections. Immediate concerns include determination of branch vessel patency for MPS assessment and risk for aortic rupture, which may necessitate surgical intervention.

Acute malperfusion is a serious complication of AD and occurs in approximately 21% of type B aortic dissections (TBAD) [3]. Data derived from the International Registry of Aortic Dissection (IRAD), encompassing over 4000 patients treated over 20 years, has provided valuable insights into the prevalence and impact of malperfusion-related complications in AD. According to this analysis, mesenteric ischemia is seen in 3.7% of type A aortic dissections (TAAD), while visceral ischemia is present in 7% of TBAD cases. Limb ischemia complicates 9.7% of all AD cases, and cerebrovascular accidents occur in 10% of TAAD cases. Additionally, patients with renal insufficiency warrant careful monitoring as they are at an increased risk for aortic branch vessel complications [3].

1.3 Importance of managing acute malperfusion

Malperfusion in AD is defined as the compromised blood supply to vital organs due to the dissection flap obstructing branch vessel inflow or diverting flow from the TL to the FL by nearly closing off the TL. MPS, chest or back pain, and hypotension at time of dissection diagnosis are predictors of increased mortality [4]. Common presentations include myocardial ischemia (MI), stroke, renal failure, bowel ischemia, lower extremity ischemia, and spinal cord ischemia (SCI) (**Figure 1**). MPS resulting in end-organ ischemia can occur acutely or over several days and weeks, since the dissection is a dynamic process. In the acute phase, the dissection flap can evolve over time. Symptomatology varies in intensity depending on the degree of branch vessel obstruction, the current clinical state of the patient, and the body's potential for angiogenesis and conditioning of collateral tributaries, complicating diagnosis and management [5]. The resulting systemic inflammatory response from ischemia and ischemia-reperfusion injury, including the generation of free radicals and cytokine release, can compromise operative success and delay postoperative recovery [5]. Therefore, early identification and management of malperfusion are essential to preserve organ function, reduce morbidity, and improve survival rates in acute AD.

2. Mechanisms of malperfusion and branch vessel obstruction

Understanding the altered hemodynamics in acute AD, especially those underlying malperfusion and branch vessel obstruction, is central for effective management. This section analyzes the pathophysiology of malperfusion, explores various clinical presentations and patterns based on associated branch vessel involvement,

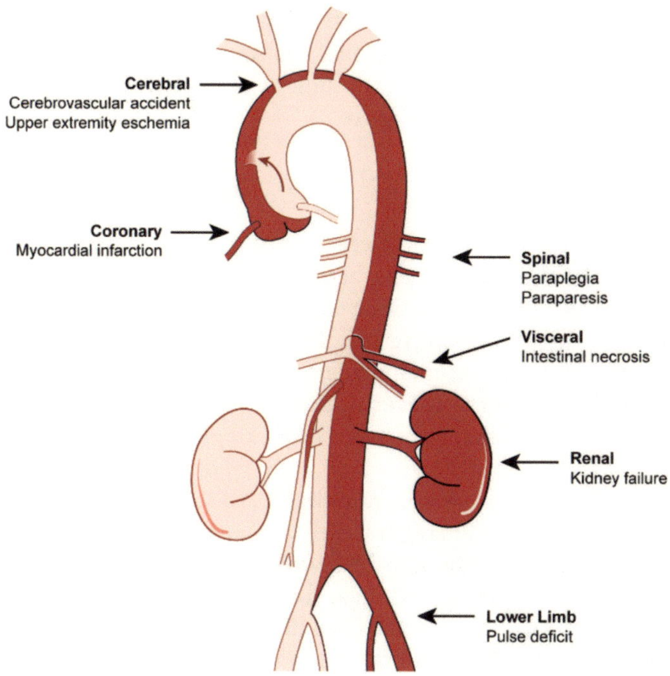

Figure 1.
Cartoon depiction of a dissected aorta. Branch vessels are labeled with common malperfusion-related complications.

and addresses the diagnostic challenges in identifying and managing malperfusion-related complications.

Blood flow through the FL alters distal perfusion. The walls of the FL inherently lack the compliance afforded by the abundant elastin in the intimal arterial layer, making it susceptible to dilation and pressurization. The pressures in the FL can

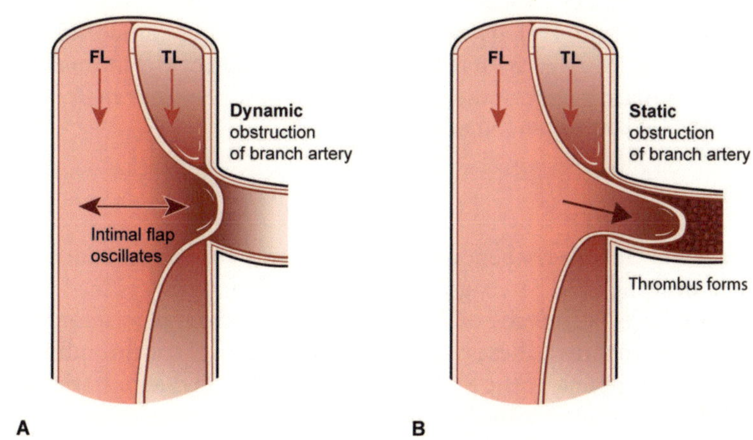

Figure 2.
Illustration of the mechanisms of static and dynamic obstruction in aortic dissection. (A) Dynamic obstruction involves the dissection flap intermittently obstructing the branch vessel due to changes in blood pressure or flow dynamics, causing variable flow. (B) Static obstruction occurs when a branch vessel is permanently blocked by the dissection flap or a thrombus, leading to constant reduction in blood flow.

compress and collapse the TL and change the relationship between the dissection septum and branch vessel ostium, hence obstructing distal blood flow to branch vessels [6]. Malperfusion can manifest through two primary mechanisms: dynamic obstruction and static obstruction (**Figure 2**).

2.1 Dynamic obstruction

Dynamic obstruction involves the oscillation of the mobile intimal flap with the pulsatile blood flow of the cardiac cycle, acting as a dynamic barrier with variable impedance (**Figure 2A**). This oscillation results in the intimal flap prolapsing into the ostia of a branch vessel, intermittently causing a physical restriction to flow. This results in a fluctuating pattern of malperfusion which can complicate the diagnostic process, as symptoms may vary in severity and duration, correlating with local hemodynamic changes in vascular tone and systemic changes in blood pressure and heart rate [7].

When the branch vessel originates from the TL, the hemodynamic impact of systole can influence blood flow, causing transient ischemia. The movement of the dissection flap can cause transient reductions in downstream perfusion pressure, increasing proximal pressurization, creating wall shear forces and pressure gradients that disrupt laminar flow and induce localized turbulence [8, 9]. The compression and narrowing of the TL by the expanding FL also restricts blood flow, contributing to MPS. This impedance causes fluctuations in the Reynolds number, which represents the ratio of inertial pressures to viscous forces within a vessel and models resulting blood flow characteristics. Factors influencing this measurement include aortic circumference, intraluminal pressures, heart rate, and peripheral vascular resistance [10].

Higher Reynolds numbers are associated with turbulent flow, most often occurring during cardiac systole when the dissection flap is more likely to obstruct the TL due to prolapse during the pressure wave. Lower Reynolds numbers, associated with laminar flow, occur during diastole when the intimal flap may only partially obstruct TL flow [11]. The extent of TL collapse can directly influence the degree of hypoperfusion, leading to ischemic episodes in affected vascular territories. Although ischemic patterns would be expected to correlate with intraluminal pathology, clinical presentation and symptomatology can vary significantly. The compression-induced narrowing of the TL, coupled with the dynamic oscillation of the intimal flap, creates a complex hemodynamic environment that exacerbates the risk of malperfusion and complicates effective management of AD.

2.2 Static obstruction

AD, in general, causes vessel endothelial injury from the exposed intimal and medial layers resulting in hypercoagulability from inflammatory cascades and ultimately thrombosis [12]. Static obstruction can result from persistent blockage of branch vessel flow. Together, these create optimal conditions for thrombosis of branch vessels and the blind pouch of the FL, causing malperfusion due to static obstruction [6, 7]. Static obstruction can also precipitate from compression of the TL by the prolapsed dissection septum from FL pressurization and along with FL thrombosis around the branch vessel inlet. Moreover, the intimal flap can protrude into a branch vessel ostium, causing thrombosis distal to the obstruction (**Figure 2B**).

The clinical presentations of patients with static obstructions are typically more severe due to the sustained nature of the blockage, leading to continuous ischemia.

These patients require urgent surgery to restore blood flow and prevent organ failure. The clinical presentations of patients with static obstructions are typically more severe due to the sustained nature of the blockage, leading to continuous ischemia. In some cases, the FL partially perfuses the branch vessel, maintaining flow despite a compressed TL. The counter pressures between the TL and FL on the dissection flap can have a shearing effect, potentially creating an opening tear. Blood can then flow from the FL directly into the branch vessel through this reentry tear, avoiding ischemia [13].

2.3 Classification of branch vessel obstruction

The pathologic anatomy of AD has been well characterized by location of entry tear and dissection propagation in the DeBakey and Stanford classification systems [2]. Obstruction of branch arteries due to acute AD causing MPS has been classified based on spatio-temporal variations with associated outcome predictions after repair [13].

Beregi and colleagues have since developed a classification system based on the physiological and morphological findings of the intimal flap on branch compromise consisting of three main categories divided into 11 distinct perfusion patterns (**Figure 3**) [14]. Nagamine and colleagues use the anatomical findings from Beregi's classification and refine it to emphasize the physiological effects of MPS (**Figure 4**). Their study demonstrated that certain branch arteries exhibited common perfusion patterns and had varied reperfusion responses after central aortic repair. For example, Class 1-b and 1-c patterns were frequently observed in abdominal aortic branches, while the Class 2-b-iii pattern was more common in cervical aortic branches. Aortic repair improved perfusion in Class 2-b-ii and Classes 1-b and 1-c obstructions. However, it was less effective in abdominal branches with Class 3-a or 2-a perfusion patterns. This classification system has significantly contributed to the development of a universal approach for treating MPSs associated with acute AD [14].

2.4 Malperfusion syndromes

Dynamic and static obstructions can lead to MPS in various vascular beds, including those supplied by the carotid, spinal, renal, visceral, and iliac arteries. The complexity of the mechanisms resulting in flow obstruction with subsequent MPS in the context of AD underscores the importance of promptly recognizing common

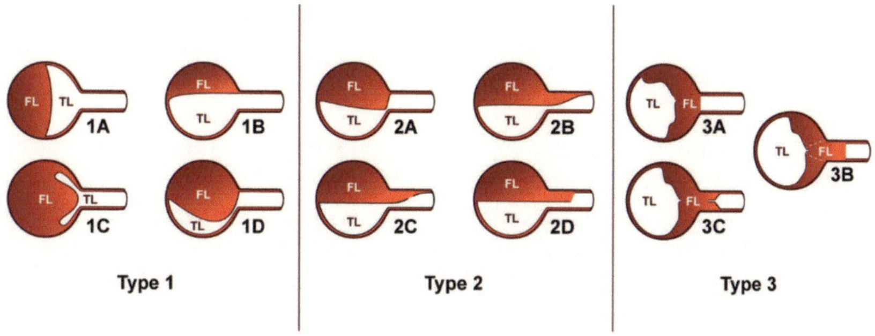

Figure 3.
Beregi's classification system based on the position and extension of the intimal flap. In type 1, the flap is positioned either along or across the origin of the compromised collateral artery. Type 2 describes the dissection propagating into the collateral vessel. Type 3 depicts whether or not a branch ostium has avulsed from the septum.

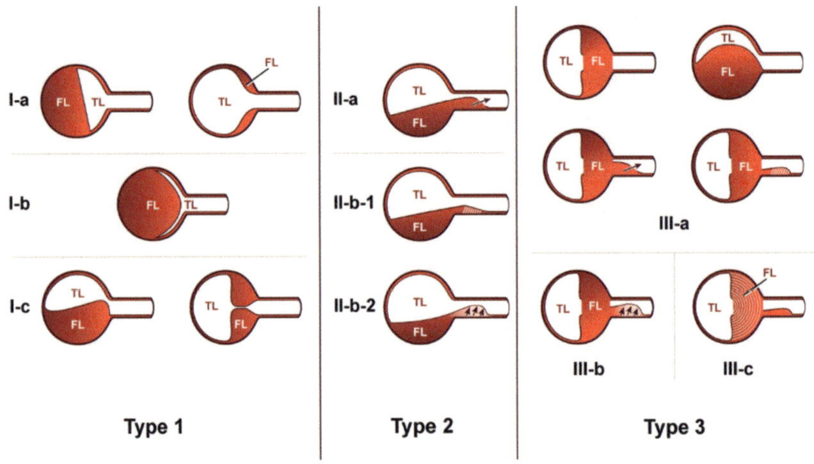

Figure 4.
Nagamine's classification system for branch artery perfusion in aortic dissection. In type 1, there is no dissection of the branch artery. In type 2, the dissection extends into the branch vessel. In type 3, there is ostial avulsion.

malperfusion patterns based on the affected organ system to tailor treatment. The clinical presentation of MPS can often assist in identifying the affected organ systems, the duration of MPS, and the chronicity of the dissection. This information can inform medical and surgical management strategies.

3. Diagnosing malperfusion syndrome in aortic dissections

Accurate and efficient diagnosis of MPS is important for improving patient outcomes due to the substantial morbidity and mortality associated with prolonged end-organ ischemia and irreversible organ damage. This diagnostic process necessitates a systematic paradigm, incorporating a detailed patient history, clinical examination, and comprehensive laboratory evaluations. The acuity of the dissection and the patient's overall clinical status can guide choice of appropriate diagnostic imaging modalities. These combined efforts ensure the timely implementation of appropriate therapeutic interventions to restore perfusion and stabilize the aorta, ultimately seeking to reduce adverse outcomes, augment end-organ perfusion and salvage, and improve survival rates.

3.1 Clinical evaluation

Initial clinical evaluation begins with a detailed patient history and physical examination to identify signs and symptoms indicative of compromised perfusion to specific organ systems. Documentation of a history of pain, the most reliable historical factor for diagnosing AD, should include the onset, duration, and nature of pain [2, 15]. Additionally, the initial sign of MPS is often pain [15]. Carefully describing the symptomatology and characteristics of pain can help differentiate acuity of presentation and stratify patient risk for MPS. Common symptoms to assess for include chest pain suggestive of MI and likely aortic root involvement, focal neurological deficits indicating cerebrovascular compromise of the great vessels of the aortic arch, abdominal pain suggestive of mesenteric ischemia from the abdominal aorta, and limb pain, paresthesias, pallor, and paresis indicative of peripheral limb ischemia. Clinicians can often predict and identify compromised aortic branch vessels at the bedside by evaluating the pattern of pain and distribution of pulse deficits [5].

A thorough history should evaluate for AD risk factors such as hypertension, atherosclerotic disease, connective tissue disorders, and a family history of aortic disease [2]. The history should also include determination of vascular health by assessing for a history of diabetes mellitus, dyslipidemia, smoking status, and menopausal status. The physical examination should include palpation of peripheral pulses to identify pulse deficits and blood pressure measurements in both arms to detect discrepancies, though these findings are present in less than half of reported cases [2]. Initial vital signs can detect hemodynamic instability and continuous vital sign monitoring is crucial as time and medical management can evolve the presentation. Persistent hypotension may suggest ongoing blood loss or cardiac tamponade, while tachycardia can be a response to pain or hypovolemia [16].

3.2 Laboratory evaluation

Laboratory tests include cardiac biomarkers such as troponins and creatine kinase-MB, which can indicate myocardial injury secondary to malperfusion. Renal function tests, including serum creatinine and blood urea nitrogen levels, should be assessed to detect acute kidney injury (AKI) due to renal artery involvement. Abnormal liver function tests (ALT, AST, ALP) may suggest hepatic ischemia or infarction. Elevated lactate levels are a nonspecific marker of tissue hypoperfusion and can indicate widespread ischemia [17]. The complete blood count provides clues about the patient's volume status and ongoing blood loss, while a coagulation profile, including PT/INR and aPTT, should be measured to assess coagulopathy, which can complicate surgical management and postoperative care.

3.3 Imaging

Despite the benefits of routine laboratory testing and a good physical exam, diagnosing MPS remains challenging due to the variable symptomatology. Symptoms of MPS overlap with other common life-threatening conditions, generating expansive differential diagnoses, making differentiation difficult without advanced diagnostic testing. Imaging with computed tomography angiography (CTA), magnetic resonance angiography (MRA), intravascular ultrasound (IVUS), doppler ultrasound (US), and transesophageal echocardiography (TEE) provide detailed insights into the extent and nature of the dissection, blood flow, and perfusion [18]. Correlating clinical state and imaging findings can confirm the diagnosis, enabling the development of an individualized management plan that incorporates endovascular or surgical interventions as indicated.

Doppler US is a non-invasive tool for assessing blood flow in peripheral vessels. IVUS offers real-time intraluminal imaging, visualization of branch vessels, and luminal configurations, information crucial during endovascular procedures [19]. TEE and transthoracic echocardiography (TTE) provide real-time imaging of the heart and aorta, detecting complications such as aortic regurgitation, pericardial effusion, and left ventricular dysfunction. TEE is particularly useful in the acute setting and during surgery to visualize the intimal flap, its relationship with branch vessel ostia, and to assess the extent of the dissection and blood flow patterns (**Figure 5**) [20].

Computed tomography angiography (CTA) is the gold standard for the accurate diagnosis of AD and associated MPS [15]. It offers high-resolution images that

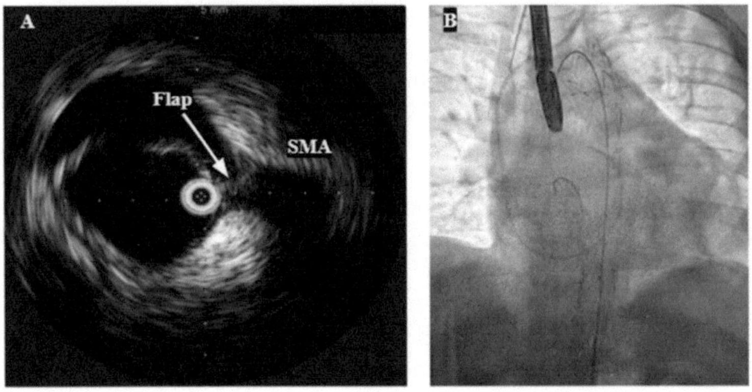

Figure 5.
Commonly used intraoperative imaging during endovascular aortic repair. (A) Intravascular ultrasound (IVUS) with visualization of a compressed true lumen, large false lumen, the dissection flap, and superior mesenteric artery (SMA) branch. (B) Fluoroscopy showing IVUS and transesophageal echocardiography used concurrently.

delineate the extent of the dissection, branch vessel involvement, and the degree and location of static obstructions. The narrowed TL and the size of the FL can also be easily visualized for operative planning [21]. CTA is also useful for the identification of MPS. For example, radiographic signs indicating TL compression are concerning for potential ischemia. For patients exhibiting clinical or laboratory inconsistencies that suggest ischemia, CTA can offer evidence to support the decision for surgical revascularization [5].

The hallmark of renal ischemia in AD has been described as asymmetrically decreased renal enhancement on CTA. A study at the University of Michigan assessing patients with AD and suspected malperfusion over 10 years determined that these radiographic findings were only 65% sensitive and 58% specific for renal malperfusion when verified by renal artery manometry measurements [22]. Further, only 48% of patients with global asymmetric renal enhancement actually had renal malperfusion during invasive angiography [22]. Given these findings, while CTA can suggest the presence of renal ischemia, it may miss it in some patients and not definitively confirm it in others.

However, the use of CTA remains controversial when assessing renal MPS and AKI. Because the kidneys are among the most commonly affected organ systems in AD-mediated MPS and their involvement is an independent predictor of operative mortality, detecting renal ischemia is paramount [23]. Iodinated contrast agents used in CTA are nephrotoxic but can provide information critical for surgical decision making on dissection anatomy and luminal architecture. Therefore, in patients with poor kidney perfusion, the need for access to this valuable information must be balanced with the imperative to protect the kidneys [5]. This issue may be exacerbated by hypotension secondary to an obstructive dissection flap at the renal branch vessel ostia or strict blood pressure regulation from preoperative medical therapy.

Magnetic resonance angiography (MRA) provides excellent soft tissue contrast and detailed flow dynamics, distinguishing blood from thrombus. However, MRA is not commonly used in acute AD or hemodynamically unstable patients because it is time-consuming and may not provide useful information that could not otherwise be obtained by CTA [24]. Doppler US and phase-contrast MRA allow visualization of dynamic processes like arterial blood flow. Doppler US can measure systolic and diastolic flow velocities and identify variations in flow patterns while phase-contrast

MRA provides information on blood flow dynamics, capturing the kinetic behavior of the flap with transient hemodynamic changes. These imaging techniques offer valuable insights into the nature of the obstruction, revealing the interaction between flap motion and blood flow [5].

Effective management of malperfusion in AD hinges on the ability to promptly identify, diagnose, and address the underlying issues. The next section will explore the various endovascular therapies available to manage these life-threatening complications.

4. Open approach to address malperfusion

Surgical management to correct malperfusion in AD focuses on restoring compromised blood flow. While this analysis primarily examines endovascular interventions for MPS, it is worth reviewing the traditionally used open operations.

4.1 Coronary

Coronary malperfusion in acute AD is potentially lethal, with poor in-hospital mortality and low long term survival rates [25]. The right coronary artery (RCA) is often affected due to the tendency of the intimal tear to involve the right side of the greater curvature of the aorta. This can also be explained by the fact that fewer cases of dissections involving the left coronary artery (LCA) survive transport to the hospital [26, 27]. However, LCA involvement in hospitalized patients demonstrates lower in-hospital mortality compared to RCA involvement [28]. Coronary malperfusion presents with electrocardiogram changes, arrhythmias, hypokinesis, and possible cardiogenic shock, necessitating emergent operative action. The classic intervention involves immediate ascending aortic repair with or without coronary artery bypass. If the dissection is limited to the base of the coronary branches from the aorta, the ostium can be repaired with aortic root salvage or replacement [29, 30].

The Bentall procedure, first introduced in 1968, is the classic technique for ascending aortic root repair, originally used for ascending aortic aneurysms [31]. Treatment involves the excision and complete replacement of the ascending aorta and aortic valve with synthetic devices and reimplantation of the coronary buttons into the graft. The Bentall procedure has satisfactory short- and long-term results in AD [32–34].

4.2 Cerebral

Cerebral malperfusion is a feared complication of acute TAAD, worsening survival and postoperative quality of life [35]. Expeditious revascularization, within 5 hours of symptom onset, is associated with improved neurologic outcomes [36]. The standard approach is open emergent ascending aortic replacement with fenestration of dissection flap. Other open methods to quickly restore cerebral perfusion include extra-anatomic revascularization with carotid-carotid or carotid-subclavian bypass [37–39].

4.3 Visceral

Visceral ischemia presents in a variety of ways including abdominal pain, worsening kidney function, bloody diarrhea, and lactic acidosis and is associated with 33.3% in hospital mortality [40, 41]. Early diagnosis and reperfusion can decrease the need for bowel resection and associated morbidity. Methods to restore visceral perfusion include open repair with dissection flap fenestration, mesenteric bypass, and renal bypass.

Traditionally, ascending aortic repair for TAAD has taken priority over managing visceral malperfusion, as central repair would relieve dynamic obstruction of the visceral arteries through septum removal. Open repair also has the benefit of intraoperative bowel assessment. However, open aortic repair alone may not reliably address static obstructions or thrombus in the visceral arteries, necessitating adjunctive open or endovascular interventions such as stenting, thrombolysis, or suction thrombectomy. Delay in reperfusion can cause operative mortality in TAAD to rise above 50% [40, 42, 43].

4.4 Lower extremity

Lower extremity MPS can result from dissection flap obstruction or propagation of the dissection into the iliac and femoral arteries. It often presents with acute limb ischemia, characterized by leg pain, pallor, paresthesia, or paralysis, and is associated with increased hospital mortality [4]. Lower extremity MPS also compels extensive abdominal examination, as these patients commonly present with concomitant renal and visceral malperfusion [44].

Before endovascular procedures, reperfusion was achieved through aortic repair, extra-anatomic bypass grafts (femoro-femoral, axillo-femoral, axillo-bifemoral), or open fenestration. Open fenestration is used for concomitant visceral malperfusion but is typically avoided in high risk surgical patients as it requires supra-celiac or supra-renal aortic cross clamping [44].

4.5 Spinal cord

Spinal cord ischemia (SCI), resulting from AD extending to the intercostal or lumbar arteries, including the artery of Adamkiewicz, causes temporary or permanent motor or sensory deficits in the lower extremities. Sandhu et al. illustrated a significant association between SCI and overall mortality, with postoperative reversal of deficits leading to improved long term outcomes [45]. The conventional framework to manage this has been immediate ascending aortic repair with flap fenestration.

5. Endovascular approach to address malperfusion

The development and refinement of endovascular devices and techniques have expanded the therapeutic options available to vascular surgeons, revolutionizing the treatment paradigm for AD. Traditional open surgical practices, while effective and necessary in certain cases, are often associated with significant morbidity, lengthy hospital admissions, and prolonged recovery times [46, 47]. In contrast, endovascular tactics offer a minimally invasive alternative, reducing the physiological stress on patients, potentially leading to better outcomes and quicker recovery [47]. Endovascular strategies include central aortic endografting, branch vessel stenting, and percutaneous septum fenestration to restore flow in MPS. By understanding the specific characteristics and applications of each endovascular intervention for MPS in AD, clinicians can adapt their operational plan to each patient's needs to optimize outcomes.

5.1 TAAD with MPS

Emergency surgical repair has long been standard management for all patients with TAAD. Emergent open surgery with aortic arch replacement, fenestration of the dissection flap, and aortic valve replacement are often necessary for life-saving treatment, especially as proximal ADs frequently involve the carotid arteries. The established treatment modality typically involves repairing the ascending aorta and various portions of the aortic arch, while leaving the descending aorta untreated (**Figure 6**). Even though the primary entry tear is repaired, there is still a significant hemodynamic effect of the FL through reentry tears in the descending aorta. Unfortunately, even when surgical repair is successful, the patient is left with the continued risk of chronic descending AD with increasing aortic diameter and subsequent aneurysmal degeneration [48].

A hybrid approach, with open repair of the ascending aorta followed by percutaneous stenting with thoracic endovascular aortic repair (TEVAR), can mitigate the consequences of an untreated descending aorta by concurrently addressing both proximal and distal aortic pathology [49]. Hybrid repair, discussed in greater detail later in this chapter, uses the reconstructed arch to extend the proximal landing zone for TEVAR to ensure satisfactory sealing of the stent graft for distal FL depressurization.

Recently, successful reports of complete endovascular repair of the aortic root and coronary revascularization, termed 'Endo-Benthall,' in TAAD with coronary malperfusion have emerged [50]. This unique application combines transcatheter aortic valve replacement with aortic and coronary endografting (**Figure 7**). As the safety and efficacy of this procedure are documented, endovascular repair of the ascending aortic arch is anticipated to play a more prominent role.

Type A aortic dissections (TAAD) is also associated with mesenteric malperfusion due to the involvement of the celiac artery. The current standard of care is prompt

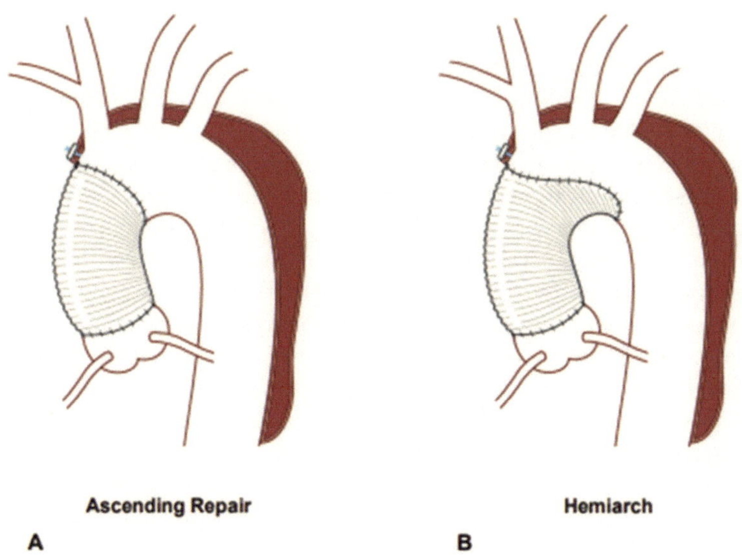

Figure 6.
Open repair and grafting of type A aortic dissections. (A) Ascending arch repair. (B) Hemiarch repair to address primary entry tears in the lower curvature of the arch.

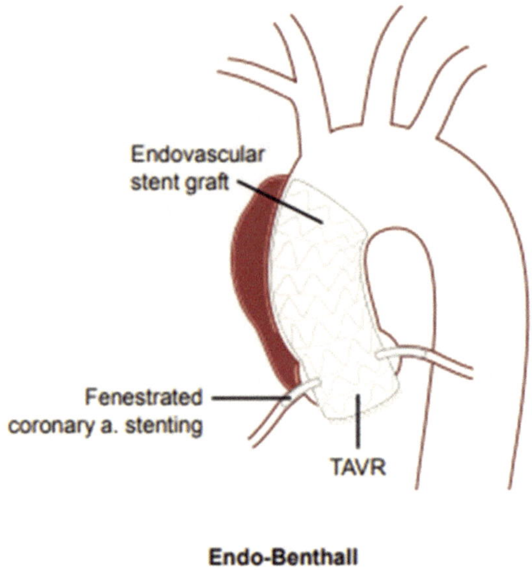

Figure 7.
Endo-Benthall procedure for endovascular aortic root repair. There is a combination of transcatheter aortic valve replacement (TAVR), endovascular stenting, and endovascular stenting of the coronary arteries.

open aortic reconstruction followed by open or endovascular mesenteric revascularization with thrombectomy or stenting [51]. A staged strategy has gained attention as a newer clinical pathway that emphasizes promptly restoring visceral perfusion before addressing the entry tear in the proximal aorta. This method, covered in a subsequent section, offers a promising alternative for managing TAAD cases complicated by mesenteric malperfusion.

5.2 TBAD with MPS

The complexity of the dissection determines the management of TBAD. According to the Society for Vascular Surgery and the Society of Thoracic Surgeons (SVS/STS), a complicated Type B aortic dissection (cTBAD) is characterized by rupture or end-organ malperfusion, while an uncomplicated Type B aortic dissection (uTBAD) does not involve these complications [52]. About 25% of TBAD cases qualify as cTBAD and about 25% of patients with uTBAD will progress to cTBAD [53, 54]. For uTBAD, medical management is generally preferred due to its association with lower mortality rates compared to open surgical repair, particularly during the acute phase [55]. However, recent evidence suggests that in addition to medical therapy, endovascular intervention with TEVAR in the acute and subacute phases can enhance long-term aortic remodeling in most AD patients [56, 57]. TEVAR can also be utilized in patients who develop complications in the chronic phase, such as aneurysmal dilation of the FL, which needs correction to prevent aortic rupture [58].

In contrast, cTBAD requires immediate intervention during the hyperacute and acute phase to correct malperfusion. Data from the Vascular Quality Initiative (VQI) has revealed that TBAD patients with MPS typically present with elevated preoperative serum creatinine levels, an ASA classification of 4 or 5, and more extensive dissection spanning from proximal aortic segments (Zones 0–2) to distal segments (Zone 9+), often involving visceral vessels (**Figure 8**) [59]. Data from the IRAD

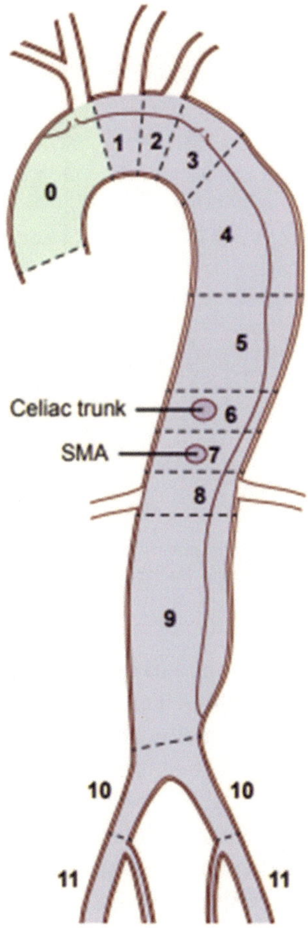

Figure 8.
The Society for Vascular Surgery/Society of Thoracic Surgeons (SVS/STS) Aortic Dissection Classification System based on the zone of the primary entry tear. The aorta is divided into 12 total sections (0–11). The location of the primary entry tear in type A aortic dissections is in zone 0. The location of the primary entry tear in type B aortic dissections is in zone 1 or thereafter.

indicate significant in-hospital mortality rates for patients undergoing open surgical repair for cTBAD with dissection septum resection [52]. Many patients may develop neurological deficits, with some suffering strokes and others developing paraplegia [60]. Key predictors of surgical mortality include advanced age and preoperative hypotension. Endovascular fenestration and branch vessel stenting offer minimally invasive alternatives to open surgery for alleviating MPS, thereby reducing the associated risks of morbidity and mortality [61]. Additionally, TEVAR can be used to optimize distal perfusion.

5.3 Fenestration

Endovascular fenestration aims to alleviate malperfusion by creating an opening in the intimal flap that allows for communication between the TL and FL, restoring branch vessel flow (**Figure 9**). This procedure equalizes pressure between the two lumens leading to quick resolution of dynamic obstructions.

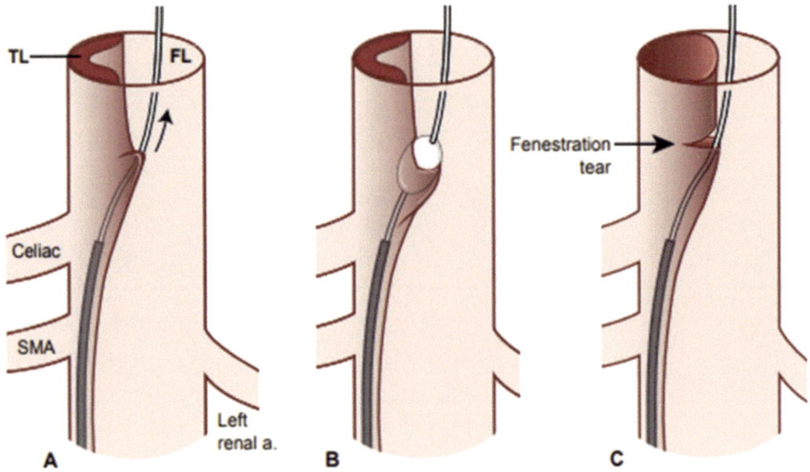

Figure 9.
Endovascular fenestration. (A) Schematic of septal puncture followed by balloon fenestration for tear formation. (B) Balloon crossing the dissection septum from true lumen (TL) to false lumen (FL). (C) Creation of an intimal tear for luminal communication.

Various methods have been developed to fenestrate the dissection septum for malperfusion correction in acute cTBAD. Traditional open surgical fenestration methods effectively eliminate malperfusion above and below the fenestration site but are poorly survivable [62]. Due to the high-risk nature of these maneuvers and advances in minimally invasive modalities, percutaneous methods for aortic fenestration have become more prevalent. The first such transfemoral technique was reported by Williams et al. in 1990. Since then, various adaptations using transseptal needle puncture, wires, and balloons have shown promising success rates [63–65].

Endovascular fenestration begins with an angiographic assessment to identify branch artery obstructions causing malperfusion. IVUS is then used to visualize the interaction of the dissection flap with branch arteries in real-time, determining the specific lumen from which each major branch originates [55]. Every action that alters aortic anatomy, like septal fenestration, can lead to hemodynamic shifts and impact the dissection flap's relationship to branch vessels. Therefore, IVUS should also be performed before and after each intervention to redefine these relationships.

Branch vessel malperfusion is confirmed by identifying a systolic pressure gradient greater than 15 mm Hg between the aortic root and the branch vessel [66]. Concurrent pressure measurements are taken in the aortic root and branch vessels of interest, such as the superior mesenteric artery, bilateral renal arteries, and bilateral external iliac arteries. In cases where the branch is involved in a dissection, pressure measurements should be taken from beyond the distal end of the dissection in the vessel. Radiographic indicators of malperfusion include failure of the branch artery to fill and diminished intensity of the vascular bed it feeds during contrast injection, IVUS detection of a 'curtain-like' occlusion at the branch vessel origin, blockage of proximal flow in the FL above the origin, or the presence of thrombosis (**Figure 5**) [55].

Often, there are natural pre-existing fenestrations in the aorta. If no pre-existing fenestrations are identified, percutaneous fenestration can be achieved by advancing a catheter through the dissection flap under fluoroscopic and IVUS guidance. The target for puncture is typically 2–4 cm above the celiac artery to create an entry tear from the TL to the FL [67]. A large diameter balloon can then be used to dilate the opening in the flap, propagating the fenestration. Importantly, this technique only requires access to the TL. In the acute phase, the dissection septum is highly pliable and can be safely and easily ruptured with a balloon. However, as the dissection becomes chronic, the septum becomes fibrotic, thickened and rubbery, meaning ballooning will not always completely open the TL unless over-ballooning is performed, which carries its own risks like aortic rupture [68]. Alternative practices to enlarge septal communications in chronic dissections, typically to create landing zones for TEVAR, use wires to cut through the septum. Although not commonly utilized in acute dissection, we will briefly review these fenestration methods.

The flossing or cheese-wire technique involves access to both the TL and FL. A snare is used to capture and guide a wire from one access point, typically the brachial artery, to another, such as the femoral artery. Alternatively, access can be obtained from the bilateral femoral arteries, resulting in femoral-femoral through-and-through wire positioning. The wire is then moved back and forth with caudal pressure across the septal fenestration, gradually tearing and enlarging it. This antegrade fenestration method can result in downstream intimal sloughing and bunching, risking occlusive filling defects and avulsion [69]. To circumnavigate these concerns, septostomy can be achieved with electrocautery attached to an insulated wire that is denuded at its contact with the septum [69, 70]. These methods offer adjunctive power to get through the noncompliant septum without the need for extra wire traction that could cause tissue trauma. Alternatively, the reverse cheese wire technique offers similar benefits without the need for electrosurgical energy. The approach involves a similar configuration to the cheese-wire technique with through-and-through wire positioning accompanied by bilateral sheaths and stiff guidewires advancing to the thoracic aorta. The stiff guidewires serve as tracks for the sheaths to be pushed cephalad rather than caudally, resulting in retrograde septostomy, lowering the risk of malperfusion by not pulling the septum across the visceral segment [71]. Successful endovascular fenestration relies on precise imaging to accurately guide the snare and wire. Key considerations for all wire-based fenestrations include securely capturing the wire without damaging surrounding tissues, selecting appropriately sized wires and sheaths to avoid vessel trauma, and ensuring the wire is stiff enough to create or enlarge the fenestration while remaining flexible for navigating the vascular anatomy.

After creating the tear, IVUS and pressure measurements are reassessed to confirm revascularization has resolved malperfusion without leading to proximal aortic TL collapse or new dynamic obstruction. Procedural success is determined by the resolution of TL collapse and significant improvement or elimination of aorto-branch-artery pressure gradients, as confirmed by IVUS, branch arteriography, and manometry.

5.4 TEVAR

Thoracic endovascular aortic repair (TEVAR) is a minimally invasive procedure that has become the preferred approach in treating a variety of thoracic aortic pathologies. Initially approved by the United States Food and Drug Administration (FDA) in 2005 for treating thoracoabdominal aortic aneurysms, TEVAR's indications have since expanded to include traumatic aortic transections, blunt aortic injuries, intramural hematomas, penetrating aortic ulcers and ADs with or without malperfusion or rupture [72]. There has also been an expanding availability of devices that are approved or under investigation to cater to various thoracic aortic anatomies [73].

These include the GORE TAG and CTAG, Zenith TX2 and Alpha, Valiant Thoracic Stent Graft System, and the Relay device.

Currently, TEVAR is the leading treatment option for cTBAD and is becoming increasingly favorable for uTBAD [57]. In acute cTBAD, TEVAR should be considered for those with life-threatening complications such as impending rupture or visceral or extremity malperfusion, having demonstrated excellent short- and long-term outcomes. A study following patients who required TEVAR for cTBAD reported no deaths attributable to aortic pathology over a seven-year follow-up period [47]. However, emergent TEVAR can result in serious complications, including AKI requiring dialysis or SCI [46].

Thoracic endovascular aortic repair (TEVAR) works by covering the entry tear with a stent graft to seal proximal flow to the FL, simultaneously depressurizing the FL, and re-expanding the TL, and (**Figure 10**). This mechanical support resolves distal dynamic obstruction by stabilizing the dissection flap. Expanding the TL and covering the entry tear markedly improves flow in the TL and branch vessels [74]. If FL pressurization persists, continued blood flow through the FL can lead to aneurysmal dilation [61]. TEVAR creates an optimal environment for FL thrombosis by excluding flow from systemic circulation, facilitating positive aortic remodeling [75, 76]. Ensuring the stent is properly placed entirely within the TL, without obstructing the visceral artery origins, is essential to prevent ischemic complications.

Among the most common long-term postoperative complications of TEVAR is continued flow into the FL [61]. This complication, termed endoleak, is classified by the presence and location of flow. The endoleak classification system after a TEVAR for AD differs from that used in TEVARs for aneurysms. Uniquely, AD repair can be complicated by type R endoleaks, which is retrograde FL flow from distal fenestrations fed by the TL [52]. If this complication persists, it can lead to dilation of the FL leading to aneurysm formation and potential rupture, which is why TEVAR is often used along fenestration [77].

5.4.1 Technique

Performing TEVAR in cTBAD involves several considerations to minimize perioperative morbidity and mortality. An algorithmic approach emphasizes wire access to the TL, coverage of the primary tear site, and assessment of any ongoing malperfusion or rupture that may require supplementary interventions. This methodology has yielded high technical success, as defined by coverage of the primary entry tear to seal the FL. It has also been associated with favorable perioperative risk when compared to open surgery [46].

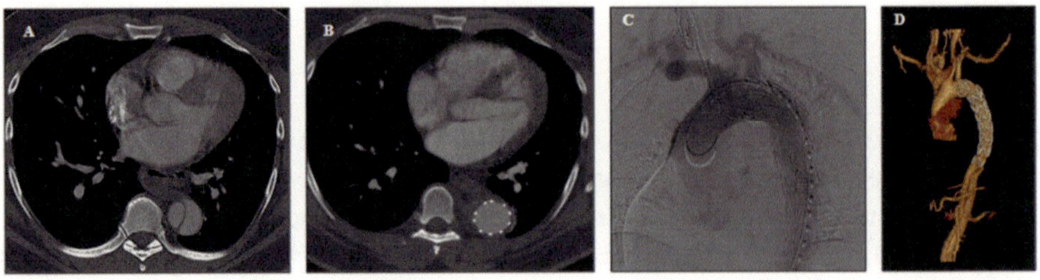

Figure 10.
TBAD repair. (A and B) Axial CTA images of aortic dissection. (A) False lumen in the descending thoracic aorta, where the contrast-filled true lumen is compressed. (B) Re-expansion of the true lumen and exclusion of the false lumen after endograft. (C) Fluoroscopy after TEVAR. (D) CT reconstruction after TEVAR.

The procedure typically begins with gaining femoral access on the side not affected by the dissection or with the best access to the TL. The access will need to accommodate a delivery sheath of 20–24F. IVUS is used to guide and confirm wire access into the TL. A proximal landing zone of 2 cm of healthy aortic tissue proximal to the entry tear is required. Since the entry tear is often near the left subclavian artery, the stent graft may need to cover this vessel, which is generally well tolerated but can cause upper extremity ischemia in some cases [78].

The stentgraft can be up-sized by 10% of the aortic diameter to secure an adequate circumferential seal with aortic wall apposition. Ballooning especially at the proximal end should be avoided in the acute and hyperacute phase to prevent retrograde dissection, since the aortic wall is acutely vulnerable, inflamed, and friable [79]. Selecting the appropriate stent graft is also important, as covered stents have been associated with a lower incidence of retrograde dissection compared to proximal bare metal stents (BMS) [59].

The extent of TEVAR coverage in TBAD often correlates with the initial presentation and may vary among institutions. For cTBAD, grafts are generally deployed from the left subclavian to the celiac artery. Extensive graft coverage has been evidenced to improve aortic remodeling through mechanical reinforcement, reducing the progression of aortic disease and aortic-specific mortality, such as FL dilation or stent-induced new entry requiring re-interventions [57, 80]. However, SCI is commonly associated with long covered grafts in the thoracic aorta, especially with coverage of the LSA, intercostal vessels, and distal extension [81, 82]. Consequently, the imperative arose to create a device that would seal the entry tear proximally and decompress the FL distally, while preserving perfusion to branch vessels.

5.4.2 PETTICOAT and STABILIZE

The Provisional Extension to Induce Complete Attachment Technique (PETTICOAT) was introduced in 2006 by Nienaber and colleagues to improve aortic remodeling, particularly in cases with large distal re-entry points where the FL is less likely to thrombose after proximal stent graft placement [83]. PETTICOAT involves deploying a BMS in the distal thoracoabdominal segment, in conjunction with the proximal covered thoracic aorta stent graft from TEVAR (**Figure 11**). This will provide the intraluminal support to compress the FL and promote thrombosis in the delaminated aortic segments where the covered stent graft does not extend to, while maintaining perfusing through its bare metal design to the visceral arteries. A modern device approved by the FDA in 2018 for PETTICOAT is the Zenith Endovascular Dissection System (Cook Medical). This includes the proximal covered Zenith TX2 dissection endovascular stent graft with pro-form and the distal uncovered Zenith dissection endovascular stent.

The distal extent of the BMS is determined by the extent of the dissection [83]. The proximal portion of the BMS is deployed within the covered stent graft to act as a scaffold, with subsequent BMSs overlapping the previous ones. To avoid complications in the friable aorta during acute dissection, balloon angioplasty is not used to oversize the stents. If static obstruction persists despite distal BMS placement, the bare metal design allows for additional stent placement in obstructed branch vessels [84]. In extended-PETTICOAT, distal placement of BMS past the visceral branches can be performed to enhance TL expansion and maximize perfusion to the bilateral iliac arteries, providing a more comprehensive solution to persistent lower extremity malperfusion. PETTICOAT has proven effective in increasing TL size, decreasing malperfusion-related mortality within 30 days of presentation, and stabilizing or

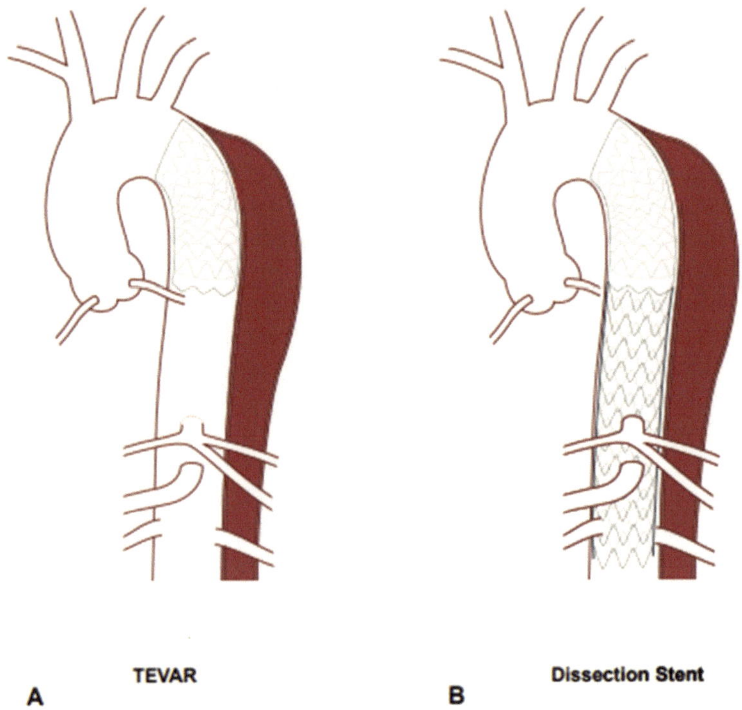

Figure 11.
Endovascular repair and endografting of type B aortic dissections. (A) TEVAR of the descending aorta. (B) PETTIOCAT stentgraft configuration with TEVAR proximally and uncovered stent distally.

reducing transaortic diameter. However, long-term follow-up (>5 years) indicates that the stent graft and BMS configuration may not protect against chronic aneurysmal degeneration, highlighting the need for lifelong surveillance [85, 86].

A variation of PETTICOAT, a technique known as stent-associated balloon-induced intimal disruption and re-lamination in AD repair (STABILIZE), may reduce the risk of malperfusion and lower the rate of reintervention [87]. STABILIZE involves ballooning the TL inside the deployed stent graft, allowing the distally deployed bare stents to intentionally rupture the septum, leading to full expansion of the stent in a single-channeled aorta. Criteria for the highest success rates with STABILIZE include a non-dissected landing zone in the descending or abdominal aorta, a total aortic diameter not exceeding 40 mm, and a distal stent graft overlapping the proximal component by more than 5 cm [88, 89].

5.5 Branch vessel stenting

Adjunctive branch vessel treatment during or after TEVAR can include target vessel stenting. Target branches commonly include the celiac, superior mesenteric, renal, and iliac arteries (**Figure 12**). After TEVAR, an angiogram is performed to assess the expansion of the TL and downstream perfusion. While TEVAR often resolves malperfusion caused by dynamic obstructions, static obstructions—where the dissection extends beyond the visceral artery ostium—may persist, leading to ongoing obstruction or thrombosis [75, 90]. It has been reported that up to 41% of patients undergoing TEVAR require branch vessel stenting, with resolution of ischemia in 93% [91].

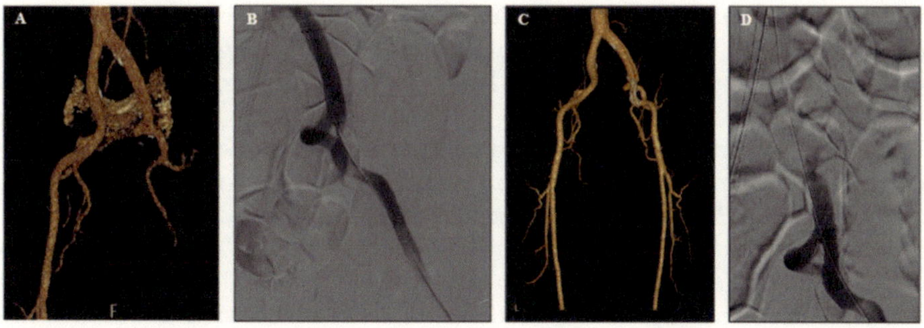

Figure 12.
Left external iliac artery (LEI) with no flow shown in (A) reconstructed CT and (B) angiography. LEI revascularization with endograft shown in (C) reconstructed CT and (D) angiography.

The placement of a covered or uncovered self-expandable stent in a side branch or iliac artery under fluoroscopy can improve flow when dynamic or static obstruction relief is inadequate from TEVAR alone (**Figure 13**). The stent is deployed at the orifice, followed by balloon angioplasty without oversizing. If there is significant static obstruction with thrombus, percutaneous suction thrombectomy can be performed

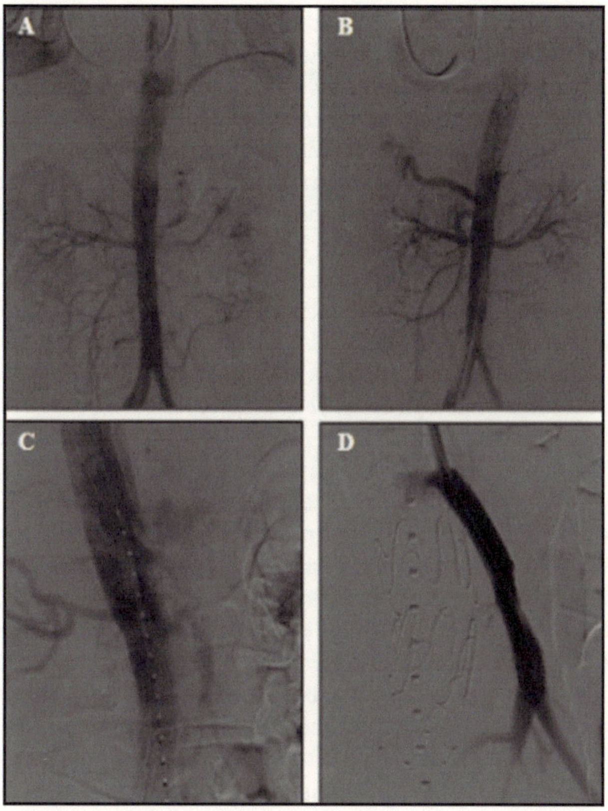

Figure 13.
CTA of insufficient alleviation of distal obstruction after TEVAR. (A) Diminished signal intensity of the left renal artery. (B) Placement of one renal stent with revascularization. (C) Diminished signal intensity of the superior mesenteric artery. (D) Superior mesenteric artery perfusion with stenting.

with the Penumbra aspiration system (Indigo Catheter CAT6 or CAT8; Penumbra, Alameda, CA, USA), although this is rarely needed [56]. An angiogram is then used to confirm flow into the branch vessels. IVUS can also be used to verify branch vessel patency [66, 67, 92].

A retrospective analysis of the VQI found that the left renal and superior mesenteric arteries were targeted the most in patients requiring branch intervention after TEVAR for acute cTBAD [93]. This is likely because ADs commonly begin with an entry tear at the greater curvature of the arch and spiral down the aorta to propagate into the left renal artery. Although these patients were subjected to increased length of procedure with more complex techniques, they did not exhibit significant differences in outcomes when compared to TEVAR patients who had not undergone adjunctive treatment. Rates of 30-day mortality, in-hospital postoperative complications such as MI, transient ischemic attack, stroke, renal or intestinal ischemia, and SCI were not significantly different. There was also no difference in overall survival at 3 years [93]. These findings highlight that branch interventions are safe and should be integrated into the treatment strategy for acute TBAD complicated by end-organ malperfusion.

6. Staged repair for TAAD: Optimizing organ perfusion through timely intervention

The conventional surgical method for addressing TAAD entails cardiopulmonary bypass and deep hypothermic circulatory arrest. These operations are physiologically stressful and poorly tolerated in patients with hemodynamic compromise and organ ischemia. Additionally, patients often present with comorbidities like hypertension, hyperlipidemia, and smoking, which further elevate mortality risks [94]. The surgeon replaces the ascending aorta with Dacron graft then the intima is meticulously re-approximated to the remaining wall to restore structural integrity and restore TL flow. However, in cases where there is significant bowel ischemia, spending extended periods of time repairing the ascending aorta may result in necrosis of the bowel. In addition, the repair of the ascending aorta does not, in every case, result in reperfusion of the bowel depending on the nature of the dissection flap as well as the anatomy of malperfusion.

Accordingly, a staged methodology has been proposed to address malperfusion secondary to aortic pathologies. In cases of extensive aortic disease or multiple comorbidities, a two-step repair may be required, allowing gradual healing and reducing strain during recovery [95]. Commonly known as the TEVAR-first, endovascular-first, and revascularization-first strategy, staged repair can be employed in cases of TAAD with distal malperfusion. In these cases, central aortic repair is delayed slightly and TEVAR is performed first to mechanically expand the thoracic aortic TL and restore distal flow and resolve MPS. Branch vessel stenting may also be necessary in this setting. The patients are then closely monitored and proceed to definitive open repair immediately after MPS resolution or if there is a change in clinical state. The TEVAR-first model protects the ischemic bowel by restoring blood flow to the visceral segment of the aorta thereby correcting acidosis before subjecting the body to circulatory arrest for definitive central repair [96, 97]. This approach can reduce operative mortality to 15%, compared to up to 35% in single-stage repairs [96]. This protocol also helps avoid otherwise unnecessary open repair when organ damage is irreversible and organ failure is present, reducing healthcare spending, improving resource allocation, and preserving quality of life [30]. It is important to note that the repair of the ascending AD should not be delayed significantly as this increases mortality.

Recent studies suggest that patients with mesenteric malperfusion secondary to TAAD have improved survival rates when malperfusion is addressed endovascularly before open central aortic repair, provided the patient's clinical presentation allows for such a delay. Patients fit for this methodology are those who are hemodynamically stable and without cardiac tamponade, aortic valve insufficiency, or coronary artery malperfusion [30, 55, 98]. Approximately 3.7–14% of acute TAAD patients present with mesenteric MPS, which has a mortality rate of 38–75% [3, 51, 97, 99]. Leshnower et al. found that ascending aorta and aortic arch replacement followed by laparotomy resulted in a 69.2% mortality rate. In contrast, the TEVAR-first strategy reduced mortality to 30% [97].

7. Hybrid repair for TAAD

Given the varying clinical presentations of ADs and the availability of multiple management strategies, repair often becomes complex, necessitating a combination of both endovascular and open strategies. Hybrid methods, utilizing both endovascular and open repair, are now recommended in the latest guidelines for treating TAAD with distal malperfusion [96]. In hybrid repair, both open and endovascular surgical strategies are performed during the same surgical session. Open intervention addresses the acute pathology and resects the intimal entry tear. Concomitant or subsequent distal endovascular aortic stenting resolves distal dynamic malperfusion and reinforces the aortic wall to decrease the risk of aneurysmal degeneration. During the second stage of the repair, percutaneous vascular access is already established for supplementary branch vessel stenting or suction thrombectomy if necessary. This hybrid approach not only addresses the immediate life-threatening aspects of AD but also offers a strategic advantage in managing the long-term risks associated with untreated portions of the aorta via immediate stabilization of the descending aorta creating favorable conditions for FL thrombosis.

The Frozen Elephant Trunk (FET) procedure is a prime example of hybrid repair. The open portion of the surgery, typically involving repair of the ascending aorta and, if necessary, the aortic arch with reimplantation of the great vessels or bypass grafting, is completed first and then a stentgraft is placed to expand the TL of the descending aorta. The Thoraflex graft is a specialized hybrid device that combines a traditional standard graft with an attached endovascular stent graft. The proximal portion, made of synthetic material like Dacron, replaces the diseased aortic arch and is sutured to the healthy aorta, restoring structural integrity. The distal portion consists of a self-expanding stent graft which is deployed into the descending thoracic aortic TL [100, 101].

The utility of hybrid repair can be easily appreciated in particular aortic pathologies. If the entry tear is in Zone 2, that is between the left common carotid artery and the left subclavian artery, hybrid repair could facilitate ascending aorta and Zone 2 arch replacement followed by retrograde TEVAR. Dracon graft replaces the entire aortic arch. The graft is designed with a single branch from the superior arch that divides into three branches for the great vessels. The arch is repaired by anastomosis to the proximal aorta in Zone 2 to minimize the risk of entrapment to the recurrent laryngeal nerve [102]. Following this, a retrograde stent is deployed, which involves placing the stent against the erection of blood flow. The retrograde deployment allows precise control over catheter navigation and stent placement, allowing for optimal alignment and reducing the risk of malposition or torsion. Combined surgical repair of the ascending aorta and transluminal stent grafting into the descending aorta has shown to achieve partial FL thrombosis, potentially minimizing the risk of further dilatation or rupture [102].

8. Conclusion

The management of MPS in acute AD has evolved with the development of endovascular strategies, offering a less invasive yet effective alternative to traditional open surgery. Clinical experience highlights the importance of understanding the underlying mechanisms of malperfusion to guide treatment choice. Techniques such as TEVAR, endovascular fenestration, and branch vessel stenting have demonstrated success in restoring perfusion and improving patient outcomes. The use of staged and hybrid repair strategies underscores the importance of utilizing various combinations of endovascular interventions to address this complex pathology. As endovascular technology continues to advance, the integration of these approaches into clinical practice promises to enhance the management of MPS in AD.

Acknowledgements

The authors would like to thank Jennifer Brumbaugh for her contribution in creating **Figures 1–4, 6–9,** and **11** for this manuscript. Publication made possible in part by support from the Thomas Jefferson University Open Access Fund.

Conflict of interest

The authors declare no conflict of interest.

Author details

Nicola Habash[1*], Jin Park[2], Natalie Lukasik[3] and Babak Abai[4]

1 Sidney Kimmel Medical College, Thomas Jefferson University, Philadelphia, PA, USA

2 Philadelphia College of Osteopathic Medicine, Philadelphia, PA, USA

3 Mercy Catholic Medical Center, Darby, PA, USA

4 Department of Surgery, Division of Vascular and Endovascular Surgery, Thomas Jefferson University Hospital, Philadelphia, PA, USA

*Address all correspondence to: nmh022@students.jefferson.edu

References

[1] Baliyan V, Parakh A, Prabhakar AM, Hedgire S. Acute aortic syndromes and aortic emergencies. Cardiovascular Diagnosis and Therapy. 2018;**8**(Suppl. 1): S82-S96

[2] Levy D, Goyal A, Grigorova Y, Farci F, Le JK. Aortic dissection. In: StatPearls. Treasure Island (FL): StatPearls Publishing; 2024

[3] Evangelista A, Isselbacher EM, Bossone E, Gleason TG, Eusanio MD, Sechtem U, et al. Insights from the international registry of acute aortic dissection: A 20-year experience of collaborative clinical research. Circulation. 2018;**137**(17):1846-1860

[4] Suzuki T, Mehta RH, Ince H, Nagai R, Sakomura Y, Weber F, et al. Clinical profiles and outcomes of acute type B aortic dissection in the current era: Lessons from the international registry of aortic dissection (IRAD). Circulation. 2003;**108**(Suppl. 1):II312-II317

[5] Crawford TC, Beaulieu RJ, Ehlert BA, Ratchford EV, Black JH. Malperfusion syndromes in aortic dissections. Vascular Medicine. 2016;**21**(3):264-273

[6] Black JH, Cambria RP. Aortic dissection: Perspectives for the vascular/endovascular surgeon. In: Rutherford's Textbook of Vascular Surgery. Philadelphia, PA: Elsevier Health Sciences; 2005

[7] Williams DM, Lee DY, Hamilton BH, Marx MV, Narasimham DL, Kazanjian SN, et al. The dissected aorta: Part III. Anatomy and radiologic diagnosis of branch-vessel compromise. Radiology. 1997;**203**(1):37-44

[8] Kazakidi A, Sherwin SJ, Weinberg PD. Effect of Reynolds number and flow division on patterns of haemodynamic wall shear stress near branch points in the descending thoracic aorta. Journal of the Royal Society Interface. 2009;**6**(35):539-548

[9] Moretti S, Tauro F, Orrico M, Mangialardi N, Facci AL. Comparative analysis of patient-specific aortic dissections through computational fluid dynamics suggests increased likelihood of degeneration in partially thrombosed false lumen. Bioengineering (Basel). 2023;**10**(3):316

[10] Chung JW, Elkins C, Sakai T, Kato N, Vestring T, Semba CP, et al. True-lumen collapse in aortic dissection: Part II. Evaluation of treatment methods in phantoms with pulsatile flow. Radiology. 2000;**214**(1):99-106

[11] Rawat DS, Pourquie M, Poelma C. Numerical investigation of turbulence in abdominal aortic aneurysms. Journal of Biomechanical Engineering. 2019;**141**(6):061001

[12] Kushner A, West WP, Khan Suheb MZ, Pillarisetty LS. Virchow triad. In: StatPearls. Treasure Island (FL): StatPearls Publishing; 2024

[13] Gaxotte V, Cocheteux B, Haulon S, Vincentelli A, Lions C, Koussa M, et al. Relationship of intimal flap position to endovascular treatment of malperfusion syndromes in aortic dissection. Journal of Endovascular Therapy. 2003;**10**(4):719-727

[14] Nagamine H, Ueno Y, Ueda H, Saito D, Tanaka N, Miyazaki M, et al. A new classification system for branch artery perfusion patterns in acute aortic dissection for examining the effects of central aortic repair. European

Journal of Cardio-Thoracic Surgery. 2013;**44**(1):146-153

[15] Hagan PG, Nienaber CA, Isselbacher EM, Bruckman D, Karavite DJ, Russman PL, et al. The international registry of acute aortic dissection (IRAD): New insights into an old disease. JAMA. 2000;**283**(7):897-903

[16] Pinsky MR. Functional hemodynamic monitoring. Critical Care Clinics. 2015;**31**(1):89-111

[17] Andersen LW, Mackenhauer J, Roberts JC, Berg KM, Cocchi MN, Donnino MW. Etiology and therapeutic approach to elevated lactate levels. Mayo Clinic Proceedings. 2013;**88**(10):1127-1140

[18] Moore AG, Eagle KA, Bruckman D, Moon BS, Malouf JF, Fattori R, et al. Choice of computed tomography, transesophageal echocardiography, magnetic resonance imaging, and aortography in acute aortic dissection: International registry of acute aortic dissection (IRAD). The American Journal of Cardiology. 2002;**89**(10):1235-1238

[19] Alagoz M, Ikeno Y, Tanaka A, Estrera AL, Afifi RO. Intraoperative antegrade intravascular ultrasound examination in acute type A aortic dissection with suspected visceral malperfusion. JTCVS Techniques. 2021;**10**:183-187

[20] Evangelista A, Maldonado G, Gruosso D, Gutiérrez L, Granato C, Villalva N, et al. The current role of echocardiography in acute aortic syndrome. Echo Research and Practice. 2019;**6**(2):R53-R63

[21] Black JH, Cambria RP. Perspectives for the vascular/endovascular surgeon. In: Rutherford RB, editor. Vascular Surgery. 6th ed. Philadelphia, PA: Elsevier Health Sciences; 2005. pp. 1512-1533

[22] van Bakel PAJ, Henry M, Kim KM, Yang B, van Herwaarden JA, Alberto Figueroa C, et al. Imaging features of renal malperfusion in aortic dissection. European Journal of Cardio-Thoracic Surgery. 2022;**61**(4):805-813

[23] Fann JI, Sarris GE, Mitchell RS, Shumway NE, Stinson EB, Oyer PE, et al. Treatment of patients with aortic dissection presenting with peripheral vascular complications. Annals of Surgery. 1990;**212**(6):705-713

[24] Miller JS. Evaluating aortic dissection: When is coronary angiography indicated? Heart. 2000;**83**(6):615-616

[25] Girdauskas E, Kuntze T, Borger MA, Falk V, Mohr F-W. Surgical risk of preoperative malperfusion in acute type A aortic dissection. The Journal of Thoracic and Cardiovascular Surgery. 2009;**138**(6):1363-1369

[26] Goldberg JB, Lansman SL, Kai M, Tang GHL, Malekan R, Spielvogel D. Malperfusion in type A dissection: Consider reperfusion first. Seminars in Thoracic and Cardiovascular Surgery. 2017;**29**(2):181-185

[27] Saito Y, Hashimoto O, Nakayama T, Sasaki H, Yumoto K, Oshima S, et al. Right versus left coronary artery involvement in patients with type A acute aortic dissection. International Journal of Cardiology. 2023;**371**:49-53

[28] Imoto K, Uchida K, Karube N, Yasutsune T, Cho T, Kimura K, et al. Risk analysis and improvement of strategies in patients who have acute type A aortic dissection with coronary artery dissection. European

Journal of Cardio-Thoracic Surgery. 2013;**44**(3):419-424; discussion 424

[29] Kawahito K, Adachi H, Murata S, Yamaguchi A, Ino T. Coronary malperfusion due to type A aortic dissection: Mechanism and surgical management. The Annals of Thoracic Surgery. 2003;**76**(5):1471-1476; discussion 1476

[30] Yang B, Rosati CM, Norton EL, Kim KM, Khaja MS, Dasika N, et al. Endovascular fenestration/stenting first followed by delayed open aortic repair for acute type A aortic dissection with malperfusion syndrome. Circulation. 2018;**138**(19):2091-2103

[31] Bentall H, De Bono A. A technique for complete replacement of the ascending aorta. Thorax. 1968;**23**(4):338-339

[32] Benke K, Ágg B, Szabó L, Szilveszter B, Odler B, Pólos M, et al. Bentall procedure: Quarter century of clinical experiences of a single surgeon. Journal of Cardiothoracic Surgery. 2016;**11**:19

[33] Gelsomino S, Morocutti G, Frassani R, Masullo G, Da Col P, Spedicato L, et al. Long-term results of Bentall composite aortic root replacement for ascending aortic aneurysms and dissections. Chest. 2003;**124**(3):984-988

[34] Al-Mudhaffar SS, Alwan A, Ouj R, Mowaffaq A, Kakamad FH, Ahmad OF, et al. Bentall procedure as a lifesaving surgery: A single center experience. Medicine International (Lond). 2023;**3**(1):8

[35] Orihashi K. Cerebral malperfusion in acute aortic dissection. Surgery Today. 2016;**46**(12):1353-1361

[36] Tsukube T, Hayashi T, Kawahira T, Haraguchi T, Matsukawa R, Kozawa S, et al. Neurological outcomes after immediate aortic repair for acute type A aortic dissection complicated by coma. Circulation. 2011;**124**(Suppl. 11):S163-S167

[37] Sasaki H, Harada T, Ishitoya H, Sasaki O. Aorto-carotid bypass for type A acute aortic dissection complicated with carotid artery occlusion: No touch until circulatory arrest. Interactive Cardiovascular and Thoracic Surgery. 2020;**31**(2):263-265

[38] Sugiyama K, Watanuki H, Futamura Y, Okada M, Oiwa T, Makino S, et al. Impact of direct carotid artery perfusion in acute type A aortic dissection involving the common carotid artery. General Thoracic and Cardiovascular Surgery. 2021;**69**(11):1467-1475

[39] Matsen SL, Chang DC, Perler BA, Roseborough GS, Williams GM. Trends in the in-hospital stroke rate following carotid endarterectomy in California and Maryland. Journal of Vascular Surgery. 2006;**44**(3):488-495

[40] Geirsson A, Szeto WY, Pochettino A, McGarvey ML, Keane MG, Woo YJ, et al. Significance of malperfusion syndromes prior to contemporary surgical repair for acute type A dissection: Outcomes and need for additional revascularizations. European Journal of Cardio-Thoracic Surgery. 2007;**32**(2):255-262

[41] Shimamoto T, Komiya T. Clinical dilemma in the surgical treatment of organ malperfusion caused by acute type A aortic dissection. General Thoracic and Cardiovascular Surgery. 2014;**62**(7):398-406

[42] Chiu P, Tsou S, Goldstone AB, Louie M, Woo YJ, Fischbein MP.

Immediate operation for acute type A aortic dissection complicated by visceral or peripheral malperfusion. The Journal of Thoracic and Cardiovascular Surgery. 2018;**156**(1):18-24.e3

[43] Yagdi T, Atay Y, Engin C, Mahmudov R, Tetik O, Iyem H, et al. Impact of organ malperfusion on mortality and morbidity in acute type A aortic dissections. Journal of Cardiac Surgery. 2006;**21**(4):363-369

[44] Gargiulo M, Bianchini Massoni C, Gallitto E, Freyrie A, Trimarchi S, Faggioli G, et al. Lower limb malperfusion in type B aortic dissection: A systematic review. Annals of Cardiothoracic Surgery. 2014;**3**(4):351-367

[45] Sandhu HK, Charlton-Ouw KM, Jeffress K, Leake S, Perlick A, Miller CC, et al. Risk of mortality after resolution of spinal malperfusion in acute dissection. The Annals of Thoracic Surgery. 2018;**106**(2):473-481

[46] Szeto WY, McGarvey M, Pochettino A, Moser GW, Hoboken A, Cornelius K, et al. Results of a new surgical paradigm: Endovascular repair for acute complicated type B aortic dissection. The Annals of Thoracic Surgery. 2008;**86**(1):87-93; discussion 93

[47] Hanna JM, Andersen ND, Ganapathi AM, McCann RL, Hughes GC. Five-year results for endovascular repair of acute complicated type B aortic dissection. Journal of Vascular Surgery. 2014;**59**(1):96-106

[48] Jubouri M, Patel R, Tan SZ, Al-Tawil M, Bashir M, Bailey DM, et al. Fate and consequences of the false lumen after thoracic endovascular aortic repair in type B aortic dissection. Annals of Vascular Surgery. 2023;**94**:32-37

[49] Kavanagh EP, Sultan S, Jordan F, et al. Hybrid repair versus conventional open repair for aortic arch dissection. Cochrane Database of Systematic Reviews. 2021;7(7):CD012920

[50] Ghoreishi M, Chahal D, Shah A, Kang J, Hirsch J, Tran D, et al. First-in-human endovascular aortic root repair (Endo-Bentall) for acute type A dissection. Circulation: Cardiovascular Interventions. 2023;**16**(10):e013348

[51] Leshnower BG, Veeraswamy RK, Duwayri YM, Chen EP. The "TEVAR-first" approach to DeBakey I aortic dissection with mesenteric malperfusion. The Annals of Thoracic Surgery. 2014;**97**(2):693-696

[52] Lombardi JV, Hughes GC, Appoo JJ, Bavaria JE, Beck AW, Cambria RP, et al. Society for Vascular Surgery (SVS) and Society of Thoracic Surgeons (STS) reporting standards for type B aortic dissections. Journal of Vascular Surgery. 2020;**71**(3):723-747

[53] Cooper M, Hicks C, Ratchford EV, Salameh MJ, Malas M. Diagnosis and treatment of uncomplicated type B aortic dissection. Vascular Medicine. 2016;**21**(6):547-552

[54] Krebs JR, Filiberto AC, Fazzone B, Jacobs CR, Anderson EM, Shahid Z, et al. Outcomes of patients with acute type B aortic dissection and high-risk features. Annals of Vascular Surgery. 2024;**106**:99-107

[55] DiMusto PD, Williams DM, Patel HJ, Trimarchi S, Eliason JL, Upchurch GR. Endovascular management of type B aortic dissections. Journal of Vascular Surgery. 2010;**52**(Suppl. 4):26S-36S

[56] Grewal S, Contrella BN, Sherk WM, Khaja MS, Williams DM. Endovascular

management of malperfusion syndromes in aortic dissection. Techniques in Vascular and Interventional Radiology. 2021;**24**(2):100751

[57] Nienaber CA, Kische S, Rousseau H, Eggebrecht H, Rehders TC, Kundt G, et al. Endovascular repair of type B aortic dissection: Long-term results of the randomized investigation of stent grafts in aortic dissection trial. Circulation: Cardiovascular Interventions. 2013;**6**(4):407-416

[58] Wheat MW. Acute dissection of the aorta. Cardiovascular Clinics. 1987;**17**(3):241-262

[59] Wang GJ, Jackson BM, Damrauer SM, Kalapatapu V, Glaser J, Golden MA, et al. Unique characteristics of the type B aortic dissection patients with malperfusion in the vascular quality initiative. Journal of Vascular Surgery. 2021;**74**(1):53-62

[60] Trimarchi S, Nienaber CA, Rampoldi V, Myrmel T, Suzuki T, Bossone E, et al. Role and results of surgery in acute type B aortic dissection: Insights from the international registry of acute aortic dissection (IRAD). Circulation. 2006;**114**(Suppl. 1):I357-I364

[61] Erbel R, Oelert H, Meyer J, Puth M, Mohr-Katoly S, Hausmann D, et al. Effect of medical and surgical therapy on aortic dissection evaluated by transesophageal echocardiography. Implications for prognosis and therapy. The European cooperative study group on echocardiography. Circulation. 1993;**87**(5):1604-1615

[62] Tsai TT, Trimarchi S, Nienaber CA. Acute aortic dissection: Perspectives from the international registry of acute aortic dissection (IRAD). European Journal of Vascular and Endovascular Surgery. 2009;**37**(2):149-159

[63] Williams DM, Brothers TE, Messina LM. Relief of mesenteric ischemia in type III aortic dissection with percutaneous fenestration of the aortic septum. Radiology. 1990;**174**(2):450-452

[64] Slonim SM, Nyman U, Semba CP, Miller DC, Mitchell RS, Dake MD. Aortic dissection: Percutaneous management of ischemic complications with endovascular stents and balloon fenestration. Journal of Vascular Surgery. 1996;**23**(2):241-251; discussion 251

[65] Chavan A, Hausmann D, Dresler C, Rosenthal H, Jaeger K, Haverich A, et al. Intravascular ultrasound-guided percutaneous fenestration of the intimal flap in the dissected aorta. Circulation. 1997;**96**(7):2124-2127

[66] Williams DM, Lee DY, Hamilton BH, Marx MV, Narasimham DL, Kazanjian SN, et al. The dissected aorta: Percutaneous treatment of ischemic complications--Principles and results. Journal of Vascular and Interventional Radiology. 1997;**8**(4):605-625

[67] Norton EL, Williams DM, Kim KM, Khaja MS, Wu X, Patel HJ, et al. Management of acute type B aortic dissection with malperfusion via endovascular fenestration/stenting. The Journal of Thoracic and Cardiovascular Surgery. 2020;**160**(5):1151-1161.e1

[68] Sherifova S, Holzapfel GA. Biomechanics of aortic wall failure with a focus on dissection and aneurysm: A review. Acta Biomaterialia. 2019;**99**:1-17

[69] Tanenbaum MT, Figueroa AV, Lee KB, Costa Filho JE, Gonzalez MS, Baig MS, et al. Early results of transcatheter electrosurgical aortic septotomy for endovascular repair of chronic dissecting aortoiliac aneurysms. Journal of Vascular Surgery

Cases and Innovative Techniques. 2024;**10**(3):101467

[70] Kabbani L, Judith Lin ME, McLaughlin D, Bendix S. A novel way to fenestrate a type B dissection flap using endovascular electrocautery. Journal of Vascular Surgery. 2019;**70**(3):e71-e72

[71] Stern JR, Pham X-BD, Lee JT. Reverse cheese-wire septotomy to create a distal landing zone for thoracic endovascular aortic repair. Journal of Endovascular Therapy. 2023;**30**(1):38-44

[72] Nation DA, Wang GJ. TEVAR: Endovascular repair of the thoracic aorta. Seminars in Interventional Radiology. 2015;**32**(3):265-271

[73] Kiguchi M, Chaer RA. Endovascular repair of thoracic aortic pathology. Expert Review of Medical Devices. 2011;**8**(4):515-525

[74] Huptas S, Mehta RH, Kühl H, Tsagakis K, Reinsch N, Kahlert P, et al. Aortic remodeling in type B aortic dissection: Effects of endovascular stent-graft repair and medical treatment on true and false lumen volumes. Journal of Endovascular Therapy. 2009;**16**(1):28-38

[75] Dake MD, Kato N, Mitchell RS, Semba CP, Razavi MK, Shimono T, et al. Endovascular stent-graft placement for the treatment of acute aortic dissection. The New England Journal of Medicine. 1999;**340**(20):1546-1552

[76] Leshnower BG, Duwayri YM, Chen EP, Li C, Zehner CA, Binongo JN, et al. Aortic remodeling after endovascular repair of complicated acute type B aortic dissection. The Annals of Thoracic Surgery. 2017;**103**(6):1878-1885

[77] Beregi J-P, Haulon S, Otal P, Thony F, Bartoli J-M, Crochet D, et al. Endovascular treatment of acute complications associated with aortic dissection: Midterm results from a multicenter study. Journal of Endovascular Therapy. 2003;**10**(3):486-493

[78] Riesenman PJ, Farber MA, Mendes RR, Marston WA, Fulton JJ, Keagy BA. Coverage of the left subclavian artery during thoracic endovascular aortic repair. Journal of Vascular Surgery. 2007;**45**(1):90-94; discussion 94

[79] Canaud L, Ozdemir BA, Patterson BO, Holt PJE, Loftus IM, Thompson MM. Retrograde aortic dissection after thoracic endovascular aortic repair. Annals of Surgery. 2014;**260**(2):389-395

[80] Davies RR, Gallo A, Coady MA, Tellides G, Botta DM, Burke B, et al. Novel measurement of relative aortic size predicts rupture of thoracic aortic aneurysms. The Annals of Thoracic Surgery. 2006;**81**(1):169-177

[81] Uchida N. How to prevent spinal cord injury during endovascular repair of thoracic aortic disease. General Thoracic and Cardiovascular Surgery. 2014;**62**(7):391-397

[82] Drinkwater SL, Goebells A, Haydar A, Bourke P, Brown L, Hamady M, et al. The incidence of spinal cord ischaemia following thoracic and thoracoabdominal aortic endovascular intervention. European Journal of Vascular and Endovascular Surgery. 2010;**40**(6):729-735

[83] Nienaber CA, Kische S, Zeller T, Rehders TC, Schneider H, Lorenzen B, et al. Provisional extension to induce complete attachment after stent-graft placement in type B aortic dissection: The PETTICOAT concept.

Journal of Endovascular Therapy. 2006;**13**(6):738-746

[84] Kazimierczak A, Rynio P, Jędrzejczak T, Samad R, Rybicka A, Gutowski P. Aortic remodeling after extended PETTICOAT technique in acute aortic dissection type III B. Annals of Vascular Surgery. 2020;**66**:183-192

[85] Lombardi JV, Cambria RP, Nienaber CA, Chiesa R, Mossop P, Haulon S, et al. Five-year results from the study of thoracic aortic type B dissection using endoluminal repair (STABLE I) study of endovascular treatment of complicated type B aortic dissection using a composite device design. Journal of Vascular Surgery. 2019;**70**(4):1072-1081.e2

[86] Nana P, Kouvelos G, Behrendt C-A, Giannoukas A, Kölbel T, Spanos K. A systematic review on PETTICOAT and STABILISE techniques for the management of complicated acute type B aortic dissection. Reviews in Cardiovascular Medicine. 2023;**24**(2):34

[87] Hofferberth SC, Nixon IK, Boston RC, McLachlan CS, Mossop PJ. Stent-assisted balloon-induced intimal disruption and relamination in aortic dissection repair: The STABILISE concept. The Journal of Thoracic and Cardiovascular Surgery. 2014;**147**(4):1240-1245

[88] Mascia D, Rinaldi E, Kahlberg A, Monaco F, De Luca M, Chiesa R, et al. The STABILISE technique to address malperfusion on acute-subacute type B aortic dissections. The Journal of Cardiovascular Surgery. 2022;**63**(2):131-136

[89] Mascia D, Rinaldi E, Salvati S, Melloni A, Kahlberg A, Bertoglio L, et al. Thoracic endovascular aortic repair with additional distal bare stents in type B aortic dissection does not prevent long-term aneurysmal degeneration. Journal of Endovascular Therapy. 2021;**28**(3):425-433

[90] Nienaber CA, Eagle KA. Aortic dissection: New frontiers in diagnosis and management: Part II: Therapeutic management and follow-up. Circulation. 2003;**108**(6):772-778

[91] Ryan C, Vargas L, Mastracci T, Srivastava S, Eagleton M, Kelso R, et al. Progress in management of malperfusion syndrome from type B dissections. Journal of Vascular Surgery. 2013;**57**(5):1283-1290; discussion 1290

[92] Barnes DM, Williams DM, Dasika NL, Patel HJ, Weder AB, Stanley JC, et al. A single-center experience treating renal malperfusion after aortic dissection with central aortic fenestration and renal artery stenting. Journal of Vascular Surgery. 2008;**47**(5):903-910; discussion 910

[93] Chia MC, Khorfan R, Eskandari MK. Adjunctive branch interventions during thoracic endovascular aortic repair for acute complicated type B dissection are not associated with inferior outcomes. Journal of Vascular Surgery. 2021;**74**(3):895-901

[94] Koba A, Yamagishi K, Sairenchi T, Noda H, Irie F, Takizawa N, et al. Risk factors for mortality from aortic aneurysm and dissection: Results from a 26-year follow-up of a community-based population. Journal of the American Heart Association. 2023;**12**(8):e027045

[95] Etz CD, Zoli S, Mueller CS, Bodian CA, Di Luozzo G, Lazala R, et al. Staged repair significantly reduces paraplegia rate after extensive thoracoabdominal aortic aneurysm repair. The Journal of

Thoracic and Cardiovascular Surgery. 2010;**139**(6):1464-1472

[96] Şulea C-M, Csobay-Novák C, Oláh Z, Banga P, Szeberin Z, Soltész Á, et al. Staged hybrid repair of a complex type B aortic dissection. Journal of Cardiovascular Development and Disease. 2022;**9**(9):297

[97] Leshnower BG, Keeling WB, Duwayri YM, Jordan WD, Chen EP. The "thoracic endovascular aortic repair-first" strategy for acute type A dissection with mesenteric malperfusion: Initial results compared with conventional algorithms. The Journal of Thoracic and Cardiovascular Surgery. 2019;**158**(6):1516-1524

[98] Deeb GM, Williams DM, Bolling SF, Quint LE, Monaghan H, Sievers J, et al. Surgical delay for acute type A dissection with malperfusion. The Annals of Thoracic Surgery. 1997;**64**(6):1669-1675; discussion 1675

[99] Yang B, Norton EL, Rosati CM, Wu X, Kim KM, Khaja MS, et al. Managing patients with acute type A aortic dissection and mesenteric malperfusion syndrome: A 20-year experience. The Journal of Thoracic and Cardiovascular Surgery. 2019;**158**(3):675-687.e4

[100] Johnson PT, Corl FM, Black JH, Fishman EK. The elephant trunk procedure for aortic aneurysm repair: An illustrated guide to surgical technique with CT correlation. AJR. American Journal of Roentgenology. 2011;**197**(6):W1052-W1059

[101] Acharya M, Sherzad H, Bashir M, Mariscalco G. The frozen elephant trunk procedure: Indications, outcomes and future directions. Cardiovascular Diagnosis and Therapy. 2022;**12**(5):708-721

[102] Czerny M, Fleck T, Zimpfer D, Kilo J, Sandner D, Cejna M, et al. Combined repair of an aortic arch aneurysm by sequential transposition of the supra-aortic branches and endovascular stent-graft placement. The Journal of Thoracic and Cardiovascular Surgery. 2003;**126**(3):916-918

Chapter 12

Safeguards and Pitfalls in the Management of Retrograde Dissection Complicating Thoracic Endovascular Aortic Repair

Ahmed Elsharkawy

Abstract

The aim of this chapter is to give hint on some special situations related to aortic dissection. Although they are not frequently encountered, these situations need a clear management strategy in mind of every aortic surgeon. The first one is retrograde proximal dissection complicating endovascular stenting of descending aortic pathologies: when to expect and how to manage. The second one is the different anatomical variations of aortic arch branches that may coexist with aortic dissection, such as aberrant subclavian artery and isolated vertebral artery. These variations, when present, add to the complexity of dissection repair and affect the management plan, either open surgical or endovascular.

Keywords: retrograde dissection, aberrant subclavian, bovine arch, Kommerell's diverticulum, isolated vertebral

1. Introduction

There is no doubt about the advantages of thoracic endovascular aortic repair (TEVAR) in the treatment of different descending thoracic aortic pathologies. However, endovascular intervention is not entirely devoid of risks. With the widespread use of endovascular stent grafts, some specific complications have been reported, such as different types of endoleak and the stent-induced retrograde type A aortic dissection (RAAD) [1].

2. Risk factors

Many risk factors have been identified for the development of RAAD following TEVAR [2–7].

2.1 Stent oversizing and ballooning

Stent oversizing by 10–20% larger than the aortic diameter of the proximal landing zone is a common practice in TEVAR deployment to ensure device stability and avoid type I endoleak or late stent migration. However, more than 20% oversizing may increase the incidence of RAAD. So, there should be a balance between stent oversizing and tension exerted on the aortic wall by the radial force of the TEVAR stent.

Stent ballooning is generally contraindicated in aortic dissection patients but may be used in aneurysm cases to minimize the risk of endoleak. However, this may favor the occurrence of retrograde dissection following stent deployment [2, 3].

2.2 Proximal bare springs of TEVAR

One of the possible causes of injury to the aortic wall is the proximal bare springs which are intended to afford proximal fixation of the TEVAR stent graft. These bare metal springs in the proximal end of stents have been frequently related to the entry tear found in the arch of operated cases of RAAD. The common site for this tear is the lesser curve of the aortic arch, probably due to the high radial force of stent graft exerted on the aortic wall at this location [4–6].

2.3 Location of the primary entry tear of initial pathology

The location of the primary entry tear in acute type B aortic dissections (ATBAD) is important. RAAD has been found to happen more when the primary entry tear was located at the concavity of the distal aortic arch, in contrast to the site of convexity, as the site of concavity is devoid of anatomical barriers such as supra-aortic vessels [6, 7].

2.4 Diameter of the ascending aorta

The shape and diameter of the ascending aorta must be considered during the treatment of complicated type B dissections. Ascending aortic diameter exceeding 40 mm in patients of ATBAD was found to be more prone to RAAD, mostly due to the generalized weakness of fragile aortic wall of dissection patients [4–6].

2.5 Timing of TEVAR and type of initial pathology

Some studies linked the occurrence of RAAD to the original indication for TEVAR being more likely to happen with the initial pathology of type B intramural hematoma (IMH) rather than descending aortic aneurysm or type B aortic dissection. Cases of acute TBAD and clinical or CT signs of rupture or immediate malperfusion are class I indicated for immediate endovascular treatment. But in the absence of the prementioned signs, careful monitoring and initial medical management are justified among other ATBAD patients that may benefit from initial medical therapy together with endovascular stent graft placement within 3 months, in the subacute phase. Recent data on a larger cohort of patients with TBAD undergoing TEVAR in the subacute phase revealed lower 30-day mortality and less TEVAR-related complications [5–7].

3. Presentation and management

Patients with RAAD usually present with new onset chest pain or pulse deficit with history of previous TEVAR. Time interval after TEVAR varies from shortly after the procedure to months, especially in patients with uncontrolled blood pressure. A detailed assessment may reveal new pericardial collection or aortic regurgitation on transthoracic or transesophageal echocardiography, new flap, or mural hematoma in ascending aorta on multi-slice computed tomography (MSCT) scan. **Figure 1** shows a MSCT reconstruction of one of our patients with a previously deployed TEVAR with subsequent occurrence of retrograde type A aortic dissection.

3.1 Surgical management

Retrograde type A aortic dissection (RAAD) following TEVAR is a potentially life-threatening complication that mandates emergency surgical replacement of the dissected ascending aorta with the high risk of rupture as well as the segment of aortic arch showing the entry tear, usually located in the lesser curvature, through median sternotomy under hypothermic circulatory arrest [4].

Arterial inflow of cardiopulmonary bypass (CPB) is established through cannulation of the axillary artery, or both the axillary and the femoral arteries connected by "y" connector, and a cannula in the right atrium is used for venous drainage. Cerebral protection was achieved by unilateral antegrade cerebral perfusion through axillary artery combined with moderate hypothermia (25°C). We prefer dual arterial cannulation through axillary and femoral arteries with balloon catheter temporary inflated within the stent lumen to allow for lower body perfusion during the period of open distal anastomosis of arch reconstruction.

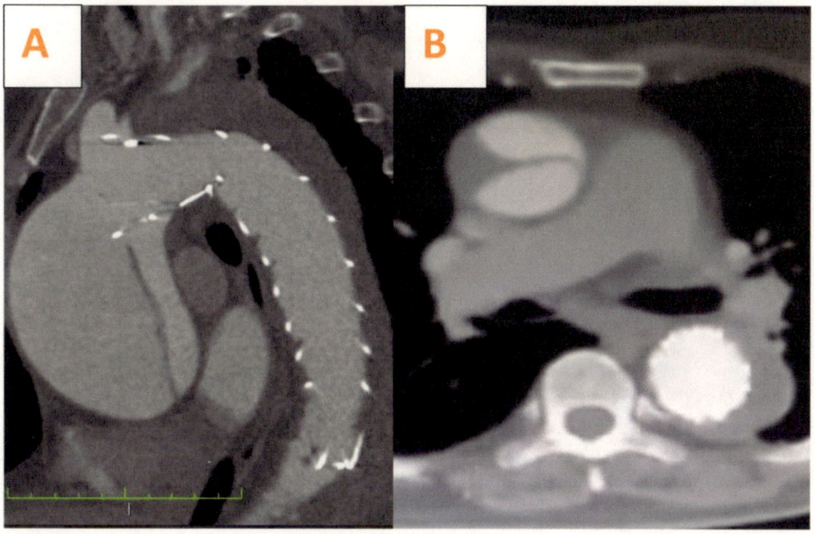

Figure 1.
CT aortography showing retrograde stanford type A aortic dissection following a previously deployed endovascular stent. (A). Protrusion of bare springs of proximal end of stent graft causing intimal tear at lesser curve of the aortic arch. (B). Axial cut revealing well-seated stent in descending aorta with complete thrombosis of false lumen but with dissection flap in ascending aorta, dividing it into true and false lumens.

3.2 Proximal aortic root reconstruction

This depends on the degree of extension of aortic dissection into the aortic root components. Usually, RAAD stops at the level of the sinotubular junction with mild affection of sinuses and aortic valve. In this situation, the ascending aorta is excised down to the level of valve commissures, followed by a supracommisural replacement of ascending aorta using Dacron tube graft anastomosed to the reconstructed sinus

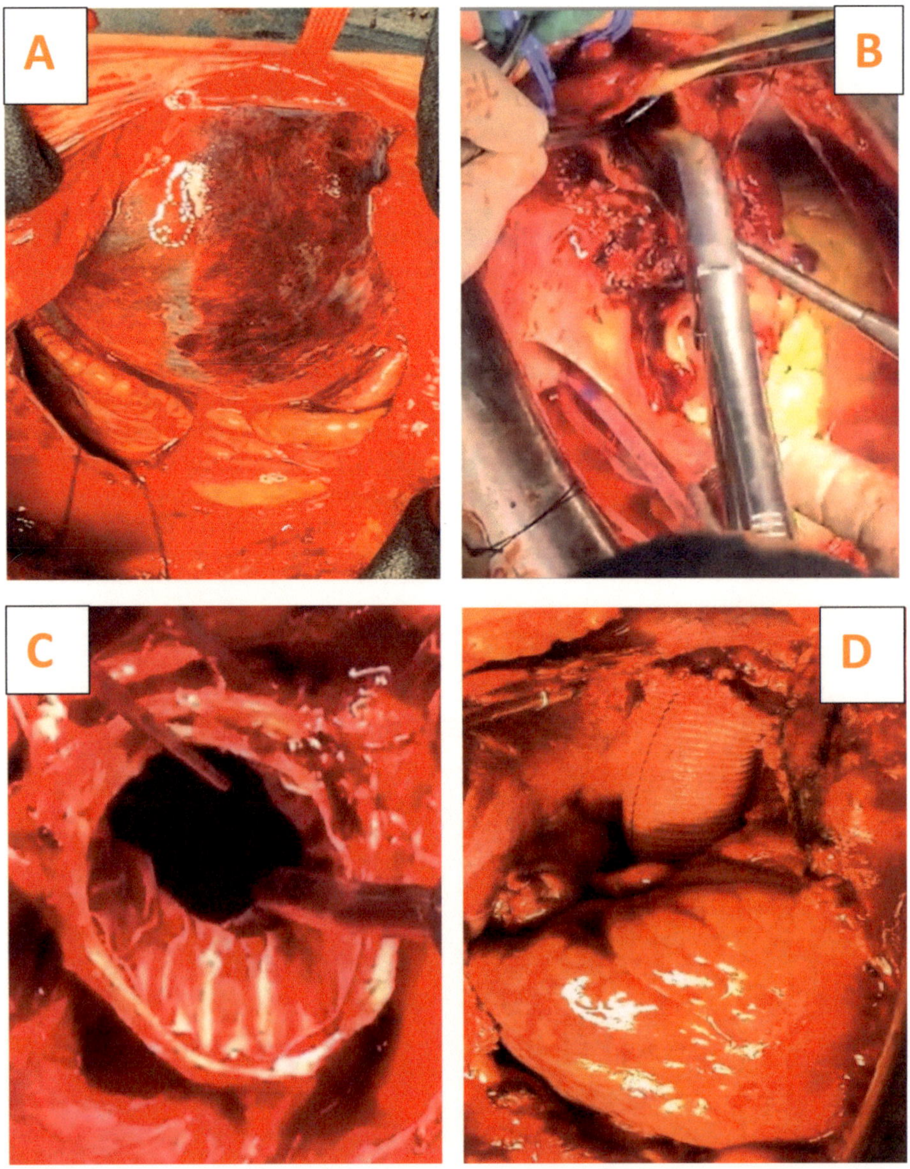

Figure 2.
Operative steps: (A) Opening the pericardium reveals extensive mural hematoma of the ascending aorta. (B) Snaring the carotid arteries and removing the cross-clamp for open distal anastomosis with trimming of metal springs of the stent using wire cutter. (C) Realignment of proximal end of endovascular stent with the native aortic wall after resection of the lesser curve and entry tear to perform Hemiarch replacement. (D) Dacron graft replacement of ascending aorta.

segment of the root using continuous 3/0 prolene suture augmented from the outer aspect with Teflon felt to support the proximal suture line. Less commonly, the aortic valve may need resuspension or valve-sparing root replacement in case of extensive affection of the aortic root.

3.3 Distal arch reconstruction

The main goal of treatment of RAAD is to completely excise the stent-induced entry tear typically located in the lesser curve of aortic arch. Total hypothermic circulatory arrest and cerebral perfusion are used for open distal anastomosis. With continuous cerebral oxygen saturation monitoring, a hemiarch replacement is usually sufficient but careful removal of some of the proximal metal springs of the endovascular stent is prudent. This allows for the inclusion of the stent as well as the native aortic wall in the distal aortic suture line all in one layer. This achieves a hemostatic repair and prevent future endoleak. Interrupted 4/0 prolene pledgeted mattress sutures and Teflon felt are used to reinforce the suture line. The proximal end of the deployed TEVAR in one of our patients with RAAD is seen in **Figure 2** with removal of the protruding metal using sternal wire cutter.

4. Discussion and follow-up

Our patient cohort includes 100 patients that received TEVAR as treatment for different descending aortic pathologies, during the period between January 2011 and January 2023. Fifty patients of our series received prosthesis with proximal bare springs. Eight patients (8%) developed RAAD with time interval ranged from 2 weeks to 6 months post TEVAR. All eight patients undergo emergency surgical replacement of ascending aorta with Hemi arch and trimming of metal springs. One patient died on the second postoperative day due to massive uncontrollable hematemesis with hemodynamic collapse 6 hours after extubation that failed to be resuscitated. One patient developed postoperative paraparesis of lower limbs that improved on insertion of spinal drain and discharged home with no residual weakness. The rest of patients had smooth uneventful postoperative course.

Gorlitzer and colleagues [6] reported in their patient cohort from August 2005 to February 2011 that retrograde aortic dissection occurred in 4 of 29 patients (13.8%) undergoing thoracic endovascular aortic repair (TEVAR) for acute complicated aortic type B dissection. In their series, a prosthesis with a proximal bare spring was used in 25 patients. The tip of the proximal bare springs induced a retrograde type A dissection in four patients. The primary entry tear was located at the concavity of the distal aortic arch. The mean duration of circulatory arrest was 56 ± 7 min. All patients survived surgery with no stroke, paraplegia, or renal failure. Postoperative CT scans revealed perigraft thrombus formation and stable aortic dimensions in all patients after 6 months.

A multicenter study of the European Registry on Endovascular Aortic Repair Complications conducted on 2009 reported on an incidence of rAAD post-TEVAR for either acute or chronic type B dissection of 1.33% (95% CI 0.75–2.4) [8].

Czerny and colleagues reported an overall RAAD incidence of 8% in a multicenter study of 66 patients with total arch de-branching and TEVAR (Zone 0), with an early (<7 days postoperatively) and delayed (>7 days postoperatively) incidence of 3 and 5%, respectively [9].

Luehr and Colleagues reported in a series of ten patients of type B aortic dissection that two patients (20%) developed retrograde type A aortic dissection on days 10 and 12 post-TEVAR. Both patients had a dilated ascending aorta and received a stent graft containing bare metal springs at the proximal end. Emergency ascending aortic replacement was performed under moderate hypothermia. In-hospital mortality was zero, and no patient developed paraplegia/paraparesis due to spinal cord ischemia. Luehr and colleagues recommended performing CT aortography 1 week after TEVAR, for the early detection of complications such as retrograde dissection as well as to assess the success of the endovascular intervention [10].

5. Impact of arch branches variations on surgical strategy of aortic dissection

5.1 Introduction

Traditionally, anatomical variations of the aortic arch and great vessels have been considered as an incidental finding of little clinical significance during routine computed tomography (CT) scanning; therefore, they were often overlooked and mostly unreported.

But from aortic surgery standpoint, the clinical significance of arch branching variations is triple-fold. First, some of these anatomical variations as aberrant subclavian artery may result in abnormal vascular ring formation around trachea and esophagus with compression symptoms as dyspnea and dysphagia. Second, these branching variations were found to occur more frequently in patients with thoracic aortic disease (TAD) than others, and therefore, these variations should be regarded as an anatomical marker for the risk of developing aortic aneurysm and dissection. Third, these variations have significant impact on the management plan whether open, endovascular, or hybrid, as well as the choice of arterial axis and cerebral protection methods in patients with aortic arch diseases and abnormal arch branching [11].

The key point for anatomical variations of arch branches is preoperative detection on multislice computed tomographic angiography (MSCTA) done to diagnose aortic aneurysm or dissection. This is a critical step in planning surgical and endovascular procedures involving the aortic arch because missing this may lead to serious problems such as branch occlusion or endoleak during endovascular treatment of type B aortic dissection, or cerebral ischemia during surgical repair of type A aortic dissection with postoperative neurological complications.

5.2 Types

The common anatomical variations related to aortic aneurysm and dissection include:

1. BOVINE ARCH (BA) or common origin of the innominate and left carotid artery (CILCA)

2. ABERRANT RIGHT SUBCLAVIAN ARTERY With left-sided aortic arch (ARSA)

3. ABERRANT LEFT SUBCLAVIAN ARTERY With right-sided aortic arch (ALSA)

4. ISOLATED LEFT VERTEBRAL ARTERY origin from aortic arch (ILVA).

5.2.1 Bovine arch (BA)

The bovine arch is defined as an aortic arch with common origin of the innominate and left carotid artery (CILCA arch). It is also called truncus bicaroticus or type I bovine arch. It represents the second most common arch configuration following the standard arch pattern of innominate trunk, left common carotid, and a left subclavian artery. Less commonly, "type 2 bovine arch" occurs when the left common carotid artery originates directly from the innominate artery rather than as a common trunk. The prevalence of the CILCA arch in the general population is around 15% [11].

- type I bovine arch [T1BA] means common origin of innominate and left common carotid artery

- type II bovine arch [T2BA], left common carotid originating from innominate artery.

The clinical relevance of the CILCA arch has become apparent in planning surgical and endovascular procedures involving the aortic arch. Also, a lot of research work has identified the CILCA arch as a potential anatomical marker for thoracic aortic disease (TAD).

Many patients who are candidate for thoracic endovascular aortic repair (TEVAR) present with this special anatomical configuration of bovine arch. Different studies reported a trend toward an increased risk of post-TEVAR complications in such patients with bovine arch, as retrograde dissection. So, further specific studies on the impact of the bovine arch configuration on TEVAR planning are needed [12].

It was proposed by certain hypothesis that in CILCA bovine arch, the peculiar anatomical configuration may entail a local biomechanical environment that adversely affects the aortic wall properties and its integrity. The relatively greater diameter of the arch vessels may alter local flow hemodynamics, leading to an increased wall shear stress, that may weaken the aortic wall [13].

During surgery for type A aortic dissection, bovine arch configuration allows for bilateral carotid perfusion when using axillary artery inflow. Also, in type B aortic dissection, the bovine configuration allows for more space in the arch for proximal landing of TEVAR.

5.2.2 Aberrant right subclavian artery (ARSA) with normal left-sided aortic arch (LSAA)

Aberrant right subclavian artery (ARSA) is a rare anatomical variant of the origin of the right subclavian artery from distal aortic arch or proximal descending aorta instead of the common origin with right carotid artery from the innominate trunk. A prevalence of 0.16–2% of ARSA has been reported. Of notice, aberrant right subclavian artery may coexist with common bicarotid trunk in some patients [14–17].

During acute type A aortic dissection surgery and arch replacement procedures, the presence of ARSA should be checked carefully in the MSCT aortography. If so, axillary cannulation will be of no value in terms of antegrade cerebral perfusion, and another axis should be selected as direct bilateral osteal carotid cannulation.

During frozen elephant trunk (FET) procedure for arch replacement, intrathoracic control of ARSA is gained by meticulous dissection of the inferolateral aspect of right carotid artery above the innominate vein, followed by division of the ARSA and end-to-end anastomosis to 8-mm Dacron graft that can be connected to separate perfusion head then to the elephant trunk graft by the end.

In case of TEVAR for type B aortic dissection with ARSA, a more detailed study of carotids and vertebral arteries by cranial CT cerebral angiography is needed to evaluate the dominance of vertebral arteries, and the integrity of the circle of Willis then to decide to go for carotid subclavian bypass on left or right side or even bilateral in case of symmetric vertebral arteries because both subclavian arteries will be covered by the stent graft affecting the perfusion of both vertebral arteries. The MSCT of some of our patients with aberrant right and left subclavian arteries is shown in **Figures 3–5**.

5.2.3 Aberrant left subclavian artery (ALSA) with right-sided aortic arch (RSAA)

Right-sided aortic arch is a rare anatomical variation resulting from persistence of the embryologic right fourth aortic arch and involution of the left, which is the reverse of what happens in most of the population. Fifty percent of the cases (0.05%) are associated with an aberrant left subclavian artery arising from an outpouching called Kommerell's diverticulum. Right-sided aortic arch is rare with prevalence of about 0.1% of the adult population. Of notice, right-sided aortic arch with aberrant left subclavian artery is much less common than left-sided aortic arch with aberrant right subclavian artery (0.5–2.0%) [18–21].

Management of aberrant left subclavian artery depends on the presentation:

a. If the main presentation is compression symptoms of vascular ring with no aneurysm formation, so the treatment is to divide the ring around the esophagus through left thoracotomy followed by interposition graft reconstruction of ALSA or left carotid subclavian bypass.

b. If the problem is Kommerell's diverticulum complicated by aneurysm formation or type B dissection, so the treatment is either open surgical repair through right thoracotomy to resect diverticulum aneurysm and replace descending thoracic aorta, or hybrid repair through median sternotomy to debranch the great vessels followed by TEVAR or to go for one-stage frozen elephant trunk procedure.

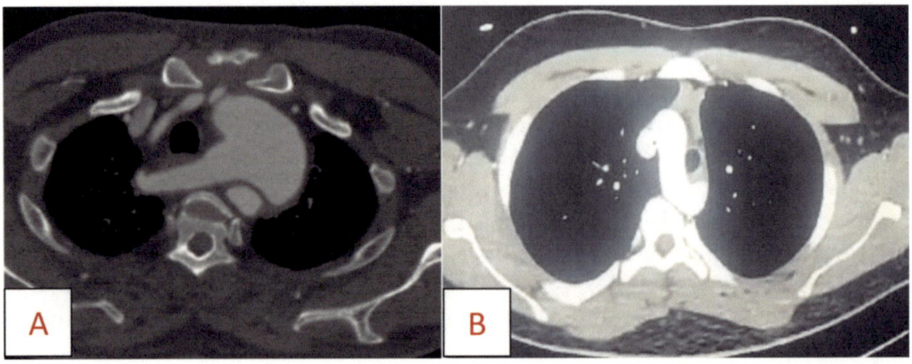

Figure 3.
A. Left-sided aortic arch with aberrant right subclavian artery retrotracheal. B. Right-sided aortic arch with aberrant left subclavian artery origin retrotracheal.

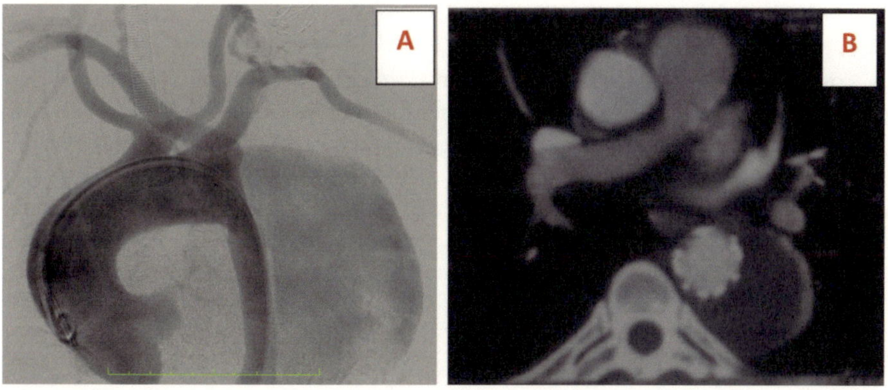

Figure 4.
A. Aortography showing type B aortic dissection with collapsed true lumen, big false lumen, aberrant right subclavian artery, and common carotid trunk. The patient had bilateral carotid subclavian bypasses followed by TEVAR. B. Follow-up MSCT showing complete thrombosis of false lumen around the stent with no endoleak.

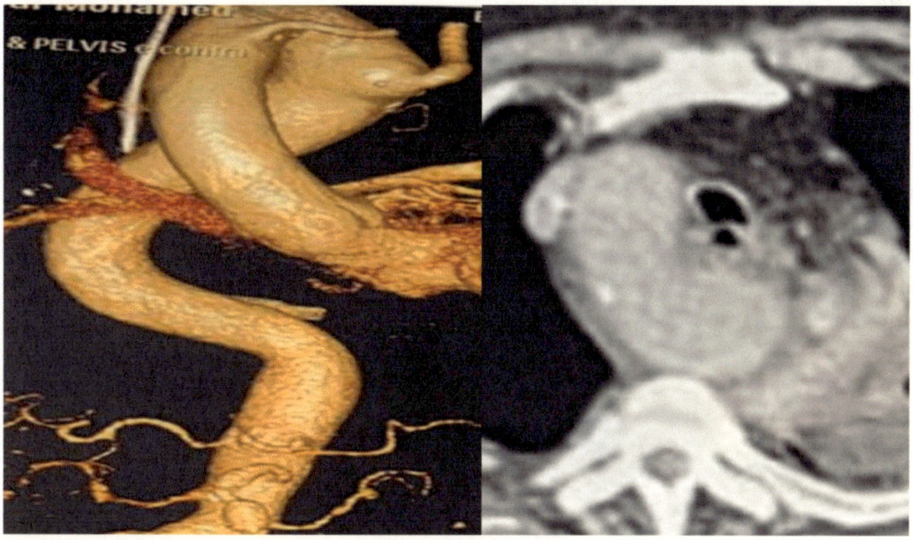

Figure 5.
MSCT aortography of one of our patients with right-sided aortic arch and aberrant left subclavian arising from Kommerell's diverticulum.

5.2.4 Kommerell's diverticulum aneurysm (KDA)

Burckhard Friedrich Kommerell (1900—1990) described his diverticulum/aneurysm of the proximal lusorian artery in 1936 [22].

Kommerell's diverticulum (KD) is defined as aneurysmal aortic dilatation at the origin of an aberrant subclavian artery (ASCA), either left or right. KD is a rare anomaly, occurring in 0.05–2.0% of the population. About 5% of patients with KD develop symptoms.While most patients with KD are asymptomatic, dysphagia is one of the common manifestations due to compression of the esophagus. KD is associated with risk of aortic rupture and/or dissection, as the tissue strength in the KD is very limited due to histological weakness, and this often leads to adverse aortic events [23].

5.2.4.1 Indication for surgery

According to the European Association of Cardiothoracic Surgery/Society of Thoracic Surgery EACTS/STS 2024 Guidelines for diagnosing and treating acute and chronic syndromes of the aortic organ, surgery for symptomatic KD is a well-established indication. However, indications for prophylactic intervention in asymptomatic patients remain based on limited reports. Observation of asymptomatic KD is generally appropriate. Current American College of Cardiology/American Heart Association guidelines recommend treatment when the orifice connecting the diverticulum to the arch is larger than 30 mm and/or the diverticulum diameter is larger than 50 mm (**Figure 6**) [7].

5.2.4.2 Operative strategy

A variety of treatment options have been reported to treat KD, including open, endovascular, or hybrid methods. The most common open approach is ligation/resection and subclavian transposition/bypass to release compression and to reestablish arterial circulation through a left thoracotomy. Open replacement of the aorta may be considered using partial heart bypass cannulating superior vena cava and distal aorta or femoral artery through a right thoracotomy. In symptomatic patients, surgery should include full decompression of the surrounding structures and fibrous bands surrounding the esophagus. Total arch replacement (TAR) through the frozen elephant trunk FET procedure may be considered if the condition is associated with aortic arch dilatation [7].

Endovascular option may be considered in patients with increased operative risk and who are anatomically convenient for stenting. This includes staged carotid-subclavian artery bypass followed by subsequent thoracic endovascular aortic repair (TEVAR). In young patients with low incidence of comorbidities, open repair through a thoracotomy is preferred due to its durability and efficacy in symptom relief. Endovascular therapy is less invasive and would be a good strategy for asymptomatic

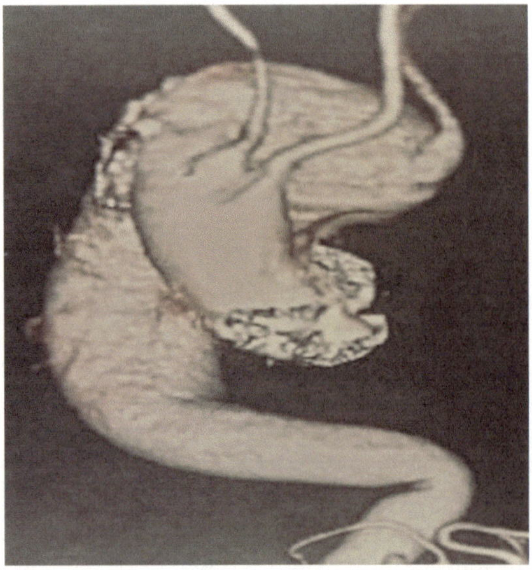

Figure 6.
Kommerell's diverticulum aneurysm with right-sided arch aneurysm and aberrant left subclavian artery.

Kommerell's aneurysm. However, in patients with symptomatic KDA, the open technique is the preferred option because relieving the compression on the esophagus would be key step. The basic concept to treat dysphagia is to remove the ASCA and all fibrous bands surrounding the esophagus through left thoracotomy [7].

During frozen elephant trunk procedure for KDA with arch aneurysm, because of the anatomical features of patients with right aortic arch + ALSA, in whom the aortic arch is sharply angulated or curved, available ready-made devices are prone to massive kinking and, therefore, modified intraoperatively assembled frozen elephant trunk works better according to the individual anatomy of arch angulation.

5.2.5 Isolated left vertebral artery origin from the arch (ILVA)

An isolated left vertebral artery (ILVA) is defined as vertebral artery which arises directly from the aortic arch. This anatomical variation has a prevalence of 0.79 to 6.1%. From surgical point of view, the preoperative diagnosis of an ILVA on CT aortography is important because missing this variation may lead to serious complications, such as occlusion or endoleak during endovascular treatment of TBAD or difficulties during the surgical approach to the aortic arch branches in type A aortic dissection with possible ischemia or infarction of the brain if the circle of Willis is incomplete. Many options, such as total arch replacement and frozen elephant trunk technique, have been reported to treat patients with aortic dissection and an ILVA. Whether an ILVA should be reconstructed or not in all cases is controversial. Most studies state that the ILVA should be reconstructed because sacrificing the ILVA may increase the risk of neurologic deficit owing to poor perfusion to the brainstem or cerebellum if arterial communication at the circle of Willis is inadequate [24].

In case of type B aortic dissection (TBAD) with an ILVA requiring endovascular therapy TEVAR, the proximal landing zone, dominance of the vertebral artery, and integrity of the circle of Willis are all studied in MSCT. Preoperative aortic CTA imaging characteristics may reveal right vertebral artery dominance, symmetric vertebral artery, or left vertebral artery dominance. The management entails ILVA reconstruction, such as ILVA-LCCA transposition of vertebral artery to left carotid artery, if the ILVA is dominant or symmetric with an incomplete circle of Willis, followed by TEVAR placement. Cerebral oximetry is used to monitor cerebral oxygen saturation during left carotid clamping period for the anastomosis.

During the treatment of Stanford type A aortic dissection (TAAD) with an ILVA, prior reconstruction of ILVA is recommended with ILVA-left common carotid artery (LCCA) transposition or bypass using saphenous vein graft segment under normothermic off-pump conditions. Median sternotomy incision is extended about 4 cm cranially to the left side of the neck for sufficient dissection of the LCCA and ILVA with enough length, and then, the ILVA is cut off. The LCCA is open with a hole puncher. The ILVA is end-side sutured to the LCCA with 6–0 Prolene line [25].

6. Conclusion

Retrograde type A aortic dissection (RAAD) following TEVAR is a life-threatening complication with potential risk of aortic rupture that needs high index of suspicion for early detection and emergency surgical intervention. Supra-commissural replacement of the dissected ascending aorta with Hemi arch procedure is usually sufficient and carries good outcome.

Congenital aortic arch variations are gaining more clinical importance with the introduction of advanced aortic therapies such as endovascular stents and the frozen elephant trunk. These anatomical variations are more common in patients with thoracic aortic disease. The key to success for case planning, whether open surgical or endovascular, is the detection of such variations on preoperative CT aortography to allow for optimum management.

Author details

Ahmed Elsharkawy
Cardiothoracic Surgery Department, Faculty of Medicine, Cairo University, Egypt

*Address all correspondence to: ahmedsharkawy.cts@hotmail.com

References

[1] Fanelli F, Salvatori F, Marcelli G, et al. Type a aortic dissection developing during endovascular repair of an acute type B dissection. Journal of Endovascular Therapy. 2003;**10**:254-259

[2] Bockler D, Schumacher H, Ganten M, et al. Complications after endovascular repair of acute symptomatic and chronic expanding Stanford type B aortic dissections. The Journal of Thoracic and Cardiovascular Surgery. 2006;**132**:361-368

[3] Neuhauser B, Greiner A, Jaschke W, et al. Serious complications following endovascular thoracic aortic stent-graft repair for type B dissection. European Journal of Cardio-Thoracic Surgery. 2008;**33**:58-63

[4] Khoynezhad A, White R. Pathogenesis and management of retrograde type A aortic dissection after thoracic endovascular aortic repair. Annals of Vascular Surgery. 2013;**27**:1201-1206

[5] Dawoud O, Omar A, Wahba M, Elsharkawy A. Management of retrograde dissection complicating thoracic endovascular aortic repair. The Egyptian Journal of Hospital Medicine. 2021;**84**:2663-2666

[6] Gorlitzer M, Czerny M, Grabenwöger M, et al. Repair of stent graft-induced retrograde type A aortic dissection using the E-vita open prosthesis. European Journal of Cardio Thoracic Surgery. 2012;**42**(2012):566-570

[7] Czerny M, Chen E, Elefteriades J, et al. Task force group (2024): EACTS/STS guidelines for diagnosing and treating acute and chronic syndromes of the aortic organ. European Journal of Cardio Thoracic Surgery. 2024;**65**(2):ezad426

[8] Eggebrecht H, Thompson M, Rousseau H, et al. Retrograde ascending aortic dissection during or after thoracic aortic stent graft placement: Insight from the European registry on endovascular aortic repair complications. Circulation. 2009;**120**:S276-S281

[9] Czerny M, Weigang EJ, Antona C, Gelpi G, et al. Targeting landing zone 0 by total arch rerouting and TEVAR: Midterm results of a transcontinental registry. The Annals of Thoracic Surgery. 2012;**94**:84-89

[10] Luehr M, Etz CD, Mohr FW, et al. Surgical management of delayed retrograde type A aortic dissection following complete supra-aortic de-branching and stent-grafting of the transverse arch. European Journal of Cardio-Thoracic Surgery. 2013;**44**(2013):958-963

[11] Marrocco-Trischitta MM, Alaidroos M, Nano G, et al. Aortic arch variant with a common origin of the innominate and left carotid artery as a determinant of thoracic aortic disease: A systematic review and meta-analysis. European Journal of Cardio-Thoracic Surgery. 2020;**57**(2020):422-427

[12] Williams JB, Andersen ND, McCann RL, et al. Retrograde ascending aortic dissection as an early complication of thoracic endovascular aortic repair. Journal of Vascular Surgery. 2012;**55**:1255-1262

[13] Marrocco-Trischitta MM, Rylski B, Schofer F, et al. Prevalence of type III arch configuration in patients with type B aortic dissection. European Journal of Cardio-Thoracic Surgery. 2019;**56**:1075-1080

[14] Kumar S. Truncus bicaroticus with aberrant right subclavian artery and

origin of right vertebral from right common carotid artery. Surgical and Radiologic Anatomy. 2014;**36**(8):829-831

[15] Chahwan S, Todd Miller M, Kim AK. Aberrant right subclavian artery associated with a common origin of carotid arteries. Annals of Vascular Surgery. 2006;**20**(6):809-812

[16] Berko NS, Jain VR, Godelman A. Variants and anomalies of thoracic vasculature on computed tomographic angiography in adults. Journal of Computer Assisted Tomography. 2009;**33**:523-528

[17] Müller M, Schmitz BL, Röhrer S, et al. Variations of the aortic arch—a study on the most common branching patterns. Acta Radiologica. 2011;**52**:738-742

[18] Hori D, Tanaka M, Yamaguchi A, Adachi H. Type A aortic dissection, right-sided aortic arch, and thoracic aortic aneurysm. Asian Cardiovascular & Thoracic Annals. 2009;**17**(6):640-642

[19] Cina CS, Arena GO, Bruin G, Clase CM. Kommerell's diverticulum and aneurysmal right-sided aortic arch: A case report and review of the literature. Journal of Vascular Surgery. 2000;**32**(6):1208-1214. DOI: 10.1067/mva.2000.108012

[20] Yang MH, Weng ZC, Weng YG, Chang HH. A right-sided aortic arch with Kommerell's diverticulum of the aberrant left subclavian artery presenting with syncope. Journal of the Chinese Medical Association. 2009;**72**(5):275-277. DOI: 10.1016/S1726-4901(09)70070-X

[21] Türkvatan A, Büyükbayraktar FG, Olçer T, Cumhur T. Multidetector computed tomographic angiography of aberrant subclavian arteries. Vascular Medicine. 2009;**14**(1):5-11. DOI: 10.1177/1358863X08097903

[22] Wolfgang GM, Wyss A. Kommerell's diverticulum images in cardio-thoracic surgery. European Journal of Cardio-Thoracic Surgery. 2009;**36**:188

[23] Hashimoto M, Nishida H, Milner R. Staged surgical intervention to treat dysphagia caused by Kommerell's diverticulum. European Journal of Cardio-Thoracic Surgery. 2020;**57**(2020):601-603

[24] Ding H, Zhu Y, Luo S, et al. Management of type B aortic dissection with an isolated left vertebral artery Guangzhou, China. Journal of Vascular Surgery. 2019;**70**(4):1065-1071

[25] Zuo Y, Zhou ZC, Ge J. Prior reconstruction of an isolated left vertebral artery for Stanford type A aortic dissection. European Journal of Cardio-Thoracic Surgery. 2021;**59**:1339-1341